£19.99

THOMAS DANBY CA

031523

C000163957

has t renew

BEAUTY & WELLNESS DICTIONARY: *for Cosmetologists, Barbers, Estheticians and Nail Technicians*

THIRD EDITION

Edited by
Catherine M. Frangie

DELMAR
CENGAGE Learning

Australia • Brazil • Japan • Korea • Mexico • Singapore • Spain • United Kingdom • United States

DELMAR
CENGAGE Learning®

Beauty & Wellness Dictionary: for Cosmetologists, Barbers, Estheticians and Nail Technicians, Third Edition

Vice President, Milady & Learning Solutions Strategy, Professional: Dawn Gerrain

Director of Content & Business Development, Milady: Sandra Bruce

Associate Acquisitions Editor: Philip I. Mandl

Senior Product Manager: Jessica Mahoney

Editorial Assistant: Elizabeth A. Edwards

Director, Marketing & Training: Gerard McAvey

Associate Marketing Manager: Matthew McGuire

Senior Production Director: Wendy Troeger

Production Manager: Sherondra Thedford

Content Project Management: PreMediaGlobal

Art Direction: PreMediaGlobal

Cover Image: Image content: various cosmetics Copyright: © Hltdelight / shutterstock.com Image content: nail polish Copyright: © kuleczka / shutterstock.com Image content: hair / beard trimmer Copyright: © Lusoimages / shutterstock.com Image content: cutting shears, thinning shears, curling iron and round brush Copyright: © Cathleen A. Clapper / shutterstock.com

Cover design: Rokusek Design, Inc.

© 2014, 2002 Milady, a part of Cengage Learning

ALL RIGHTS RESERVED. No part of this work covered by the copyright herein may be reproduced, transmitted, stored, or used in any form or by any means graphic, electronic, or mechanical, including but not limited to photocopying, recording, scanning, digitizing, taping, Web distribution, information networks, or information storage and retrieval systems, except as permitted under Section 107 or 108 of the 1976 United States Copyright Act, without the prior written permission of the publisher.

For product information and technology assistance, contact us at
Cengage Learning Customer & Sales Support, 1-800-354-9706
For permission to use material from this text or product, submit all requests online at **www.cengage.com/permissions.**
Further permissions questions can be e-mailed to
permissionrequest@cengage.com

Library of Congress Control Number: 2012946518

ISBN-13: 978-1-133-68698-9

ISBN-10: 1-133-68698-2

Milady
5 Maxwell Drive
Clifton Park, NY 12065
USA

Cengage Learning is a leading provider of customized learning solutions with office locations around the globe, including Singapore, the United Kingdom, Australia, Mexico, Brazil, and Japan. Locate your local office at: **international.cengage.com/region.**

Cengage Learning products are represented in Canada by Nelson Education, Ltd.

For your lifelong learning solutions, visit **milady.cengage.com**

Purchase any of our products at your local college store or at our preferred online store **www.cengagebrain.com**. Visit our corporate website at **cengage.com**

Notice to the Reader
Publisher does not warrant or guarantee any of the products described herein or perform any independent analysis in connection with any of the product information contained herein. Publisher does not assume, and expressly disclaims, any obligation to obtain and include information other than that provided to it by the manufacturer. The reader is expressly warned to consider and adopt all safety precautions that might be indicated by the activities described herein and to avoid all potential hazards. By following the instructions contained herein, the reader willingly assumes all risks in connection with such instructions. The publisher makes no representations or warranties of any kind, including but not limited to, the warranties of fitness for particular purpose or merchantability, nor are any such representations implied with respect to the material set forth herein, and the publisher takes no responsibility with respect to such material. The publisher shall not be liable for any special, consequential, or exemplary damages resulting, in whole or part, from the readers' use of, or reliance upon, this material.

Printed in the United States of America
1 2 3 4 5 6 7 16 15 14 13 12

PREFACE

In today's fast-paced and ever-changing world of beauty and technology, understanding terms and the language of the beauty industry is essential for all professionals who interact with and inform clients every day. It is imperative that students and professionals of the beauty and wellness industry understand the technical terms of their profession and use them correctly when consulting with clients. As the industry changes and expands, professionals must also become proficient in the terminology used in all areas of the related sciences. For this reason, the *Beauty & Wellness Dictionary: for Cosmetologists, Barbers, Estheticians and Nail Technicians,* Third Edition, is written.

This dictionary includes words and phrases that are used in the arts and sciences of cosmetology, nail technology, barbering, and esthetics, with specific definitions pertinent to the industry and defined in their sense of relationship to anatomy, cosmetic chemistry, dermatology, electricity, esthetics, hair structure and chemistry, massage therapy, nail technology, nutrition, and professional skills. Utilizing the "as it sounds" pronunciation guide will ensure that you "speak the language" of the industry.

This dictionary, revised from requests by industry professionals and updated to today's most recent terminology, includes labeled neuromuscular and skeletal charts and detailed diagrams of the circulatory, digestive, endocrine, integumentary, lymphatic, nervous, and respiratory systems. Charts on vitamins, minerals, the pH scale, and a table of the elements are designed to assist students, instructors, and professionals on product knowledge and nutrition. Accuracy in measuring chemicals is critical and oftentimes is given in metrics. Therefore, we have included an easy-to-read metric conversion chart.

We wish to express our sincere appreciation to the many industry educators and professionals who contributed their valued advice during the preparation of this dictionary:

- Jane Barrett, Instructor, Chisholm Institute, Australia
- Yota Batsaras, Cosmetologist/makeup artist & business owner, CA
- Linda Burmeister, Undergraduate Education Manager, International Dermal Institute/Dermalogica, CA

- Shari Golightly, Owner, Intuitive Touch & the Hair Studio, CO
- Maria Lynch, Independent beauty contractor, NY
- Sandra Alexcae Moren, Owner, Chiron Marketing Inc.—Kyronspaconsulting, Canada
- Sandra Peoples, Cosmetology Instructor, Counselor, Pickens Technical College, CO
- Lisa Reinhardt, Owner, Rhine Institute, CA
- Amy Fields Rumley, Owner & Esthetician, Merle Norman Cosmetics and Skin Care Services, NC
- Denise Sauls, Cosmetology/Esthetics Instructor, Lurleen B. Wallace Community College, AL
- Linda Schoenberg, Technical Director, Regency Beauty Institute, MN
- Jennifer Schrodt, University of Nebraska, NE
- Donna Simmons, Master Cosmetology Instructor, Tulsa Tech Broken Arrow, OK
- Patricia Stander, Licensed Aesthetician, LPN, BA, Hampshire Dermatology & Skin Health Center, MA
- Rebecca Udwary, Advisor, San Francisco Institute of Esthetics and Cosmetology, CA
- Tina Marie Zillmann, Owner, Manufacturer, Educator, Skin Rejuvenation Clinique/Advanced Rejuvenating Concepts, TX

LIBRARY ✓

CLASS NO.	646.7203 FRA
ACC.	031523

A

A

abdomen (AB-duh-men)—the belly; the cavity in the body between the thorax and the pelvis that contains the stomach, intestines, liver, and kidneys.

abdominoplasty (ab-DOM-un-oh-plas-tee)—procedure that removes excessive fat deposits and loose skin from the abdomen to tuck and tighten the area.

abducent (ab-DOOS-int)—drawing away from the midline of the body, as muscles draw away.

abducent nerve (ab-DOOS-int NURV)—either of the six cranial nerves; small motor nerves supplying the external rectus muscle of the eye.

abductor digiti minimi (ab-DUK-tor dij-it-ty MIN-eh-mee)—muscles that flex and separate the fingers and the toes.

abductor hallucis (ab-DUK-tor huh-LU-sis)—muscle located on the outer portion of the foot, running alongside the big toe; it moves the big toe and helps maintain balance while walking and standing.

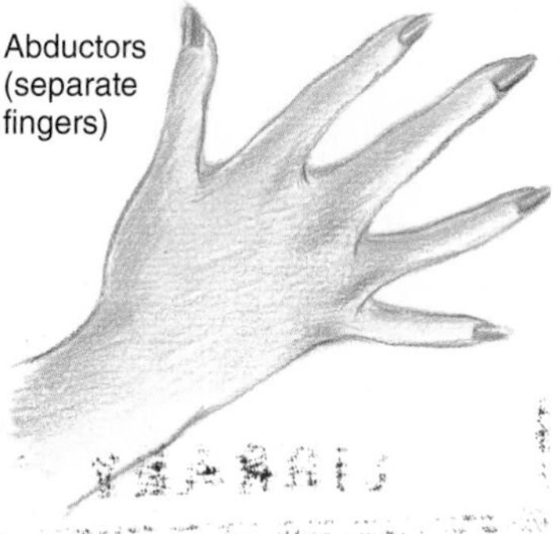

© Milady, a part of Cengage Learning

abductors

abductors (ab-DUK-turz)—muscles that draw a body part, such as a finger, arm, or toe, away from the midline of the body or of an extremity. In the hand, abductors separate the fingers.

abnormal (ab-NOR-mul)—irregular; contrary to the natural law or customary order.

aboral (ah-BOHR-ul)—located or situated opposite to or away from the mouth.

abrade (uh-BRAYD)—to remove, wear away, or roughen by friction or rubbing.

abrasion (uh-BRAY-zhun)—scraping of the skin; excoriation; rubbing or wearing off of the surface; an irritation; a scraped or scratched area of the skin.

A

abrasive (uh-BRAY-siv)—a substance used for roughing or smoothing, as in dermabrasion and in nail files when filing the nail.

abscess (AB-ses)—a localized collection or pocket of pus in any part of the body, characterized by dead tissue and inflammation.

absorb (ab-SORB)—to take in and make part of an existing whole; to suck up or take up, as a towel absorbing water.

absorption (ub-SORP-shun)—act of absorbing, as in nutrients; the transport of fully digested food into the circulatory system to feed the tissues and cells.

acanthosis nigricans (ak-an-THOH-sis NEG-rih-kanz)—skin condition that causes the skin in body folds and creases to become dark, thick, and velvety.

acarid (AK-uh-rud)—infestation of mites causing a dermatitis.

acceleration (ak-SELL-uh-ray-shun)—an increase in speed; the process of moving or developing faster.

accelerator (ak-SELL-uh-rayt-ur)—also known as *activator*, any agent that hastens or quickens action.

accent (AK-sent)—to give special force or emphasis to; to highlight or give added color tone.

accentuate (ak-SEN-choo-ayt)—to emphasize; to heighten effect; in makeup, to enhance the features of the face.

accessory nerve (ak-SESS-uh-ree NURV)—the eleventh cranial nerve; conveys motor impulses to muscles of the head, neck, and shoulder.

acellular (ay-SEL-yuh-lur)—containing no cells.

acetic acid (uh-SEET-ik AS-ud)—a colorless, pungent, liquid; the chief acid of vinegar.

acetone (AS-uh-tohn)—also known as *nail polish remover*; a colorless, volatile, extremely flammable liquid that is widely used as a solvent and, when used properly, is considered safe for salon use.

acetylated lanolin (uh-SEET-ul-ayt-ed LAN-ul-un)—considered water resistant; used in cosmetics to reduce water loss from the skin; an emollient.

acetylcholine (uh-SEET-ul-koh-leen)—a neurotransmitter (chemical that transmits signals from a neuron to a target cell) that plays a role in muscle contraction.

ache (AYK)—a dull, distressing, and often persistent pain.

achromasia (ak-roh-MAY-zhuh)—a lack of normal pigmentation; a condition such as albinism or vitiligo in which there is loss of normal color or lack of melanin in the skin.

acid(ic) (AS-ud)—substances that have a pH below 7.0 and turn litmus paper from blue to red.

acid-alkali neutralization reactions (AS-ud AL-ka-lye Nuu-tral-eye-zay-shun Re-ack-shunz)—when an acid is mixed with an alkali in equal proportions to neutralize each other and form water (H_2O) and a salt.

acid balanced (AS-ud BAL-anst)—describes a product with a stabilized pH level; commonly used to refer to products such as shampoos and conditioners balanced to the pH of skin and hair (4.5 to 5.5).

acid-balanced waves (AS-ud BAL-anst wayvz)—permanent waves that have a 7.0 or neutral pH; because of their higher pH, they process at room temperature, do not require the added heat of a hair dryer, process more quickly, and produce firmer curls than true acid waves.

acid-balanced shampoos (AS-ud BAL-anst sham-poos)—shampoos that are balanced to the pH of hair and skin (4.5 to 5.5).

acidic (uh-SID-ik)—containing a high percentage of acid; having properties of an acid.

acidic solution (uh-SID-ik so-LUU-shon)—a solution that has a pH below 7.0 (neutral).

acidify (uh-SID-ih-fy)—to change into an acid; to lower the degree of alkalinity.

acid mantle (AS-ud MAN-tul)—protective barrier of lipids and secretions on the surface of the skin.

acid peel (AS-ud PEEL)—also known as *peel*; an exfoliating treatment or process using a diluted acidic substance.

acid rinse (AS-ud RINS)—a solution or emulsion that has acidic properties such as lemon juice; commonly used to close the cuticle of the hair after shampooing or chemical services.

acid wave (AS-ud WAYV)—permanent wave with lotion that has a pH of 7.0 or below and requires heat or another form of activator to speed processing.

acne (AK-nee)—also known as *acne simplex* or *acne vulgaris*; skin disorder characterized by chronic inflammation of the sebaceous glands from retained secretions and *Propionibacterium acnes* (*P. acnes*) bacteria. Chronic inflammatory skin disorder of the sebaceous glands, characterized by comedones and blemishes; commonly known as acne simplex or acne vulgaris.

acne albida (AK-nee AL-bih-duh)—a type of acne caused by milia.

A

A

acne artificialis (AK-nee ar-tih-fish AL-is)—acne resulting from external irritants, or as a result of drugs taken internally such as iodines or bromides.

acne atrophica (AK-nee uh-TRO-Fih-kuh)—acne in which the lesions leave a slight amount of scarring.

acne cachecticorum (AK-nee kah-KEK-tih-kor-um)—pustular eruptions that sometimes occur when anemia or some debilitating constitutional disease is present.

acne conglobata (AK-nee kon-gloh-BAY-tuh)—a highly inflammatory type of acne; symptoms include comedones, nodules, abscesses, and draining sinus tracts.

acne cream (AK-nee KREEM)—a facial cream containing medicinal substances or agents used in the treatment of acne.

acne cystica (AK-nee SIS-tih-kuh)—a form of acne with cysts.

acne excoriee (ak-nee ek-SKOR-ee)—disorder where clients compulsively scrape off acne lesions, causing scarring and discoloration.

acne hypertrophica (AK-nee hy-pur-TRAHF-ih-kuh)—acne vulgaris in which the lesions, upon healing, leave hypertrophic or rosacea-type scars.

acne indurata (AK-nee in-dyoo-RAH-tuh)—a progression of papular acne, with deep-seated and destructive lesions that may produce severe scarring.

acne keratosa (AK-nee kair-uh-TOH-sa)—an eruption of papules consisting of horny plugs projecting from the hair follicles, accompanied by inflammation.

acne miliaris (AK-nee mil-ee-AIR-us)—a condition marked by excessive whiteheads (milia).

acne pits (AK-nee PITS)—pitlike scars produced by acne.

acne punctata (AK-nee punk-TAH-tuh)—a form of acne containing blackheads in all the lesions.

acne pustulosa (AK-nee pus-tyuh-LOH-suh)—acne in which pustular lesions predominate.

acne simplex (AK-nee SIM-pleks)—acne vulgaris; simple uncomplicated pimples.

acne vulgaris (AK-nee vul-GAIR-is)—chronic acne, usually occurring in adolescence, with comedones, papules, nodules, and pustules on the face, neck, and upper part of the trunk.

acoustic nerve (uh-KOO-stik NURV)—eighth cranial nerve controlling the sense of hearing.

acquired immune deficiency syndrome (AIDS) (uh-KWY-erd ih-MYOON di-FISH-en-see sin-drohm)—also known as *acquired immunodeficiency syndrome*; an epidemic, transmissible retroviral (virus containing an enzyme which allows the virus's genetic information to become part of the genetic information of the host cell upon replication) disease caused by infection with the human immunodeficiency virus, manifested in severe cases as profound depression of cell immunity.

acquired immunity (uh-KWY-erd ih-MYOO-nih-tee)—immunity that the body develops after overcoming a disease, through inoculation (such as flu vaccinations), or through exposure to natural allergens.

acromial process (uh-KROH-mee-al PRAH-ses)—the outward extension of the spine of the scapula that forms the point of the shoulder.

acronyx (AK-roh-niks)—an ingrown nail.

acrylates (AHK-ra-latez)—a specialized acrylic monomer (cross-linking) that has good adhesion to the natural nail plate and polymerizes in minutes; used to make UV gels.

acrylic (uh-KRIL-ik)—the name for an entire family of chemicals used to make all types of nail enhancements and adhesives, including wraps, glues, UV gels, and liquid/powder systems.

acrylic acid (uh-KRIL-ik AS-ud)—unsaturated aliphatic acid used to make plastics, such as combs, brushes, and capes.

acrylic nails (uh-KRIL-ik NAYLS)—a commonly used, but professionally incorrect term for monomer liquid and polymer powder nail enhancements.

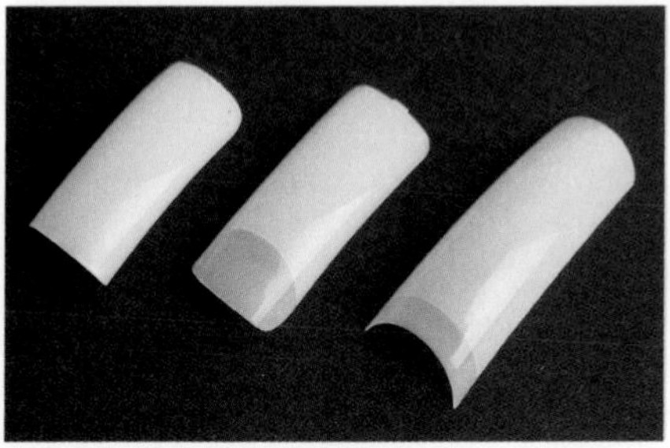

© Milady, a part of Cengage Learning. Photography by Dino Petrocelli.

acrylonitrile butadiene styrene

acrylonitrile butadiene styrene (ABS) (ak-ruh-loh-NAHY-tril byoo-tah-DAHY-een STAHY-reen)—a common thermoplastic used to make light, rigid, molded nail tips.

actinic (ak-TIN-ik)—1. producing chemical action; said of rays of light beyond the violet end of the spectrum. 2. Damage or condition caused by sun exposure.

actinic dermatosis (ak-TIN-ik der-muh-TOH-sis)—a condition in which the skin becomes inflamed, particularly in areas that have been exposed to sunlight or artificial light.

actinic keratoses (ak-TIN-ik Kara-toe-sis)—pink- or flesh-colored precancerous lesions that feel sharp or rough; result from sun damage.

actinic ray (ak-TIN-ik RAY)—an invisible ray that produces chemical action; a ray of light beyond the violet spectrum that is capable of bringing about chemical changes.

actinodermatitis (ak-tin-oh-dur-muh-TY-tus)—dermatitis caused by overexposure to sunlight or X-rays.

actinomycosis (ak-tin-oh-my-KOH-sus)—a chronic, infectious disease that affects animals and people; caused by bacteria and characterized by lesions and tumors formed around the jaws.

actinotherapy (ak-tin-oh-THAIR-uh-pee)—the treatment of disease by use of sunlight, X-rays, and ultraviolet rays.

activators (AK-tih-vay-terz)—also known as *boosters*, *protinators*, or *accelerators*; powdered persulfate salts added to hair color to increase its lightening ability.

active electrode (AK-tiv ih-LEK-trohd)—the electrode used on the area being treated.

active immunity (AK-tiv ih-MYOO-nih-tee)—a form of acquired immunity in which the body produces its own antibodies against disease-causing agents.

acupressure (AK-yoo-presh-ur)—an ancient healing art by using fingers to gradually press key healing points, which stimulate the body's natural self-curative abilities.

acupuncture (AK-yoo-pun-chur)—an alternative medicine originating in ancient China that treats patients by insertion and manipulation of solid, generally thin, needles in the body.

acute (uh-KYOOT)—coming to a crisis quickly, as opposed to chronic; a disease with a rapid onset, severe symptoms, and short course.

additive (AD-ut-iv)—a substance that is added to another product.

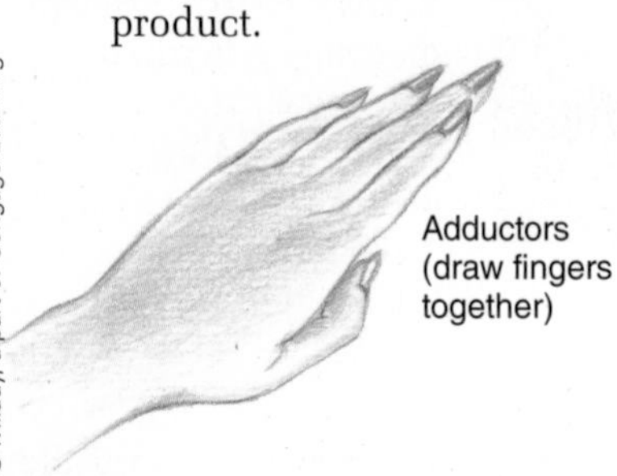

© Milady, a part of Cengage Learning

adductors

adductors (ah-DUK-turz)—muscles that draw a body part, such as a finger, arm, or toe, in toward the median axis of the body or of an extremity. In the hand, adductors draw the fingers together.

adenitis (ad-un-ITE-us)—inflammation of the lymph nodes and glands.

adenoid (AD-un-oyd)—as *pharyngeal tonsil*, or *nasopharyngeal tonsil*; a mass of lymphoid tissue situated posterior to the nasal cavity, in the roof of the nasopharynx, where the nose blends into the throat.

adenology (ad-uh-NAHL-uh-jee)—the branch of anatomy concerned with glands.

adenoma (ad-un-OH-muh)—a tumor of glandular origin.

adenosine diphosphate (ADP) (uh-DEN-uh-seen dy-FAHS-fayt)—formed when a muscle contracts and a phosphate splits from ATP, releasing energy.

adenosine triphosphate (ATP) (uh-DEN-uh-seen try-FAHS-fayt)—a multifunctional nucleotide that transports chemical energy within cells for metabolism and converts oxygen to carbon dioxide.

adermogenesis (ay-dur-moh-JEN-uh-sus)—imperfect development or healing of the skin.

adhesion (add-hee-shun)—chemical reaction resulting in two surfaces sticking together.

adhesive (add-hees-ive)—agent that causes two surfaces to stick together.

adhesive nail enhancement (add-hees-ive NAYL en-hans-ment)—a nail enhancement that is strengthened using nail adhesive.

adiaphoretic (ay-dy-uh-foh-RET-ik)—any agent, drug, or cosmetic preparation that reduces, checks, or prevents perspiration.

adipose (AD-uh-pohs)—relating to fat.

adipose tissue (AD-uh-pohs TISH-oo)—technical term for a specialized connective tissue considered fat; gives smoothness and contour to the body.

adjustable wig (ad-JUST-uh-bul WIG)—a wig designed for ready-to-wear use, constructed with an elastic insert at the back to make it easily adjustable for various head sizes.

adrenal glands (uh-DREN-ul-un glanz)—glands that sit atop the kidneys and secrete about 30 steroid hormones and control metabolic processes of the body, including the fight-or-flight response.

adrenaline (uh-DREN-ul-un)—epinephrine; a hormone secreted under stress by the adrenal glands; it stimulates the nervous system, raises metabolism, increases cardiac pressure and output, and increases blood pressure to prepare the body for maximum exertion.

adrenocorticotripic hormone (ACTH) (uh-dren-a-kor-ti-ka-TRIP-ik HOR-mohn)—stimulates the adrenal cortex to produce cortical hormones; aids in protecting the body in stressful situations.

adsorption (ad-SORP-shun)—the adhesion of an extremely thin layer of one substance (a gas or liquid) to the surface of a solid body or liquid with which it is in contact.

advertising (ADD-ver-ty-sing)—promotional efforts that are paid for and are directly intended to increase business.

adynamia (ad-ih-NAY-mee-uh)—loss of physical strength; weakness.

aerate (AIR-ayt)—to supply or charge with air or gas; to oxygenate.

aeration (air-AY-shun)—exposure to air; saturating a fluid with air or gas; conversion of venous to arterial blood in the lungs.

aerification (air-ih-fih-KAY-shun)—the process of converting into gas, air, or vapor.

aerobe (AIR-ohb)—a microorganism that can live and grow in the presence of oxygen.

aerobic (air-ROH-bik)—living or occurring in the presence of oxygen; a term applied to modern dance exercises; aerobic exercises improve cardiovascular and respiratory fitness.

aerobic cellular respiration (air-ROH-bik SEL-u-lar res-puh-RAY-shun)—takes place in the mitochondria of cells and is responsible for the sustained energy supply needed for synthesis of ATP.

aerosol (AIR-uh-sahl)—colloidal suspension of liquid or solid particles in a gas; container filled with liquified gas and dissolved or suspended in ingredients that can be dispersed as a spray; used for cosmetic and food preparations.

aesthetician (es-the-TISH-un)—also known as *medical aesthetician*; a specialist who performs esthetic treatments integrated with surgical and medical procedures.

aesthetics (es-THET-iks)—a branch of esthetics that integrates esthetic treatments with surgical and medical procedures.

afferent nerves (AAF-eer-ent NURVS)—nerves that convey stimulus from receptors or sense organs to the brain.

agent (AY-jent)—an active ingredient that can produce a physical, chemical, or medicinal effect.

aging skin (AY-jing SKIN)—skin that has lost its elasticity, and has developed lines or wrinkles.

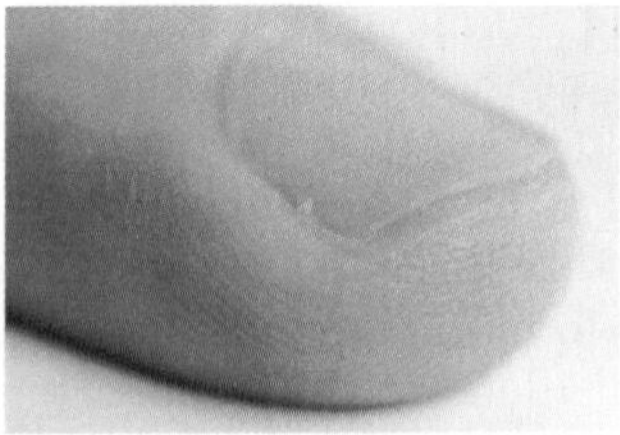
© F.C.G./www.Shutterstock.com

agnail

agnail (AG-nayl)—also known as *hangnail*; the condition in which the cuticle splits around the nail. Can be caused by dryness, removing too much, or improper removal of cuticle.

air (AYR)—the gaseous mixture that makes up the earth's atmosphere. It is odorless, colorless, and generally consists of about 1 part oxygen and 4 parts nitrogen by volume.

air purifier (AYR PYOOR-ih-fy-ur)—an apparatus that removes impure substances from the air.

airbrush (AYR-brush)—a tool used with an air compressor to spray liquids.

airbrush stencil (AYR-brush sten-sill)—a precut sheet of clear, thin plastic with a sticky backing that is cut by a machine into various shapes or designs. Any variety of paper, lace, mesh, fabric, or other material can be used as a stencil.

ala nasi (AY-lee NAY-zy)—the wing cartilage of the nose.

albinism (AL-bi-niz-em)—absence of melanin pigment of the body, including the skin, hair, and eyes. The technical terms for albinism are *congenital leukoderma* or *congenital hypopigmentation*.

albino (al-BY-noh)—an individual affected with albinism; the result of an absence of coloring matter in the hair shaft, accompanied by a lack of pigment coloring in the skin or irises of the eyes.

albumin (al-BYOO-min)—any of a class of proteins occurring naturally; soluble in water, coagulated by heat, and found in eggs, milk, muscle tissue, blood, and in many vegetable tissues.

albumose (AL-byuh-mohs)—a substance formed from protein during digestion; chemical compounds derived from albumin by the action of certain enzymes.

alcohol (AL-kuh-hawl)—a readily evaporating, colorless liquid; obtained by the fermentation of starch, sugar, and other carbohydrates.

alcohol-based makeup—also known as *waterproof makeup*; a makeup product containing alcohol as its primary ingredient, rendering it waterproof, smudge-proof, and completely nontransferable.

aldosterone (al-DA-ster-ohn)—steroid hormone that regulates the sodium/potassium balance in the extracellular fluid and in the blood.

algae (AL-jee)—a marine plant, used as an ingredient in products that remineralize and revitalize the skin.

algin (AL-jun)—the dried gelatinous form of various seaweeds, especially kelp; used as an emulsifier, thickening, and ripening agent.

A

aliment (AL-uh-ment)—nourishment; food or anything that allows a substance to grow.

alimentary canal (al-uh-MENT-uh-ree ka-NAL)—consists of the mouth, pharynx, esophagus, stomach, and small and large intestines.

alipidic (al-ah-PIDD-ic)—lack of oil or "lack of lipids"; describes skin that does not produce enough sebum, indicated by absence of visible pores.

alkali (AL-kuh-ly)—also known as *base*; a class of compounds (hydrogen, a metal, and oxygen) that reacts with acids to form salts; turns red litmus blue; used to make soap and hair relaxers; has a pH number above 7.0.

alkaline (AL-kuh-line)—having the qualities of, or pertaining to, an alkali; an aqueous (water-based) solution with a pH greater than 7.0; opposite of acidic; bitter tasting.

alkaline solution (AL-kuh-line sah-LUU-shon)—a solution that has a pH above 7.0 (neutral).

alkaline waves (AL-kuh-line WAYVZ)—also known as *cold waves*; have a pH between 9.0 and 9.6, use ammonium thioglycolate (ATG) as the reducing agent, and process at room temperature without the addition of heat.

alkalis (AL-kuh-lyz)—also known as *bases*; compounds that react with acids to form salts.

alkalinity (al-kuh-LIN-ut-ee)—the quality or state of being alkaline.

alkaloid (AL-kuh-loyd)—any organic base containing nitrogen; a substance containing alkaline properties.

alkalosis (al-kuh-LOH-sus)—excessive alkalinity of the blood, other body fluids, and tissues of the body.

alkanolamines (al-kan-oh-LAH-mynz)—alkaline substances used to neutralize acids or raise the pH of many hair products.

allantoin (al-ahn-toyn)—an anti-inflammatory compound from the herb comfrey. Used in cold cream, hand lotion, hair lotion, aftershave, and other skin-soothing cosmetics because of its ability to help heal wounds and skin ulcers and to stimulate the growth of healthy tissue.

allergic contact dermatitis (ACD) (AL-ur-jic con-tact der-muh-TIT-us)—an allergy to an ingredient or a chemical, usually caused by repeated skin contact with the chemical.

allergy (AL-ur-jee)—a hypersensitivity disorder of the immune system. Allergic reactions occur when a person's immune system reacts negatively to normally harmless substances in the environment.

aloe vera (AL-oh VAIR-uh)—most popular botanical used in cosmetic formulations; emollient and film-forming gum resin with hydrating, softening, healing, antimicrobial, and anti-inflammatory properties.

alopecia (al-uh-PEE-she-a)—abnormal hair loss.

alopecia androgenetic (al-uh-PEE-she-a andro-je-NET-ik)—also known as *male pattern baldness* or *androgenic alopecia*; the most common form of hair loss, possibly caused by hereditary factors.

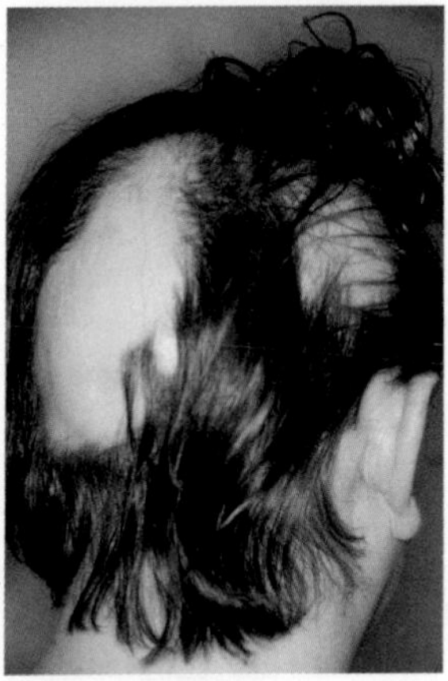

Courtesy of www.dermnet.com

alopecia areata

alopecia areata (al-uh-PEE-she-a ay-reh-AH-tuh)—autoimmune disorder that causes the affected hair follicles to be mistakenly attacked by a person's own immune system; usually begins with one or more small, round, smooth bald patches on the scalp.

alopecia cicatrisata (al-uh-PEE-she-a sih-kah-trih-SAH-tah)—irreversible loss of hair, usually on the scalp; scarring results.

alopecia dynamica (al-uh-PEE-she-a dy-NAM-ih-kuh)—loss of hair due to destruction of the hair follicle by ulceration or disease process.

alopecia follicularis (al-uh-PEE-she-a fol-ik-yoo-LAIR-is)—loss of hair due to inflamed hair follicles.

alopecia localis (al-uh-PEE-she-a loh-KAY-lis)—loss of hair occurring in patches along the course of a nerve or at the site of an injury.

alopecia maligna (al-uh-PEE-she-a muh-LIG-nuh)—a term applied to a form of alopecia that is severe and persistent.

alopecia prematura (al-uh-PEE-she-a pree-muh-TOO-ruh)—baldness in males beginning before middle age.

alopecia seborrheica (al-uh-PEE-she-a seb-or-EE-ih-kah)—baldness caused by diseased sebaceous glands.

alopecia senilis (al-uh-PEE-she-a seh-NIL-is)—baldness occurring in old age.

A

alopecia syphilitica (al-uh-PEE-she-a sif-il-IT-ih-kuh)—loss of hair resulting from syphilis, occurring in the second stage of the disease.

alopecia totalis (al-uh-PEE-she-a toe-TAL-is)—total loss of scalp hair.

alopecia traction (al-uh-PEE-she-a TRAK-shun)—hair loss caused by holding the hair tight and under tension for long periods of time.

alopecia universalis (al-uh-PEE-she-a yoo-nih-vur-SAA-lis)—complete loss of body hair.

alpha helix (AL-fah HEE-liks)—the spiral of the polypeptide chains within the hair cortex in the first or unstretched position.

alpha hydroxy acids (AHAs) (al-FAH HY-drok-see-AS-udz)—acids derived from plants (mostly fruit) that are often used to exfoliate the skin; mild acids: glycolic, lactic, malic, and tartaric acid. AHAs exfoliate by loosening the bonds between dead corneum cells and dissolving the intercellular matrix. Alpha hydroxy acids also stimulate cell renewal.

alpha lipoic acid (al-FAH LIP-oh-ic ASs-ud)—a natural molecule found in every cell in the body; it is a powerful antioxidant and is soluble in water and oil.

alphosis (al-FOH-sis)—pertaining to lack of skin pigmentation, as in albinism.

alternating current (AC) (AWL-tur-nayt-ing KUR-rent)—rapid and interrupted current, flowing first in one direction and then in the opposite direction; produced by mechanical means and changes directions 60 times per second.

alum (AL-um)—compound made of aluminum, potassium, or ammonium sulfate with strong astringent action.

aluminum (uh-LOO-mih-num)—silver-white metal with low specific gravity, noted for its lightness and resistance to oxidation; often used in the manufacture of combs and rollers.

aluminum acetate solution (uh-LOO-mih-num AS-uh-tayt suh-LOO-shun)—a solution diluted with water and used as an antiseptic and astringent.

aluminum chloride (uh-LOO-mih-num KLOHR-yd)—a crystalline powder soluble in water; used as an astringent, antiseptic, or deodorant.

aluminum sulfate (uh-LOO-mih-num SUL-fayt)—used in antiseptics, astringents, and in some deodorant preparations.

alveola (al-VEE-oh-lah); pl–, alveolae (-lie)—a small cavity, cell, or pit on the surface of an organ.

alveolar ducts (al-VEE-oh-lar DUKTS)—tiny end ducts of the branching airways that fill the lungs.

alveolar process (al-VEE-oh-lar PRAH-ses)—the ridge of bone in the maxilla and mandible containing the alveolar of the teeth.

alveoli (al-VEE-oh-lye)—microscopic air sacs in the lungs.

alymphia (ay-LIM-fee-uh)—absence or deficiency of lymph.

amino acids (uh-MEE-noh AS-udz)—organic acids that form the building blocks of protein. Units that are joined together end to end like pop beads by strong, chemical peptide bonds (end bonds) to form the polypeptide chains that comprise proteins.

amino dye (uh-MEE-noh DY)—a synthetic, organic tint produced from a coal tar derivative known as analine.

amitosis (ay-my-TOH-sus)—cell multiplication by direct division of the nucleus in the cell.

ammonia (uh-MOH-nee-uh)—colorless gas with a pungent odor that is composed of hydrogen and nitrogen.

ammonia-free waves (uh-MOH-nee-uh FREH WAYVZ)—perms that use an ingredient that does not evaporate as readily as ammonia, so there is very little odor associated with their use.

ammonium hydroxide (uh-MOH-nee-um hy-DRAHKS-yd)—an alkaline base formed from ammonia and water; used in products such as permanent hair color, lightener preparations, hair relaxers, and cleansing solutions.

ammonium persulfate (uh-MOH-nee-um pur-SUL-fayt)—ammonium salt; soluble in water; used as an oxidizer and bleach in some hair and skin cosmetics; an ingredient used in some disinfectants and deodorants.

ammonium sulfide (uh-MOH-nee-um SUL-fyd)—a combination of ammonia and sulfur.

ammonium sulfite (uh-MOH-nee-um SUL-fyt)—a combination of ammonia and salt of sulfuric acid.

ammonium thiocyanate (uh-MOH-nee-um thy-oh-SY-ah-nayt)—a combination of ammonia and thiocyanic acid.

A

ammonium thioglycolate (ATG) (uh-MOH-nee-um thy-oh-GLY-kuh-layt)—active ingredient or reducing agent in alkaline permanents.

ampere (A) (AM-peer)—also known as *amp*; unit that measures the strength of an electric current (quantity of electrons flowing through a conductor).

ampholytic surfactant (AM-foh-lih-tik sur-FAK-tent)—a base surfactant found in shampoos; does not sting eyes; behaves as an anionic or cationic substance depending on the pH of the solution.

amphoteric (am-fuh-TAIR-ik)—having the characteristics of both an acid and an alkali; a substance used in cleaning agents.

ampoules (AM-pyoolz)—small, sealed vials containing a single application of highly concentrated extracts in a water or oil base.

anabolism (uh-NAB-o-liz-em)—constructive metabolism; the process of building up larger molecules from smaller ones.

anaerobic (AN-uh-roh-bik)—cannot survive in the presence of oxygen.

anaerobic respiration (AN-uh-roh-bik res-puh-RAY-shun)—consists of breaking down of glucose in the absence of oxygen, releasing energy for synthesis of ATP, and production of lactic acid.

anagen phase (AN-uh-jen FAYZ)—also known as *growth phase*; phase during which new hair is produced.

analine derivative tint (AN-ul-ine duh-RIV-uh-tiv TINT)—a synthetic, organic hair tint produced from a coal tar product.

analogous (an-AL-uh-gus)—similar or comparable in certain respects.

analogous colors (uh-NAL-O-gus colorz)—colors that are located beside each other on the color wheel.

analysis (uh-NAL-uh-sis)—the process by which the nature of a substance is recognized, and its chemical or physical composition is determined; for example, to examine hair to determine condition and natural color.

analysis, hair (uh-NAL-uh-sis, HAYR)—examination to determine the condition and natural color of the hair prior to a hair treatment.

anaphase (AN-uh-fayz)—a stage in cell division in which centromeres divide, and chromatids move apart to form the next generation of chromosomes.

anaphoresis (an-uh-for-EES-sus)—process of infusing an alkaline (negative) product into the tissues from the negative pole toward the positive pole.

anatomy (ah-NAT-ah-mee)—branch of biology that deals with the form and structure of organisms, animals, and plants.

anaplasty (an-uh-PLAS-tee)—an operation for the restoration of lost parts; plastic surgery.

anatripsis (an-ah-TRIP-sis)—in massage, the use of friction as treatment or therapy.

androgen (AN-druh-jen)—any of various hormones that control the development of masculine characteristics.

androgenic alopecia (an-druh-JEN-ik al-oh-PEE-shah)—also known as *androgenetic alopecia,* or *male pattern baldness*; hair loss characterized by miniaturization of terminal hair that is converted to vellus hair.

androsterone (an-DRAHS-tuh-rohn)—a male sex hormone.

anemia (uh-NEE-mee-uh)—a condition in which the blood is deficient in, or produces inadequate amounts of, red corpuscles; deficient in hemoglobin, or both.

anesthesia (an-us-THEE-zhuh)—partial or complete loss of sensation with or without loss of consciousness; can be result of disease, injury, or administration of an anesthetizing agent.

aneurysm (an-yuh-RIH-zm)—a localized abnormal dilation of a blood vessel.

angiectasis (an-jee-ek-TAY-sis)—abnormal dilation of the blood vessels causing tension and tenderness in the skin.

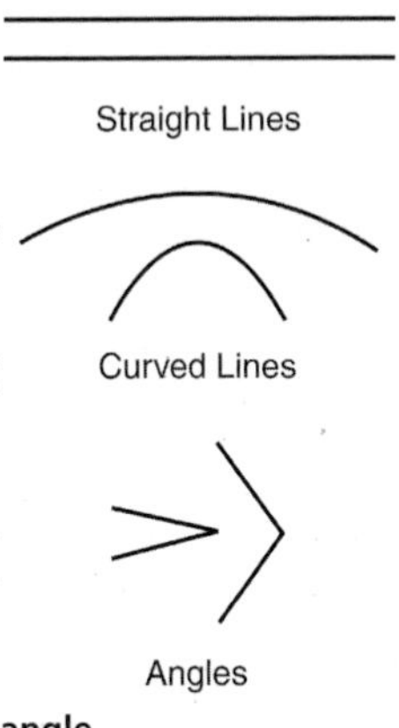

© Milady, a part of Cengage Learning
angle

angiodermatitis (an-jee-oh-dur-muh-TY-tus)—inflammation of the blood vessels of the skin.

angiology (an-jee-AHL-uh-jee)—the study of the blood vessels and the lymphatic system.

angioma (an-jee-OH-muh)—a tumor formed of blood or lymph vessels.

angle (ANG-gul)—space between two lines or surfaces that intersect at a given point; in haircutting, the hair is held away from the head to create an angle of elevation.

angular artery (ANG-yoo-lur ART-ur-ee)—supplies blood to the side of the nose.

A

angular chelitis (ANG-yoo-lur KEE-ly-tus)—an acute or chronic inflammation of the skin around the corners of the mouth.

anhidrosis (an-hy-DROH-sis)—deficiency in perspiration, often a result of fever or certain skin diseases that require medical treatment.

anhydration (an-hy-DRAY-shun)—dehydration; removal of water; lacking moisture.

anhydrous (an-HY-drus)—describes products that do not contain any water.

aniline (AN-ul-un)—a colorless liquid with a faint characteristic odor obtained from coal tar and other nitrogenous substances; combined with other substances, it forms the aniline colors or artificial dyes derived from coal tar.

aniline derivatives (AN-ul-un DUR-ive-it-ivez)—contain small, uncolored dyes that combine with hydrogen peroxide to form larger, permanent dye molecules within the cortex.

aniline dye (AN-ul-un DY)—any dye produced synthetically from coal tar; used in the manufacture of hair-coloring products and fragrances.

anion (AN-eye-on)—an ion with a negative electrical charge.

anionic (an-eye-AHN-ik)—a base surfactant found in shampoos producing rich foam that rinses easily.

ankle bone (ANG-kul BOHN)—the talus; the proximal bone of the foot.

annular (AN-yuh-lur)—ring-like.

annular finger (AN-yuh-lur FING-gur)—the ring finger or third finger of the left hand.

anode (AN-ohd)—positive electrode; the anode is usually red and is marked with a *P* or a plus (+) sign.

anodermous (an-uh-DUR-mus)—lacking skin.

anomalous (uh-NAHM-uh-lus)—abnormal; unusual; irregular.

antacid (ant-AS-ud)—a substance that relieves or neutralizes acidity.

antagonist (an-TAG-uh-nust)—in anatomy, a muscle that acts counter to another muscle.

anterior (an-TEER-ee-ur)—situated before or in front of; the ventral or belly-side of the body.

anterior auricular artery (an-TEER-ee-ur aw-RIK-yuh-lur ART-uh-ree)—supplies blood to the front part of the ear.

anterior auricular muscle (an-TEER-ee-ur aw-RIK-yuh-lur MUS-uhl)—the muscle in front of the ear.

anterior auricular nerve (an-TEER-ee-ur aw-RIK-yuh-lur NURV)—nerve found in the skin anterior to the external ear.

anterior cardiac vein (an-TEER-ee-ur KARD-ee-ak VAYN)—vein located in front of the right ventricle.

anterior facial veins (an-TEER-ee-ur FAY-shul VAYNZ)—veins located on the anterior sides of the face and which drain into the internal jugular vein located on the sides of the neck.

A

anterior interosseous artery (an-TEER-ee-ur in-tur-AHS-ee-us ART-uhree)—supplies blood to the anterior part of the forearm.

anterior jugular vein (an-TEER-ee-ur JUG-yuh-lur VAYN)—vein located near the midline of the neck that drains into the external jugular or subclavian veins.

anterior tibial artery (an-TEER-ee-ur TIB-ee-al ART-uh-ree)—artery that supplies blood to the lower leg muscles and to the muscles and skin on the top of the foot and adjacent sides of the first and second toes. This artery continues to the foot where it becomes the dorsalis pedis artery.

anthrax (ahn-thraks)—an acute disease caused by the bacterium *Bacillus anthracis*. Most forms of the disease are lethal, and it affects both humans and other animals. There are effective vaccines against anthrax, and some forms of the disease respond well to antibiotic treatment.

antibacterial soap (an-ti-bak-TEER-ee-ul SOHP)—a detergent destructive to or preventing the growth of bacteria; used to clean hands.

antibiotic (ant-ih-by-AHT-ik)—a compound or substance that kills or slows down the growth of bacteria.

antibody (ANT-ih-bahd-ee)—a protein produced by B-cells that is used by the immune system to identify and neutralize foreign objects such as bacteria and viruses.

anticatalyst (an-tih-KAT-uh-list)—a substance that stops or inhibits a chemical reaction.

anticathode (an-tih-KATH-ohd)—the electrode in an electron or X-ray tube that receives and reflects rays emitted from a cathode.

antidote (ANT-ih-doht)—an agent preventing or counteracting the action of poison.

A

antifungal (ant-ih-FUN-gal)—pertaining to a substance that stops or inhibits the growth of fungi.

antigen (ANT-ih-jin)—any of several substances such as toxins, enzymes, or foreign proteins that cause the development of antibodies.

antioxidant (ant-eye-AHK-sih-dent)—a molecule capable of inhibiting the oxidation of other molecules. Oxidation reactions can produce free radicals. In turn, these radicals can start chain reactions in a cell that can cause damage or death to the cell. Antioxidants terminate these chain reactions by removing free radical intermediates, and inhibit other oxidation reactions.

antiperspirant (ant-ih-PUR-spih-rent)—a strong astringent liquid or cream used to stop the flow of perspiration in the region of the armpits, hands, or feet.

antisepsis (ant-ih-SEP-sis)—a method by which a substance, item, or organism is kept sterile by preventing the growth of pathogenic bacteria.

antiseptics (ant-ih-SEP-tiks)—chemical germicides formulated for use on skin; registered and regulated by the Food and Drug Administration (FDA).

antitoxin (ant-ih-TAHK-sun)—a substance in serum that binds and neutralizes toxin (poison).

aorta (ay-ORT-uh)—the largest artery in the body, originating from the left ventricle of the heart and extending down to the abdomen, where it branches off into two smaller arteries. The aorta distributes oxygenated blood to all parts of the body through the systemic circulation.

aortic valve (ay-ORT-ik VALV)—heart valve that permits the blood to be pumped from the left ventricle into the aorta.

apex (AY-peks)—also known as *arch*; highest point on the top of the head; the area of the nail that has all of the strength; usually oval-shaped and is located in the center of the nail.

apocrine glands (AP-uh-krin GLANZ)—coiled structures attached to hair follicles found in the underarm and genital areas that secrete sweat.

aponeurosis (ap-uh-noo-ROH-sus)—a broad, flat tendon that serves to connect muscle to the part that it moves; a tendon that connects the occipitalis and the frontalis.

apparatus (ap-uh-RAT-us)—a collection of instruments or devices adapted for a specific purpose.

appendage (uh-PEN-dij)—an outgrowth attached to an organ or part of the body and dependent on it for growth; a limb or limb-like structure.

appendicular skeleton (ap-pen-DIK-yoo-lur SKEL-uh-tun)—consists of bones of the shoulder, upper extremities, hips, and lower extremities.

appendix (uh-PEN-diks)—a small appendage of the intestine.

applicator (AP-lih-kay-tur)—an instrument or item used to apply products such as brushes, combs, and spatulas.

apprentice (uh-PREN-tis)—one who learns a trade by working and studying under the direction of others who are already skilled in that trade.

aqueous (AY-kwee-us)—watery; pertaining to water; descriptive term for a water solution or any medium that is largely composed of water.

arc (ARK)—part of the circumference of a circle; an incomplete circle; in hairstyling, the first half of a shaping is referred to as base direction and the last half of the shaping is called the arc.

arc base pin curls (ARK BAS PIN CURLZ)—also known as *half-moon* or *C-shape base pin curls*; are carved out of a shaping.

arching technique (ARE-ching tek-neek)—method used to cut around the ears and down the sides of the neck.

aromatherapy (uh-ROH-muh-THAIR-uh-pee)—a form of alternative medicine that uses volatile plant materials, known as essential oils, and other aromatic compounds for the purpose of altering a person's mind, mood, cognitive function, or health.

arrector pili muscles (ah-REK-tohr-PY-leh MUS-uhls)—also known as *goose bumps*; small, involuntary muscles in the base of the hair follicle that cause goose flesh.

arrectores pili (ur-REK-tohr pi-li [plural])—the minute involuntary muscle fibers in the skin inserted to the base of the hair follicles; contraction of the arrectores pili causes skin hair to stand on end, resulting in "goose bumps."

arteries (AR-tuh-reez)—thick-walled, muscular, flexible tubes that carry oxygenated blood away from the heart to the capillaries throughout the body.

arteriole (ar-TEER-ee-ohl)—a minute artery; a terminal artery continuous with the capillary network that deliver blood to capillaries.

arteriosclerosis (ar-teer-ee-oh-skluh-ROH-sus)—an abnormal condition characterized by an accumulation of fatty deposits on the inner walls of the arteries; the affected arteries tend to thicken, become fibrous, and lose their elasticity.

arthritis (ar-THRIT-is)—inflammation and/or stiffening of the joints, causing pain.

articular (ar-TIK-yuh-lur)—pertaining to the junction of two or more skeletal parts, or to the muscle or ligament associated with a joint.

ascorbic acid (uh-SKOR-bik AS-ud)—one form of vitamin C; scurvy-preventing vitamin found in fruits and vegetables.

asepsis (ay-SEP-sis)—freedom from disease-causing germs.

aseptic (ay-SEP-tik)—free from pathogenic bacteria.

aseptic procedures (ay-SEP-tik pro-ceed-yures)—a process of properly handling sterilized and disinfected equipment and supplies to reduce contamination.

ash (ASH)—a drab shade containing no red or gold tones; dominated by greens, blues, violets, or grays. May be used to counteract unwanted warm tones.

asphyxic skin (as-FIK-sik SKIN)—skin lacking oxygen.

assimilate (uh-SIM-ih-layt)—to absorb; to incorporate into the body; to digest.

assimilation (uh-sim-ih-LAY-shun)—the incorporation of materials prepared by digestion of food into the tissues of the body.

asteatosis (as-tee-ah-TOH-sis)—dry and scaly skin due to a deficiency or absence of sebum; due to aging, body disorders, alkalis of harsh soaps, or by exposure to cold.

astringent (uh-STRIN-jent)—a chemical compound that tends to shrink or constrict body tissues; used in skin care to help remove excess oil on the skin.

asymmetrical balance (A-sym-et-rical BAL-antz)—typically off-center or created with an odd or mismatched number of disparate elements; when the left and right sides of the design are unequal but still pleasing to the eye.

asymptomatic (A-symp-toe-mat-ic)—showing no symptoms.

atlas (AT-lis)—in anatomy, the first cervical vertebra in the spinal column.

atomize (AT-uh-myz)—to reduce to minute particles or to a fine spray.

atoms (AT-umz)—the smallest chemical components (often called particles) of an element; structures that make up the element and have the same properties of the element.

atopic dermatitis (UH-top-ick DERM-uh-tit-is)—excess inflammation; dry skin, redness, and itching from allergies and irritants.

atria (AY-tree-ah)—the upper chambers of the heart through which blood is pumped to the ventricles.

atrichosis (uh-TRI-koh-sis)—absence of hair; congenital or acquired.

atrioventricular valves (ATV) (at-rio-ven-trick-u-lar VALVz)—valves which are designed to prevent the blood from flowing back into the pumping chamber.

atrium (AY-tree-um)—thin-walled, upper chamber of the heart through which blood is pumped to the ventricles. There is a right atrium and a left atrium.

atrophy (A-truh-fee)—a wasting away of the cells organs, or tissues of the body, or a part of the body, from lack of nutrition, injury, or disease.

attenuate (uh-TEN-yoo-ayt)—to make thin; to increase the fluidity or thinness of the blood or other fluids; to lessen the effect of an agent.

attolens aurem (AT-oh-lenz OH-rem)—auricularis superior; muscle that elevates the ear slightly.

attrahens (AT-ruh-henz)—a muscle that draws or pulls forward.

attrahens aurem (AT-ruh-henz OH-rem)—a muscle that pulls the ear forward.

auditory nerve (AWD-uh-tohr-ee NURV)—either of the eighth pair of cranial nerves controlling hearing and balance.

aurantiasis cutis (oh-ran-TY-ah-sus KYOO-tis)—a condition of the skin that renders it a golden yellow; sometimes caused by excessive intake of carotene.

auricular anterior artery (aw-RIK-yuh-lur an-TEER-ee-ur ART-uh-ree)—artery that supplies blood to the anterior part of the ear.

auricularis anterior (aw-rik-yuh-LAIR-is, an-TEER-ee-ur)—the muscle in front of the ear that draws the ear forward.

auricularis posterior (aw-rik-yuh-LAIR-is poh-STEER-ee-ur)—the muscle behind the ear that draws the ear backward.

auricularis superior (aw-rik-yuh-LAIR-is soo-PEER-ee-ur)—the muscle above the ear that draws the ear upward.

auricular nerve (aw-RIK-yuh-lur NURV)—nerve that receives stimuli from the skin around the ear.

auricular posterior artery (aw-RIK-yuh-lur poh-STEER-ee-ur ART-ur-ee)—posterior artery that supplies blood to the scalp and parotid (salivary) gland.

auriculotemporal nerve (aw-RIK-yuh-loh-TEM-puh-rul NURV)—affects the external ear and skin above the temple, up to the top of the skull.

autoclave (AW-toh-klayv)—a device used for sterilization by steam under pressure.

autolysis (aw-TAHL-uh-sis)—the disintegration of cells and tissues by the action of enzymes already present; self-digestion of tissues within a living body.

A

automatic (aw-toh-MAT-ik)—acting from forces within; self-acting; largely or entirely involuntary.

autonomic; autonomous (aw-toh-NAHM-ik; aw-TAHN-uh-mus)—independent in origin, action, or function; self-governing.

autonomic nervous system (ANS) (aw-toh-NAHM-ik NURV-us SIS-tum)—the part of the nervous system that controls the involuntary muscles; regulates the action of the smooth muscles, glands, blood vessels, heart, and breathing.

avant-garde (av-vahnt guard)—French term meaning advance guard, and refers to things that are unique and new; experimental or innovative in nature.

avant-garde style (av-vahnt guard STY-uhl)—a look that represents pushing the boundaries, resulting in a very edgy, high-voltage look.

avitaminosis (ay-vyt-uh-muh-NOH-sus)—a disease that results from lack of vitamins in the diet such as scurvy (vitamin C) or rickets (vitamin D).

axial skeleton (AK-see-ul SKEL-uh-tun)—bones of the skull, thorax, vertebral column, and hyoid bone.

axilla (ag-ZIL-uh)—armpit; the region between the arm and the thoracic wall.

axillary artery (AK-suh-lair-ee AR-tur-ee)—artery associated with the region of the muscles of the upper arm, chest, shoulder, and the skin of the pectoral region.

axillary glands (AK-suh-lair-ee GLANZ)—the lymph nodes of the armpit.

axillary nerves (AK-suh-lair-ee NURVZ)—nerves located in the shoulder and armpit regions that stimulate deltoid muscles.

axillary veins (AK-suh-lair-ee VAYNZ)—veins located within the regions of the armpits.

axon (AK-sahn)—the extension of a neuron through which impulses are sent away from the cell body to other neurons, glands, or muscles.

axon terminal (AK-sahn TER-min-al)—distal (furthest away) terminations of the branches of an axon.

Ayurveda (ah-yur-VAY-dah)—Indian philosophy of balancing life and the body through various methods ranging from massage to eating habits. It is based on three *doshas*, or mind and body types. One of the world's oldest holistic healing systems, it originated in India and is thought to be as much as 5,000 years old. Ayurveda translates from Sanskrit as "science of health and wellness."

azulene (azz-U-leen)—derived from the chamomile plant and characterized by its deep-blue color; has anti-inflammatory and soothing properties.

B

b vitamins (BEE vy-ta-minz)—these water-soluble vitamins interact with other water-soluble vitamins and act as coenzymes (catalysts) by facilitating enzymatic reactions. b vitamins include niacin, riboflavin, thiamine, pyridoxine, folacin, biotin, cobalamine, and pantothenic acid.

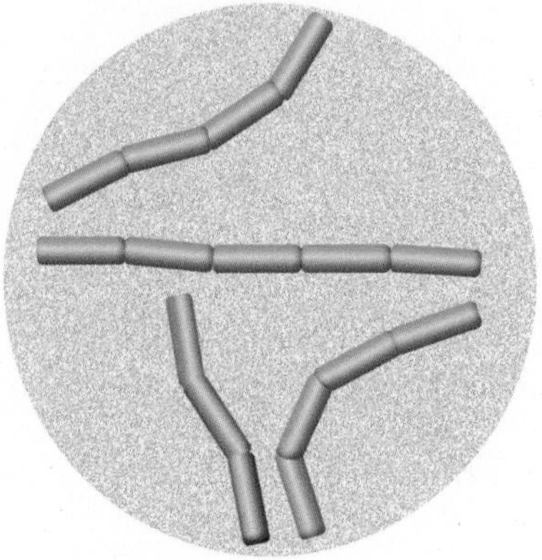
© Milady, a part of Cengage Learning

bacilli

bacilli (bah-SIL-ee)—short rod-shaped bacteria. They are the most common bacteria and produce diseases such as tetanus (lockjaw), typhoid fever, tuberculosis, and diphtheria.

back bubble (BAK BUHB-uhl)—a technique that is used to clean an airbrush or to blend colors.

backbone (BAK-bohn)—the spinal or vertebral column.

backbrushing (BAK BRUSH-ing)—also known as *ruffing*; technique used to build a soft cushion or to mesh two or more curl patterns together for a uniform and smooth comb out.

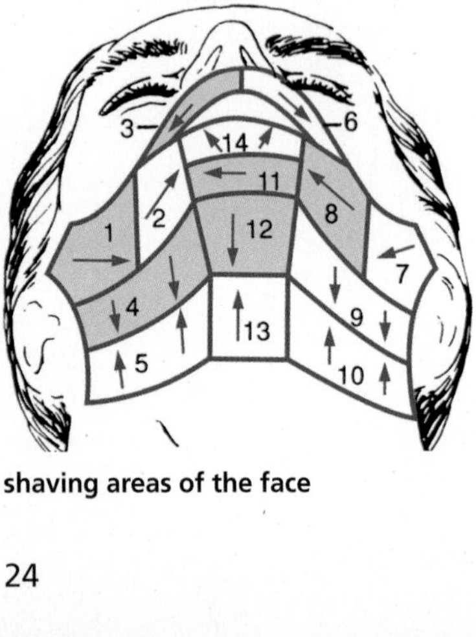

© Milady, a part of Cengage Learning

shaving areas of the face

backcombing (BAK KOHM-ing)—also known as *teasing, ratting, matting,* or *French lacing*; combing small sections of hair from the ends toward the scalp, causing shorter hair to mat at the scalp and form a cushion or base.

backhand position/stroke (BAK-hand POZ-ish-un/STROW-k)—razor position and stroke used in 4 of the 14 basic shaving areas: numbers 2, 6, 7, and 9.

backsweep (BAK-sweep)—sweeping the hair backward with a comb or brush; also, upsweep (hair is swept upward into the desired style).

backward curls (BAK-ward KURLZ)—curls wound in a counterclockwise direction on the left side of the head or curls wound in a clockwise direction on the right side of the head; curls with stems directed toward the back of the head.

backward direction (BAK-ward dih-REK-shun)—movement used when brushing, combing, winding, or wrapping the hair away from the face.

bacteria (bak-TEER-ee-ah); pl., bacterium (bak-TEER-ee-uhm)—also known as *microbes* or *germs*; one-celled microorganisms that have both plant and animal characteristics.

bacterial spores (bak-TEER-ee-ul SPOORZ)—reproductive cells, usually unicellular, produced by plants and some protozoa; they are remarkably resistant to heat, drying, and the action of disinfectants.

bactericidal (bak-TEER-uh-syd-uhl)—capable of destroying bacteria.

bacteriology (bak-teer-ee-AHL-uh-jee)—the science that deals with microorganisms (bacteria).

balance (BAL-uns)—establishing equal or appropriate proportions to create symmetry. In hairstyling, it is the relationship of height to width.

balancing shampoo (BAL-uns-ing SHAM-poo)—shampoo that washes away excess oiliness from hair and scalp, while preventing the hair from drying out.

baldness (BALD-nes)—a deficiency of hair; hair loss.

baliage (BAHL-ee-ahj)—also known as *free-form technique*; painting a lightener (usually a powdered off-the-scalp lightener) directly onto clean, styled hair.

ball-and-socket joint (BAL-and-SOK-et JOYNT)—one bone that is rounded and fits into the socket of another bone such as the hip or shoulder joints.

balneology (bal-nee-AHL-uh-jee)—the science of immersion of the body (or parts of the body) in the waters of mineral springs for therapeutic purposes.

balneotherapy (bal-nee-oh-THAYR-uh-pee)—body water treatments that use mud or fango, Dead Sea salt, seaweed, enzymes, or peat baths. Many of these treatments originated in ancient Greek and Roman bathhouses. Although water treatments were originally used primarily for medicinal purposes, they eventually evolved into relaxation treatments as well.

band lashes (BAND lash-ez)—also known as *strip lashes*; eyelash hairs on a strip that are applied with adhesive to the natural lash line.

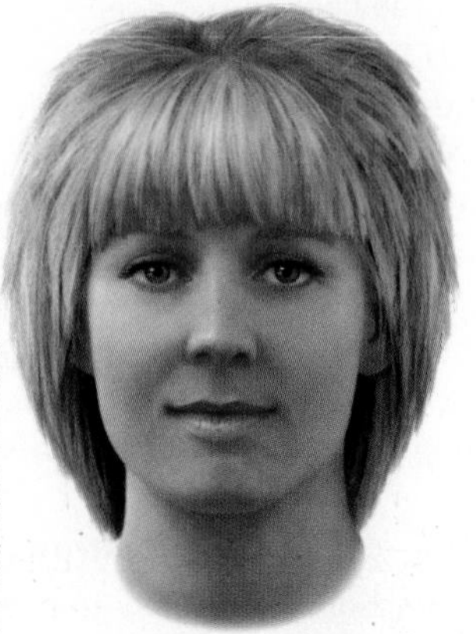

© Milady, a part of Cengage Learning

bangs or fringe

bang area (BAYNG air-ee-ah)—also known as *fringe area*; triangular section that begins at the apex, or high point of the head, and ends at the front corners.

barber (BAR-bur)—one whose occupation includes haircutting, hairdressing, shaving and trimming beards, and related services.

barber chair (BAR-bur CHAYR)—a specially designed chair for barber clients; a hydraulic, reclining chair with adjustable footrest and headrest.

barber comb (BAR-bur KOHM)—a comb of plastic or hard rubber with a three-quarter inch wide set of teeth tapering to a narrow end about one inch wide with a set of fine teeth; an implement for combing and styling hair.

barber pole (BAR-bur POHL)—most often a red-, white-, and blue-striped pole that is the iconic symbol of the barbering profession.

barber science (BAR-bur SY-ens)—the study of the beard and hair, and their treatment.

barbering (BAR-bur-ingh)—the performance of techniques and arts of haircutting, shaving, massaging, facial treatments, and the trimming and styling of facial hair.

barber-surgeons (BAR-bur SIR-genz)—early practitioners of barbering who cut hair, shaved, and performed bloodletting and dentistry.

barbershop (BAR-bur-SHOP)—the barber's place of business; where barbers' clients receive services.

barber's itch (BAR-burz ITCH)—also known as *tinea barbae*; a disease that mainly affects adult males, usually in the beard and moustache areas. Infections caused by zoophilic (having to do with animals or insects) species are responsible for the great majority of cases; the two main species involved are *T.*

mentagrophytes and *T. verrucosum*. Clinically, tinea barbae displays deep folliculitis with red inflammatory papules and pustules and exudation or crusting. Hair shaft loss is also present.

barrel (BAYR-ul)—the part of a thermal heating iron or curling iron that contains the heating element.

barrel curls (BAYR-ul KURLZ)—pin curls with large center openings, fastened to the head in a standing position on a rectangular base.

barrier function (BEAR-ee-ore FUNK-shun)—protective barrier of the epidermis; the corneum and intercellular matrix protect the surface from irritation and dehydration.

basal cell carcinoma (BAY-zul CEL kar-si-NOO-mah)—most common and least severe type of skin cancer; often characterized by light or pearly nodules.

basal layer (bay-ZUL LAY-ur)—the layer of cells at the base of the epidermis closest to the dermis.

base (BAYS)—a cosmetic preparation applied to the face to form a foundation on which to apply other cosmetics such as powder and cheek color; in hairstyling, the stationary, or nonmoving, foundation of a pin curl (the area closest to the scalp); in chemistry, the chief substance of a compound; an electropositive element that unites with an acid to form a salt; an alkali.

base coat (BAYS KOHT)—a colorless liquid applied to the natural nail and/or nail enhancement to improve adhesion of colored polish.

base color (BAYS KUL-ur)—predominant tone of a color.

base control (BAYS KUL-ur CON-troll)—position of the tool in relation to its base section, determined by the angle at which the hair is wrapped.

base cream (bays creem)—also known as *protective base cream*; oily cream used to protect the skin and scalp during hair relaxing.

base direction (BAYS dy-REK-shun)—angle at which the rod is positioned on the head (horizontally, vertically, or diagonally); also, the directional pattern in which the hair is wrapped.

base of a curl (BAYS UV UH KURL)—that portion of the hair strand being curled that is nearest the scalp.

base part (BAYS PART)—the working part of the hair toward which the curl is rolled.

base placement (BAYS PLAYS-ment)—refers to the position of the rod in relation to its base section; base placement is determined by the angle at which the hair is wrapped.

B

base, protective (BAYS, proh-TEK-tiv)—oily cream used to protect the skin and scalp during hair relaxing.

base relaxers (BAYS RE-lax-ors)—relaxers that require the application of protective base cream to the entire scalp for the application of the relaxer.

base sections (BAYS SEK-shuns)—subsections of panels into which hair is divided for perm wrapping; one rod is normally placed on each base section.

base substance (BAYS SUB-stans)—a supporting or carrying ingredient in a preparation that serves as a vehicle for active ingredients in some medicinal and cosmetic preparations.

B

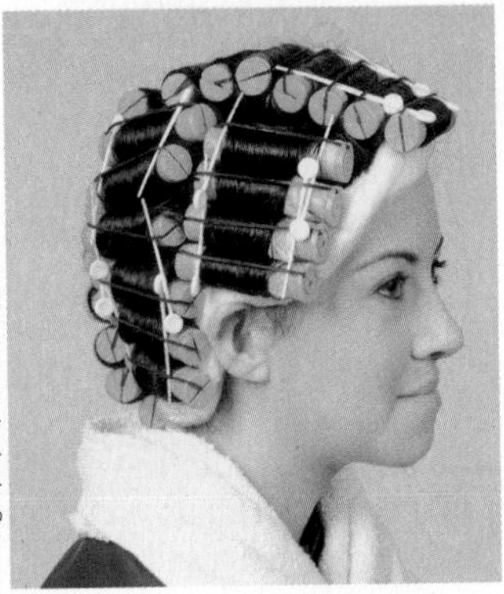

© Milady, a part of Cengage Learning. Photography by Yanik Chauvin.

basic perm wrapping pattern

basic permanent wrap (BAY-sik PER-muh-nant RAP)—also known as *straight set wrap*; perm wrapping pattern in which all the rods within a panel move in the same direction and are positioned on equal-sized bases; all the base sections are horizontal and are the same length and width as the perm rod.

basify (BAYS-if-eye)—to change into a base by chemical means; to make alkaline.

beard (BEERD)—the hair on a man's face, especially on the chin (the hair over the upper lip is usually called a mustache, which may be a part of a full beard).

beating (BEE-ting)—in massage, heaviest and deepest form of percussion, and is used over the denser areas of the body.

Beau's lines (BOWZ LYNEZ)—visible depressions running across the width of the natural nail plate; usually a result of major illness or injury that has traumatized the body.

bed epithelium (BED ep-ih-THEE-lee-um)—thin layer of tissue that attaches the nail plate and the nail bed.

belly (BELL-ee)—the middle part of a muscle; as in a brush, the midsection of the brush bristles; the area of the brush that retains the most paint.

benign (bih-NYN)—mild in character; in relation to tumors, not harmful or dangerous.

bentonite (BENT-un-ite)—a porous clay from volcanic ash; a type of facial mask used to absorb oil on the face; used in a variety of cosmetic products to thicken lotions, emulsify oils, and suspend pigments.

benzine (BEN-zeen)—an inflammable liquid derived from petroleum and used as a cleaning fluid.

benzoyl peroxide (BEN-zoyl puh-RAHK-syd)—a type of peroxide that reduces bacteria, a drying ingredient with antibacterial properties commonly used for blemishes and acne.

beta helix (BA-ta HEE-lix)—term indicating that the spiral of the body of the polypeptide chains within the cortex of the hair are in the second position; the spiral is stretched but can return to its alpha or first position when released.

beta-glucans (BA-ta GLOO-canz)—derived from plants and yeast; ingredients used in antiaging cosmetics to help reduce the appearance of fine lines and wrinkles by stimulating the formation of collagen.

beta hydroxy acids (BHAS) (BA-ta hi-droxy asudz)—exfoliating organic acid; salicylic acid; milder than alpha hydroxyl acids (AHAs). BHAS dissolve oil and are beneficial for oily skin.

bevel (BEV-ul)—to slope the edge of a surface; in haircutting, to taper the ends of the hair.

bevel cut (BEV-ul KUT)—holding the shears at an angle to the hair strand other than 90 degrees.

beveling (BEV-ul-ing)—technique using diagonal lines by cutting hair ends with a slight increase or decrease in length.

bicep (BY-sep)—muscle that produces the contour of the front and inner side of the upper arm; lifts the forearm and flexes the elbow.

bicuspid valve (by-KUS-pid VALV)—the heart valve located between the left atrium and the left ventricle that regulates blood backflow between the two chambers.

bilateral (by-LAT-uh-rul)—pertaining to or having two sides.

bile (BYL)—a bitter alkaline fluid, greenish yellow to brown, secreted by the liver; it aids in the emulsification, digestion, and absorption of fats.

bi-level haircut (by-LEV-ul HAYR-kut)—a style that divides the head into two separate design lines.

binary fission (BYN-airey FISH-in)—the division of bacteria cells into two new cells called *daughter cells*.

binder (BYND-ur)—substances such as glycerin that bind, or hold, products together.

bioburden (BY-oh-burr-den)—the number of viable organisms in or on an object or surface or the organic material on a surface or object before decontamination or sterilization.

biocatalyst (by-oh-KAT-ul-est)—a substance that acts to promote or modify some physiological process, especially an enzyme, vitamin, or hormone.

biochemistry (by-oh-KEM-is-tree)—the chemistry of living organisms, and the study of the chemical compounds and processes occurring within them.

biodegradable (by-oh-dee-GRAYD-uh-bul)—the ability of a substance to decay organically or naturally.

bioelectricity (by-oh-ee-lek-TRIHS-ih-tee)—electric phenomena occurring in living tissues; effects of electric current on living tissues.

bioflavonoids (BY-oh-FLAYV-en oydz)—biologically active antioxidant, derived from plants and found abundantly in the human diet; considered an aid to healthy skin.

biology (by-AHL-uh-jee)—the study of life and living things.

biorhythm (BY-oh-rith-um)—any regular pattern or cycle in an organism with accompanying variations such as body temperature, blood pressure, heart rate, and the like.

biostimulant (by-oh-STIM-yoo-lant)—an agent used to stimulate activity in living tissue.

biotin (BY-uh-tihn)—a vitamin B complex, found in small amounts in plant and animal tissue.

biphosphate (by-FAHS-fayt)—a salt of phosphoric acid in which one of the three hydrogen atoms of the acid is replaced by a base.

bipolar (by-POH-lar)—of or having two poles; characterized by opposite natures.

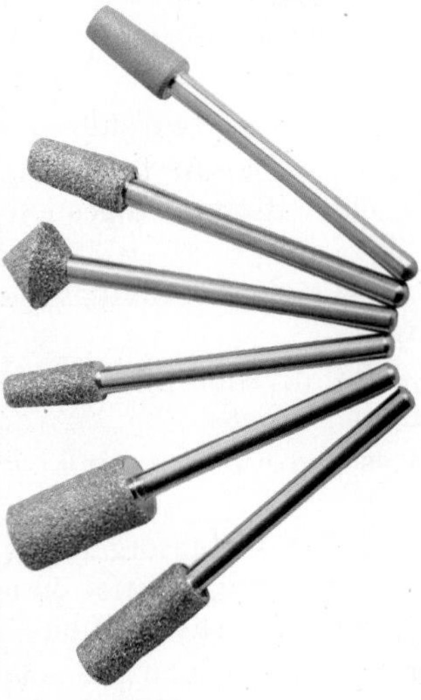
© Milady, a part of Cengage Learning. Photography by Dino Petrocelli.
diamond bits

bipolarity (by-poh-LAIR-ih-tee)—the use of two electrodes in the stimulation of muscles or nerves; the condition of having two processes extending from opposite poles.

birthmark (BURTH-mark)—a mark on the skin due to abnormal pigmentation.

bisulfate (by-SUL-fayt)—an acid sulfate.

bisulfide (by-SUL-fyd)—a compound containing two atoms of sulfur; a disulfide.

bisulfite (by-SUL-fyt)—an acid sulfite.

bit (BIT)—in nail technology; filing tool that inserts into the handpiece of an electric file and that actually does the filing of the nail enhancement.

biterminal (by-TUR-mih-nul)—two terminals or poles of an electric source.

blackhead (BLAK-hed)—also known as *open comedone*; small mass of hardened sebaceous matter that has darkened when exposed to air, appearing most frequently on the face, shoulders, chest, and back.

bladder (BLAD-ur)—a membranous sac that serves as a reservoir for holding urine.

blades (BLAYDZ)—the cutting parts of the clippers, usually manufactured from high-quality carbon steel and available in a variety of styles and sizes.

bleach (BLEECH)—to make lighter or whiten; to remove color or stains. A chemical preparation used to remove the color from hair; also used in some preparations to lighten skin pigmentation; as in disinfecting; hydrogen peroxide with the addition of ammonia.

bleeding (BLEED-ing)—in haircoloring; seepage of tint/lightener from foil or cap due to improper application.

blemish (BLEM-ish)—a mark, spot, or defect on the skin.

blemish cover (BLEM-ish KUV-ur)—also known as *concealer*; a cosmetic in stick or cream form based on alcohol, oil, wax, and pigments; used to conceal minor blemishes.

blend (BLEND)—to meet or join; in haircoloring, to mix or blend colors to achieve various hair colors; in haircutting, to graduate from shorter to longer lengths; in makeup, to mix together so there is no line of demarcation.

blending (BLEND-ing)—the physical act of merging one tint or tone with another during haircolor and lightening applications; mixing of makeup colors; connection between two or more shapes in hair design.

blepharitis (BLEFF-uhr-eye-tiz)—eye condition characterized by chronic inflammation of the eyelid.

blepharoplasty (BLEF-uh-roh-plas-tee)—also known as *eye lift*; cosmetic surgery that removes the fat and skin from the upper and lower lids.

blister (BLIS-tur)—a vesicle; a collection of serous fluid causing an elevation of the skin.

block (BLAHK)—in wigs, head-shaped form, usually made of canvas-covered cork or Styrofoam, on which the wig is secured for fitting, cleaning, coloring, and styling; in parting, to mark off or indicate sections in an outline to be followed when sub-sectioning the hair.

block holder (BLAHK HOLD-ur)—a clamping device used to hold the block to a table.

blocking (BLAHK-ing)—also known as *parting*; subdividing of panels of hair into uniform, individual, rectangular rod sections.

blog (BLOHG)—an on-line journal or newsletter reflecting your knowledge, talent, and skills.

blond (BLAHND)—a term used to describe hair shades and tints that range from light yellowish-brown to platinum or silver-white.

blonding (BLAHND-ing)—term applied to lightening the hair, sometimes in preparation for the application of a toner, and sometimes as an end result in itself.

blond on blond (BLAHND ON BLAHND)—two shades or colors used to create lighter and darker strands of hair to achieve a natural sun-bleached look.

blood (BLUD)—nutritive fluid circulating through the circulatory system (heart and blood vessels) to supply oxygen and nutrients to cells and tissues and to remove carbon dioxide and waste from them.

bloodborne (BLUD born)—transmitted through direct blood-to-blood contact, such as by sharing needles or through a blood transfusion.

blood clot (BLUD KLOT)—a coagulated mass that forms in the circulatory system, and which consists of the elements in the blood such as platelets, red blood cells, and the like.

blood plasma (BLUD PLAZ-ma)—the fluid part of the blood in which red and white blood cells and blood platelets flow.

blood platelets (BLUD PLATY-lehts)—thrombocytes; colorless, irregular bodies, much smaller than red corpuscles that play an important role in the clotting of blood.

blood poisoning (BLUD POY-zun-ing)—also known as *septicemia*; an infection in the bloodstream.

blood pressure (BLUD PREHSH-ur)—the pressure exerted by the circulatory blood on the walls of the blood vessels.

blood spill (BLUD SPIYL)—also known as *exposure incident*; a situation occurring when a cosmetologist, nail technician, esthetician, or barber or client sustains an injury that results in bleeding.

blood vascular system (BLUD VAS-kyoo-lur SIS-tum)—consists of the heart, arteries, veins, and capillaries that distribute blood throughout the body.

blood vessels (BLUD VES-ul)—tube-like structures that include arteries, arterioles, capillaries, venules, and veins.

bloodborne pathogens (BLUD-boorn PATH-o-genz)—disease-causing microorganisms carried in the body by blood or body fluids, such as hepatitis and HIV.

bloodstream (BLUD-STREEM)—the flowing of blood throughout the body.

blotting paper (BLOTTING PAY-pur)—a highly absorbent, thin paper used to absorb excess oil from the surface of the skin, leaving a smooth, matte finish.

blowdry (BLOH-dry)—to use an electrical apparatus called a *blowdryer* to dry and style hair in a single process, usually without presetting.

blowdry styling (BLOH-dry stihyl-ing)—technique of drying and styling damp hair in a single operation.

blowdryer (BLOH-dry-ur)—a small, handheld hair dryer used when styling and blowdrying hair. Parts of the blowdryer include the handle, air-directional nozzle, small fan, heating element, and controls.

blue light (BLOO LYT)—a light-emitting diode for use on clients with acne.

bluing rinse (BLOO-ing RINS)—a temporary coloring used to neutralize the unbecoming yellowish tinge in gray or white hair.

blunt (BLUNT)—having a thick or rounded edge or end.

blunt haircut (BLUNT HARE-cut)—also known as a *one-length haircut, or bob cut*; haircut in which all the hair comes to one hanging level, forming a weight line or area; hair is cut with no elevation or overdirection.

blusher (BLUSH-ur)—a powdered substance, also called *rouge*, used to add color or highlights to the cheeks or to shade areas of the face.

boar bristle brush (BOHR BRIS-ul BRUSH)—a brush made with the short, stiff hairs from a wild boar; considered to be less damaging to hair than other types of bristles.

bobby pin (BAHB-ee PIN)—a long "U" shaped clamp or clasp-like pin with the ends pressing close together; used to hold the hair in place in a style or hair set.

body (BAHD-ee)—in anatomy, the human or animal frame and its organs; in cosmetology, the consistency or solidarity of texture or quality of liveliness and springiness the hair possesses.

body image (BAHD-ee IM-ij)—the conscious and unconscious concept a person has of his or her body as it may be perceived by others.

body masks (BAHD-ee masks)—application of clay, mud, gel, or seaweed mixtures that remineralize and detoxify the body.

body scrubs (BAHD-ee scrubz)—use of friction and products to exfoliate, hydrate, increase circulation, and nourish the skin.

B

body substance isolation (BSI) (BAHD-ee sub-stanz iso-lay-shun)—a system of precautions developed by a Seattle hospital in 1987 to prevent contact with bodily substances and fluids by using protective apparel to prevent the spread of communicable disease.

body surface area (BAHD-ee SUR-fus AIR-ee-uh)—the area covered by a person's skin expressed in square meters.

body systems (BAHD-ee SYS-tims)—also known as *systems*; groups of body organs acting together to perform one or more functions. The human body is composed of 11 major systems.

body wave (BAHD-ee WAYV)—a large wave pattern created by a permanent wave as a foundation for a style.

body wrap (BAHD-ee RAP)—the use of such products as aloe, gels, lotions, oils, seaweed, herbs, clay, or mud, applied to the body and usually covered with plastic; used to remineralize, hydrate, stimulate, or promote relaxation.

boil (BOYL)—also known as *furuncle*; a collection of pus, caused by an acute staphylococci infection of a hair follicle that causes constant pain, redness, swelling, and heat.

bond (BAHND)—the force that binds one atom to another in a molecule, resulting from the transfer or sharing of one or more electrons.

bond breaker (BAHND BRAYK-ur)—a substance that has the ability to disrupt or destroy the bond units of chemical compounds.

bonding (BAHND-ing)—method of attaching hair extensions in which hair wefts or single strands are attached with an adhesive or bonding agent.

bone (BOHN)—hard tissue of the body comprised of connective tissues consisting of cells, blood, calcium carbonate, and calcium phosphate that form the framework of the body.

bone tissue (BOHN TISH-oo)—the substance forming the layers of bone and dentin of the teeth; connective tissue in which the intercellular substance is rendered hard by mineral salts, chiefly calcium carbonate and calcium phosphate.

bookend wrap (BOOK END RAP)—perm wrap in which one end paper is folded in half over the hair ends like an envelope.

booster (BOOST-ur)—also known as *activator* or *catalyst*, oxidizer such as ammonium persulfate or percarbonate added to hydrogen peroxide to increase its chemical action.

booth rental (BOO-th ren-tal)—also known as *chair rental*; renting a booth or station in a salon; a form of self-employment, business ownership, and tax designation with certain responsibilities for bookkeeping, taxes, insurances, etc.

B

boric acid (BOR-ik AS-ud)—used as a mild antiseptic and in liquid form as a healing agent.

botanicals (bow-tan-ee-calz)—ingredients derived from plants.

botox® (Bow-tocks)—neuromuscular-blocking serum (botulinum toxin) that paralyzes nerve cells on the muscle when this serum is injected into it.

brachial artery (BRAY-kee-ul ART-uh-ree)—located in the upper arm, the brachial artery is a major blood vessel which runs down the arm and ends by dividing into the radial and ulnar arteries, which run down through the forearm.

brachial plexus (BRAY-kee-ul PLEX-us)—composed of four lower cervical nerves and the first pair of thoracic nerves which control arm movements.

brachialis (bray-kih-AY-lis)—the muscle that flexes the elbow joint.

brachioradialis (bray-kih-oh-ray-dih-AL-us)—a flexor muscle located in the posterior compartment of the forearm.

brachium (BRAY-kih-um)—the part of the arm above the elbow.

braid (BRAYD)—three interwoven strands of hair that form a repetitive pattern; a braided or coiled hair switch that is used to create different hairstyles; a three-stemmed switch joined with a loop at the top; to weave, entwine, or interlace hair strands.

braid-and-sew method (BRAYD ahnd SOO meth-id)—attachment method in which hair extensions are secured to client's own hair by sewing braids or a weft onto an on-the-scalp braid or cornrow, which is sometimes called the track.

brain (BRAYN)—part of the central nervous system contained in the cranium; largest and most complex nerve tissue and controls sensation, muscles, gland activity, and the power to think and feel emotions.

brain stem (BRAYN STEM)—intricate masses of nerve fiber that relay and transmit impulses from one part of the brain to another consisting of the midbrain, pons, and the medulla oblongata.

branding (BRAND-ING)—the character of your business and the personality and image you are projecting to potential clients and employers.

brassy tone (BRAS-ee TOHN)—in hair coloring, a harsh color quality exhibiting excess red, orange, or gold.

B

Brazilian bikini waxing (BRA-zill-ee-on bi-KI-ni WAKS-ing)—a waxing technique that involves the removal of all the hair from the front and the back of the bikini area.

breakage (BRAYK-ij)—a condition in which hair splits and breaks off; caused by damage to the hair.

breastbone (BREST-bohn)—the sternum; the flat bone located in the middle of the chest.

bricklay permanent wrap (BRIK-lay PERM-ahn-ent RAP)—perm wrap similar to actual technique of bricklaying; base sections are offset from each other row by row to prevent noticeable splits and to blend the flow of the hair.

briefing (BREEF-ing)—usually fifteen to thirty minutes before the start of the (hair, nail, or makeup) competition during which the competition director or head judge will review the rules and guidelines to ensure everyone understands and is able to comply.

brightening (BRYT-un-ing)—adding highlights and luster to hair by lightening or toning its natural shade.

brittle (BRIT-ul)—easily broken, fragile.

brittle hair (BRIT-ul HAYR)—hair that is dry and fragile and is easily broken.

bromhidrosis (bro-mih-DROH-sis)—foul-smelling perspiration, usually noticeable in the armpits or on the feet, that is caused by bacteria.

bromoacid (broh-moh-AS-ud)—a soluble dye used to impart a red indelible color in lipsticks and similar cosmetics.

bronchial (BRAHNG-kee-ul)—pertaining to or involving the bronchi and their branches in the lungs.

bronchus (BRAHNG-kus); pl., bronchi (BRAHNG-kai)—one of the two main branches of the windpipe.

brow **(BROW)**—the upper anterior portion of the head; the forehead; the supraorbital ridge; the hair above the eyes called the eyebrows.

bruise **(BROOZ)**—a superficial injury without laceration caused by a blow or impact with an object that produces capillary hemorrhage beneath the surface of the skin causing a bluish discoloration.

bruised nails **(BROOZ-ed NAYLZ)**—condition in which a blood clot forms under the nail plate, causing a dark purplish spot. These discolorations are usually due to small injuries to the nail bed.

brush **(BRUSH)**—a grooming tool with a handle and rows of bristles embedded in the other end.

brush electrode **(BRUSH ih-LEK-trohd)**—an electrode resembling a brush that is used for the application of electricity.

brushing machine **(BRUSH-ing muh-SHEEN)**—a rotating electric appliance with interchangeable brushes that can be attached to the rotating head, used to exfoliate dead skin cells during a facial.

bucca **(BUK-uh)**—the cheek.

buccal artery **(BUK-ul ART-uh-ree)**—the artery that supplies blood to the cheeks.

buccal nerve **(BUK-ul NURV)**—affects the muscles of the mouth.

buccinator muscle **(BUK-sih-nay-tur MUS-uhl)**—the thin, flat muscle of the cheek between the upper and lower jaw, which compresses the cheeks and expels air between the lips.

buffer **(BUF-ur)**—a manicuring implement used buffing cream to impart a sheen to the nails; an abrasive tool used to blend a nail enhancement product; a system that resists changes in pH.

buffer activity **(BUF-ur ak-TIV-ih-tee)**—the action of a buffer solution that has a tendency to resist changes in its pH when treated with strong acids or bases.

buildup **(BILD-up)**—repeated coatings on the hair shaft. In hairstyling, an accumulation of excess foreign matter deposited in the hair shaft; in manicuring, an accumulation of substance to create artificial nails.

bulb **(BULB)**—the lowest area or part of a hair strand.

bulk **(BULK)**—in haircutting and hairstyling, the density, thickness, textured length, and volume of the hair.

bulla **(BULL-uh)**—large blister containing a watery fluid; similar to a vesicle but larger.

bullous pemphigoid (BULL-us PEM-fih-goyd)—a chronic skin disorder characterized by large blisters **(bulla)** that heal without leaving scars.

bundle (BUN-dul)—a structure composed of a group of fibers, either muscular or nervous.

bunion (BUN-yun)—a swelling of a bursa of the foot, generally affecting the joint of the great (big) toe.

burrowing hair (BUR-oh-ing HAYR)—a condition in which the hair does not emerge from the skin but grows beneath the surface and may become infected.

bursa (BUR-sah)—a fibrous sac lined with a synovial membrane and lubricated with synovial fluid functioning as a cushion in areas of pressure.

bursitis (bur-SY-tis)—inflammation and swelling of the bursae.

business plan (BIZ-nez plahn)—strategy for understanding key elements in developing business; also serves as a guide to making informed business decisions; a written description of your business as you see it today, and as you foresee it in the next five years (detailed by year).

business regulations and laws (BIZ-nez reg-U-lay-shuns AND LAWZ)—any and all local, state, and federal regulations and laws that you must comply with when you decide to open your salon or rent a booth.

butterfly clamp (BUT-ur-fly KLAMP)—also known as *jaw clamp or clip*; a clamping device designed to hold the hair in place while sectioning, subsectioning, or during other procedures.

butyl alcohol (BYOOT-ul AL-kuh-hawl)—any of four isomeric alcohols obtained from petroleum products; used as a clarifying agent in shampoos.

butylene glycol (BYOOT-ul-een GLY-kawl)—a substance made from acetylene formaldehyde and hydrogen used in hair sprays and hair setting preparations.

butyl stearate (BYOOT-ul STEER-uh-ayt)—stearic acid; butyl ester; used as emollient in nail polish, lipstick, creams, and bath oils.

C

cadmium sulfide (KAD-mee-um SUL-fyd)—a yellow-orange powder, used in shampoo for the treatment of dandruff.

cake makeup (KAYK MAYK-up)—also known as *pancake makeup*; a heavy-coverage makeup pressed into a compact and applied to the face with a moistened cosmetic sponge.

cake mascara (KAYK mas-KAR-ah)—a makeup for the eyelashes applied with a moistened brush or applicator; comes in dry molded form or a liquid product in a cylinder or tube.

calcaneus bone (kal-KAY-nee-us bohn)—the largest of the tarsal bones, it forms the heel.

calcium (KAL-see-um)—the most abundant mineral in the body; is found in some foods, added to others, available as a dietary supplement, and present in some medicines (such as antacids). Calcium is required for vascular contraction and vasodilation, muscle function, nerve transmission, intracellular signaling, and hormonal secretion.

calendula (ca-LEND-yoo-lah)—a variety of the daisy plant, anti-inflammatory plant extract.

callus (KAL-us)—also known as *keratoma*; thickening of the skin caused by continued, repeated pressure on any part of the skin, especially the hands and feet.

callus softeners (KAL-us soff-en-erz)—products designed to soften and smooth thickened tissue (calluses), especially on heels and over pressure points.

calories (cal-ore-eez)—a measure of heat units; measures food energy for the body.

camouflage makeup (KAM-oh-flaj MAYK-up)—the strategic layering of various colors and textures to hide pigmentation issues.

cancer (KAN-sur)—a large class of diseases in which a group of cells display uncontrolled growth, invasion that intrudes upon and destroys adjacent tissues, and often metastasizes, wherein the tumor cells spread to other locations in the body via the lymphatic system or through the bloodstream.

candida (KAN-dih-duh)—a genus of yeastlike fungi commonly found in the mouth, intestinal tract, and vagina.

candidate information booklet (CAN-di-date IN-for-may-shun BOOK-let)—in barbering, literature provided to examination candidates by the barber board.

candidiasis (kan-dih-dy-AY-sus)—also known as *thrush*, a type of fungal infection of the tongue; can range from superficial to life-threatening.

caninus (kay-NY-nus)—the levator anguli oris muscle which raises the angle of the mouth.

canities (kah-NISH-ee-eez)—technical term for gray hair; results from the loss of the hair's natural melanin pigment.

canities, accidental (kah-NISH-ee-eez ak-sih-DEN-tul)—grayness of hair caused by fright.

canities, congenital (kah-NISH-ee-eez kahn-JEN-uh-tul)—a type of grayness or whiteness of the hair that is hereditary.

canities, premature (kah-NISH-ee-eez pree-muh-CHOOR)—early graying of the hair.

canities, senile (kah-NISH-ee-eez SEN-yl)—grayness of hair associated with advanced age.

C

canker sore (KANG-kur SOAR)—an ulceration usually affecting the mucous membranes of the mouth.

canthus (KAN-thus)—the corner of each side of the eye where the upper and lower lids meet.

canvas strop (can-viss strohp)—used in barbering, made of high-quality linen or silk and woven into a fine or coarse texture; used to remove small metal particles from the blade, smooth the edge, and polish the razor.

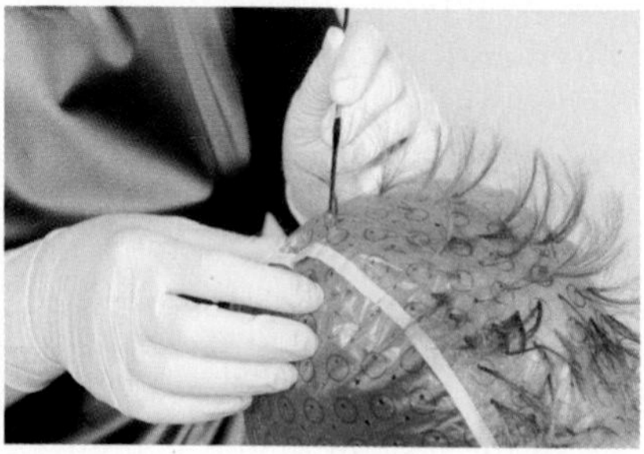

© Milady, a part of Cengage Learning. Photography by Yanik Chauvin.

cap technique

cap technique (KAP tek-NEEK)—lightening technique that involves pulling clean, dry strands of hair through a perforated cap with a thin plastic or metal hook, and then combing them to remove tangles.

cap wigs (KAP WHIGZ)—wigs constructed of elasticized, mesh-fiber bases to which the hair is attached.

cape (KAYP)—a sleeveless garment of cloth or plastic used to protect the client's clothing during cosmetology services.

capillaries, pl. (KAP-ih-lair-eez) capillary s., (KAP-uh-lair-ee)—tiny, thin-walled blood vessels that connect the smaller arteries to the veins. Capillaries enable the exchange of nutrients to the cells and carry away waste materials.

capillaritis (KAP-ih-lair-eye-tis)—inflamed capillaries.

capillary hemangioma (KAP-uh-lair-ee hee-man-jee-OH-muh)—a benign vascular tumor made up largely of capillaries.

capital (KAP-uh-tal)—money needed to invest in or start a business.

capitate (KAP-uh-tayt)—shaped like or forming a head as the rounded end of a bone; the large bone of the wrist; the largest carpal bone.

capless wigs (KAP-less WHIGZ)—also known as *caps*; machine-made from human or artificial hair, which is woven into rows of wefts. Wefts are sewn to elastic strips in a circular pattern to fit the head shape.

capsule (KAP-sool)—a membranous or sac-like structure enclosing a part of an organ; a small case to enclose substances of disagreeable taste.

carbohydrates (kahr-boh-HY-draytz)—a category of food; enzymes break down carbohydrates into the basic chemical sugars and supply energy for the body.

C

carbolic acid (kahr-BAHL-ik AS-ud)—phenol; a caustic and corrosive poison found in coal tar that is used in dilute solution as an antiseptic.

carbomers (KAHR-boh-murz)—ingredients used to thicken creams; frequently used in gel products.

carbon (KAHR-bun)—an abundant nonmetallic element found in all organic compounds, the symbol for carbon is the capital letter C.

carbon dioxide (KAHR-bun dy-AHK-syd)—carbonic a naturally occurring chemical compound composed of two oxygen atoms bonded to a single carbon atom. It is a gas at standard temperature and pressure and exists in Earth's atmosphere in this state.

carbon monoxide (KAHR-bun mahn-AHK-syd)—a colorless, odorless, and poisonous gas; its toxic action is due to its strong affinity for hemoglobin.

carbon tetrachloride (KAHR-bun tet-ruh-KLOHR-yd)—a nonflammable, colorless liquid used as a solvent in cleaning mixtures.

carbuncle (KAHR-bung-kul)—cluster of boils; large inflammation of the subcutaneous tissue caused by staphylococci bacterium; similar to a furuncle (boil) but larger.

carcinogen (kahr-SIN-uh-jin)—a cancer-causing agent or substance.

carcinoma (kahr-sin-OH-muh)—a malignant (cancerous) tumor; malignant new growth of epithelial or gland cells infiltrating the surrounding tissues.

cardiac cycle (KAHRD-ee-ak SY-kul)—the rhythmic cycle of contraction, dilation, and relaxation of all four chambers of the heart (atria and ventricles).

cardiac glands (KAHRD-ee-ak GLANZ)—glands of the stomach that primarily secrete mucus.

cardiac muscle (KAHR-ee-ak MUS-uhl)—the involuntary muscle that is the heart. This type of muscle is not found in any other part of the body.

© Milady, a part of Cengage Learning

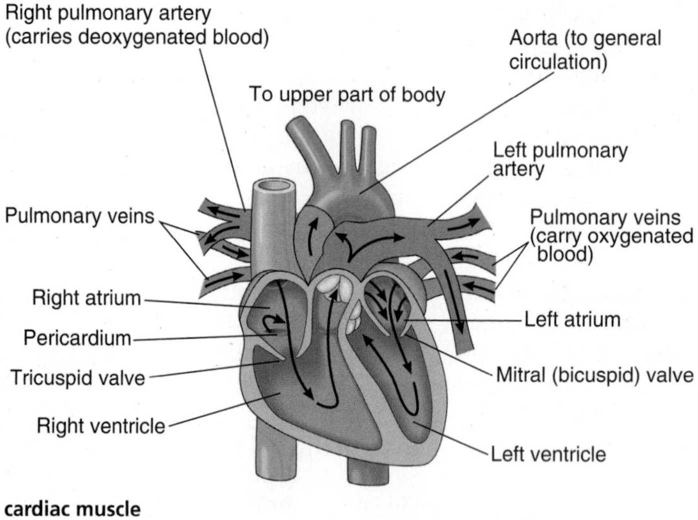

cardiac muscle

cardiac nerves (KAHRD-ee-ak NURVZ)—nerves affecting the heart.

carotid artery (kuh-RAHT-ud ART-uh-ree)—the artery that supplies blood to the head, face, and neck; the principal artery on either side of the neck.

carotid nerves (kuh-RAHT-ud NURVZ)—sympathetic nerves (functioning without cognitive thought) associated with glands and smooth muscles of the head.

carpal tunnel syndrome (KAR-pul TUN-nul SIN-drom)—compression of the median nerve as it passes through the wrist, causing pain and weakness in the fingers; most common cumulative trauma disorder affecting the wrist.

carpus (KAR-pus)—also known as *wrist*; flexible joint composed of eight small, irregular bones (carpals) held together by ligaments.

cartilage (KAR-ti-ledg)—a flexible connective tissue found in the bodies of humans and other animals, including the joints between bones, the rib cage, the ear, the nose, the elbow, the knee, the ankle, and the bronchial tubes. It is as hard and rigid as bone but is stiffer and less flexible than muscle.

cartilaginous joints (kar-tuh-la-JIN-us JOYNTS)—joints held together with cartilage, with no joint cavity.

carve (KARV)—in hair setting, to pick up or slice a strand of hair from a shaping.

carved curls (KARV-ed CURLZ)—also known as *sculptured curls* or *molded curls*; pin curls sliced from a shaping and formed without lifting the hair from the head.

carving (KARV-ing)—haircutting technique done by placing the still blade into the hair and resting it on the scalp, and then moving the shears through the hair while opening and partially closing the shears.

cascade (kas-KAYD)—a hair piece with an oblong-shaped base, offering endless styling possibilities.

cascade curls (kas-KAYD KURLZ)—also known as *stand-up curls*; pin curls fastened to the head in a standing position to allow the hair to flow upward and then downward.

cast (KAST)—a method of manufacturing shears; a metal-forming process whereby molten steel is poured into a mold and, once the metal is cooled, takes on the shape of the mold.

catabolism (kuh-TAB-uh-liz-um)—the phase of metabolism that involves the breaking down of complex compounds within the cells into smaller ones. This process releases energy that has been stored.

catagen phase (KAT-uh-jen FAYZ)—the brief transition period between the growth and resting phases of a hair follicle. It signals the end of the growth phase.

catalyst (KAT-ul-est)—substances that speed up chemical reactions.

cataphoresis (kat-uh-fuh-REE-sus)—process of forcing an acidic (positive) product into deeper tissues using galvanic current from the positive pole toward the negative pole; tightens and calms the skin.

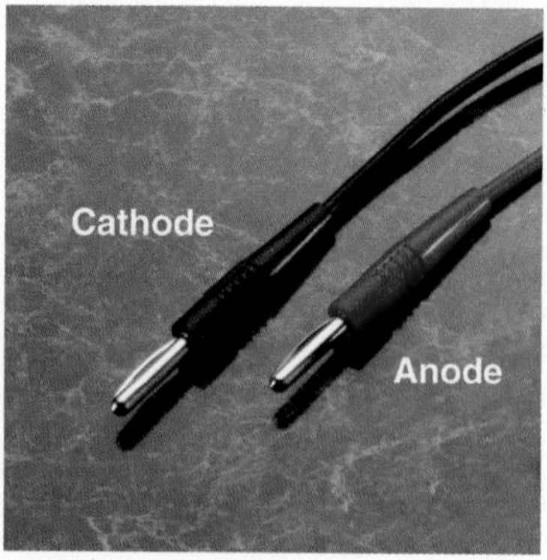

© Milady, a part of Cengage Learning. Photography by Larry Hamill.
anode and cathode

cathode **(KATH-ohd)**—negative electrode; the cathode is usually black and is marked with an *N* or a minus (–) sign.

cation **(KAT-ee-un)**—an ion with a positive electrical charge.

Caucasian race **(kaw-KAY-zhun RAYCE)**—also known as *Caucasoid*; a term used to denote the general physical type of some or all of the populations of Europe, North Africa, the Horn of Africa, West Asia, Central Asia, and South Asia. Historically, the term has been used to describe the entire population of these regions, without regard necessarily to skin tone.

C

caustic **(KAW-stik)**—an agent that damages proteins or tissues by burning; capable of eating away by chemical action.

cauterize **(KAWT-uh-ryz)**—to burn or sear with a caustic substance, or with heat.

cell division **(SELL dih-VIZH-un)**—the reproduction of cells by the process of each cell dividing in half and forming two cells.

cell membrane **(SELL mem-brain)**—cell part that encloses the protoplasm and permits soluble substances to enter and leave the cell.

cell renewal factor **(sell re-new-uhl fack-tor) (CRF)**—cell turnover rate.

cells **(SELLZ)**—basic units of all living things from bacteria to plants to animals, including human beings.

cellular pathology **(SEL-yuh-lur puh-THAHL-uh-jee)**—the study of changes in cells as the basis of disease.

cellular physiology **(SEL-yuh-lur fiz-ee-AHL-uh-jee)**—the physiology of individual cells as compared with entire tissues or organisms.

cellulite **(SEL-yoo-lyt)**—gel-like lumps composed of fat, water, and residues of toxins beneath the skin, usually around the hips and thighs of overweight people.

cellulitis **(sel-yuh-LYT-us)**—a diffuse inflammation of connective tissues, especially the subcutaneous tissues.

cellulose **(SEL-yuh-lohs)**—the principal carbohydrate constituent of the cell membranes of plants; absorbent cotton is a pure form of cellulose.

cellulose paper (SEL-yuh-lohs PAY-pur)—also known as *end paper*; a transparent, insoluble paper used to confine the ends of the hair before winding onto a rod in preparation for permanent waving.

Celsius (SEL-see-us)—in metric measurement, a temperature scale in which the freezing point of water at normal atmospheric pressure is zero degrees and the boiling point is 100 degrees; the centigrade scale.

Centers for Disease Control and Prevention (CDC)—a federal agency that establishes guidelines and makes recommendations for ensuring public health.

centigrade (SENT-uh-grayd)—consisting of 100 divisions or degrees; pertaining to a temperature scale in which the freezing point of water is zero degrees and the boiling point is 100 degrees.

centigram (SENT-ih-gram)—one-hundredth of a gram.

centimeter (SENT-ih-mee-tur)—in the metric system, one hundredth of a meter.

central nervous system (CNS) (SEN-trul NUR-vus SIS-tum)—consists of the brain, spinal cord, spinal nerves, and cranial nerves.

centric (SEN-trik)—relating to or having a center; of or relating to a nerve center.

centrifugal movement (sen-TRIF-ih-gul MOOV-ment)—movement directed away from the center part or point; in massage, the directing of massage movement away from the heart; moving outward from a nerve center.

centriole (SEN-tree-ohl)—a minute body, rod, or granule usually found within the centrosome of the cell; considered to be the active, self-perpetuating division center of the cell.

centripetal movement (sen-TRIP-ut-ul MOOV-ment)—movement directed toward a center; in massage, a movement directed toward the heart; afferent; toward the central nervous system.

centrosome (SEN-tro-sohm)—a small, round body in cytoplasm. Controls the transportation of substances in and out of cells and affects reproduction of cells.

cephalic vein (suh-FAL-ik VAYN)—the vein of the arm.

ceramides (SARA-mydes)—glycolipid (lipids with a carbohydrate attached; provide energy and also serve as markers for cellular recognition) materials that are a natural part of skin's intercellular matrix and barrier function.

cerebellum (sair-uh-BEL-um)—lies at the base of the cerebrum and is attached to the brain stem; this term is Latin for "little brain."

cerebral (suh-REE-brul)—pertaining to the brain or the cerebrum.

cerebral allergy (suh-REE-brul AL-ur-jee)—symptoms of cerebral disturbances associated with certain allergies.

cerebral hemisphere (suh-REE-brul HEM-ih-sfeer)—one of the two halves of the brain.

cerebrospinal fluid (ser-ree-bro-SPY-nahl FLU-id)—a liquid that is comparable to serum and functions as a shock absorber for the brain and spinal cord.

cerebrospinal system (ser-ree-bro-SPY-nahl SIS-tum)—consists of the brain, spinal cord, spinal nerves, and the cranial nerves.

cerebrovascular (suh-ree-broh-VAS-kyoo-lur)—pertaining to the blood vessels of the cerebrum (brain).

cerebrovascular accident (suh-ree-broh-VAS-kyoo-lur AKS-sid-dent)—a stroke, caused by a blood clot or ruptured blood vessel in or around the brain.

cerebrum (suh-REE-brum)—the upper, larger part of the brain considered to be the seat of consciousness controlling speech, sensation, communication, memory, reasoning, will, and emotions.

C

certified color (SUR-tih-fyd KUL-ur)—inorganic color agents known as metal salts; listed on ingredient labels as d&c (drug and cosmetic).

cerumen (suh-ROO-mun)—the medical term for earwax.

cervical (SUR-vih-kul)—pertaining to the neck or the neck of any organ or structure.

cervical artery (SUR-vih-kul ART-uh-ree)—deep artery that supplies blood to the muscles of the neck and the spinal cord.

cervical cutaneous nerve (SUR-vih-kul kyoo-TAY-nee-us NURV)—located at the side of the neck, affects the front and sides of the neck as far down as the breastbone.

cervical glands (SUR-vih-kul GLANZ)—the lymph nodes of the neck.

cervical nerves (SUR-vih-kul NURVZ)—affect the side of the neck and the platysma muscle.

cervical plexus (SUR-vih-kul PLEX-us)—the four upper cervical nerves supplying the skin of the neck and controlling the movement of the head, neck, and shoulders.

cervical vertebrae (SUR-vih-kul VURT-uh-bray)—the seven bones of the top part of the vertebral column located in the neck region.

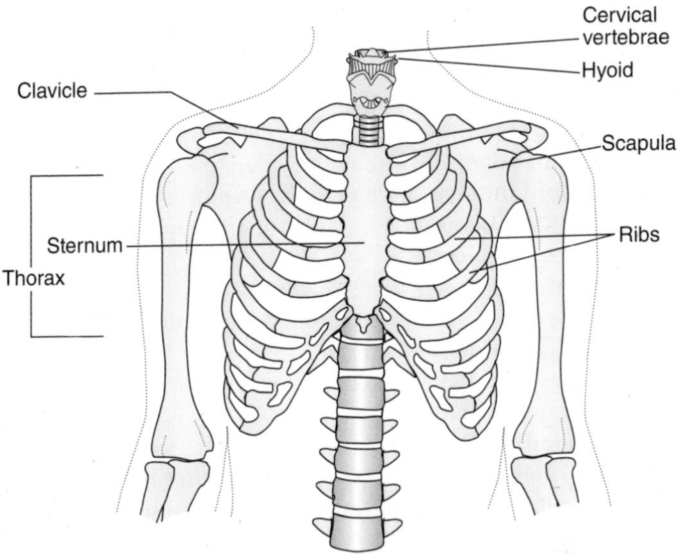

© Milady, a part of Cengage Learning

cervical vertebrae

C

cervicofacial (SUR-vih-koh-FAY-shul)—pertaining to the face and neck.

cervix (SUR-viks)—the neck; any necklike structure.

chain reaction (CHAYN RE-act-shun)—also known as *polymerization reaction*; process that joins together monomers to create very long polymer chains.

changeable-blade straight razor (CHAYNJE-able BLAYD STRAYT RAY-zor)—a type of straight razor that uses changeable, disposable blades.

channel (CHAN-ul)—in anatomy, a passage for liquids such as blood and lymph.

chapped (CHAPT)—pertaining to a skin condition characterized by rough, red, and cracked areas, generally caused by exposure to cold wind and moisture.

cheek (CHEEK)—the fleshy part of the sides of the face below the eyes and above the sides of the mouth.

cheek color (CHEEK KUL-ur)—also known as *blush* or *rouge*; used primarily to add a natural looking glow to the cheeks.

cheekbone (CHEEK-bohn)—zygomatic bone.

chelating agent (KEE-layt-ing AY-jent)—a chemical added to cosmetics to improve the efficiency of the preservative.

chelating soaps (KEE-layt-ing SOAPZ)—also known as *chelating detergents*; detergents that break down stubborn films and remove the residue of pedicure products such as scrubs, salts, and masks.

chelators (KEE-lay-tuhrs)—also known as *clarifiers*; pretreatments that neutralize metallic elements in or on the hair that could interfere with chemical processes.

chemical (KEM-uh-kul)—relating to chemistry; a substance of chemical composition.

chemical action (KEM-uh-kul AK-shun)—the molecular change produced in a substance through the action of electricity, heat, light, or another chemical.

chemical blow-out (KEM-uh-kul blow out)—combination of a relaxer and hairstyling used to create a variety of styles.

chemical bond (KEM-uh-kul BAHND)—the force exerted by shared electrons that holds atoms together in a molecule.

chemical cauterization (KEM-uh-kul KAWT-uh-ryz-ay-shun)—the process by which tissue is destroyed by use of a caustic substance.

C

chemical change (KEM-uh-kul CHAYNJ)—a change in the chemical composition or makeup of a substance.

chemical composition (KEM-uh-kul kom-poh-ZIH-shun)—the balance and proportion of elements that make up a given substance; the formation of compounds.

chemical compound (KEM-uh-kul KOM-pownd)—a combination of elements chemically united in definite proportions; compounds formed by the chemical combination of the atoms of one element and the atoms of another element or elements.

chemical damage (KEM-uh-kul DAM-ihj)—the destruction of the protein structure of the hair produced by reactive chemicals during the process of permanent waving, coloring, or bleaching.

chemical exfoliants (KEM-uh-kul EX-foley-antz)—chemical agents that dissolve dead skin cells and the intercellular matrix, or "glue," that holds them together.

chemical hair relaxing (KEM-uh-kul HAYR re-lax-ing)—also known as *hair straightening, relaxing, hair relaxing,* or *chemical straightening*; a process or service that rearranges the structure of curly hair into a straighter or smoother form.

chemical properties (KEM-uh-kul PROP-er-teez)—characteristics that can only be determined by a chemical reaction and a chemical change in the substance.

chemical texture service (KEM-uh-kul TEKS-chur SER-vicez)—hair services that cause a chemical change that alters the natural wave pattern of the hair.

chemistry (KEM-uh-stree)—the science that deals with the composition, structures, and properties of matter, and how matter changes under different conditions.

chevron (SHEV-run)—in hairstyling, the inverted V shape that forms the base curve of the hair shaping.

chignon (SHEEN-yahn)—also known as *knot* or *coil*, popular method of styling long hair with a simple ponytail.

chin (CHIN)—the anterior prominence of the lower jaw below the mouth; the lower part of the face between the mouth and neck.

chin bone (CHIN BOHN)—the anterior part of the human mandible; the bone beneath the fleshy part of the chin.

chloasma (kloh-AZ-ma)—also known as *liver spots*; condition usually caused by hormonal imbalance, characterized by flat, discolored brownish patches, mainly on the face.

chlorine (KLOHR-een)—a powerful oxidant used in bleaching and disinfectants, as well as an essential reagent in the chemical industry.

chlorophyll (KLOHR-uh-fil)—the green coloring matter of plants by which photosynthesis is accomplished; preparations of water-soluble chlorophyll derivatives are used in deodorants, in some medicinal preparations, and as coloring agents.

cholesterol (koe-LEST-er-awl)—a waxy substance found in the liver, that is needed to produce hormones, vitamin D, and bile; also important for protecting nerves and for the structure of cells.

chromatic vision (kroh-MAT-ik VIZH-un)—vision pertaining to the sense of color.

chromatics (kroh-MAT-iks)—the science of color.

chromhidrosis (krohm-hi-DROH-sus)—the excretion of colored sweat.

chromophore (krohma-for)—the colored cells or target in the epidermis or dermis that absorbs the laser beam's thermal energy, causing the desired injury or destruction of the material.

chromosome (KROH-muh-sohm)—tiny, dark-stained bodies in the cell nucleus that transmit hereditary characteristics during cell division.

chronic (KRAHN-ik)—long; continued; the opposite of acute.

chucking (CHUK-ing)—massage movement accomplished by grasping the flesh firmly in one hand and moving the hand up and down along the bone while the other hand keeps the arm or leg in a steady position.

chunking shear (CHUNK-ing sheer)—a texturizing shear used for removing large sections of hair due to the space between the teeth of the shear.

cicatrix (SIK-uh-triks); pl., cicatrices (sik-uh-TRY-seez)—also known as *scar*; the skin or film that forms over a wound which later contracts to form a scar.

cilia (SIL-ee-uh)—hairlike extensions that protrude from cells and help sweep away fluids and particles.

circle (SUR-kul)—the part of the pin curl that forms a complete circle; also, the hair that is wrapped around the roller.

circuit (SUR-kit)—the path of an electric current.

circuit breaker (SUR-kit BRAYK-ar)—switch that automatically interrupts or shuts off an electric circuit at the first indication of overload.

C

circuit, complete (SUR-kit, kum-PLEET)—the path of negative and positive electric currents moving from the generating source through the conductors and back to the generating source.

circuit, short (SUR-kit, SHORT)—a term used when electrical current is diverted from its regular circuit.

circular movements (SUR-kyoo-lur MOOV-ments)—in massage, movements (circulatory friction) using the fingers or palm, employed to increase circulation and glandular activity of the skin.

circulation, general (sur-kyoo-LAY-shun, JEN-ur-ul)—blood circulation from the heart throughout the body and back again.

circulation, pulmonary (sur-kyoo-LAY-shun, PUL-muh-nair-ee)—blood circulation from the heart to the lungs and back to the heart.

circulatory system (SUR-kyoo-lah-tohr-ee VAS-kyoo-lar SIS-tum)—also known as *cardiovascular system* or *vascular system*; controls the steady circulation of the blood through the body by means of the heart and blood vessels.

circulatory vessels (SUR-kyoo-luh-tohr-ee VES-ulz)—the blood vessels of the circulatory system consisting of the large arteries, small arteries (arterioles), capillaries, and veins and venules.

circumference (sur-KUM-fur-ens)—the outside boundary of a circle.

citric acid (SIT-rik AS-ud)—acid found in fruits such as lemons, limes, oranges, and grapefruit; often added to finishing rinses to smooth tangles and increase the sheen of the hair.

clamp (KLAMP)—a small device used to hold a wave in place; in medicine, a surgical instrument for holding or compressing. A table-top clamp is a device employed to hold another object, such as a mannequin head, or for compressing something within its parts; used in wig styling to hold or steady the wood or canvas wig block.

clapping (KLAP-ing)—a movement in body massage accomplished by striking the area of skin with the palm of the hand slightly cupped.

clarify (KLARE-if-eye)—to make clear.

clarifying shampoo (KLARE-if-eye-ing SHAM-poo)—also known as *chelating shampoo*; shampoo containing an active chelating agent that binds to metals (such as iron and copper) and removes them from the hair; contains an equalizing agent that enriches hair, helps retain moisture, and makes hair more manageable.

C

clavicle (KLAV-ih-kul)—also known as *collarbone*; bone that joins the sternum and scapula.

clay (KLAY)—an earthy substance containing kaolin; used for facial masks and packs.

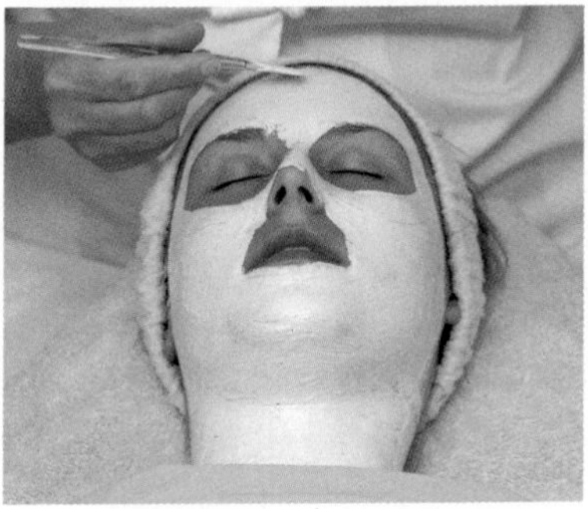

© Milady, a part of Cengage Learning. Photography by Rob Werfel.

clay mask

clay masks (KLAY MASKZ)—oil-absorbing cleansing masks used in facial treatments to draw impurities to the surface of the skin as they dry and tighten. Have an exfoliating effect and an astringent effect on oily and combination skin, making large pores temporarily appear smaller.

clean (cleaning) (KLEEN)—a mechanical process (scrubbing) using soap and water or detergent and water to remove dirt, debris, and many disease-causing germs. Cleaning also removes invisible debris that interferes with disinfection.

clean-cut (KLEEN-KUT)—neatly groomed; in hairstyling, hair that is sharply defined; to cut smooth and even.

cleansers (KLENZ-erz)—soaps and detergents that clean the skin.

cleansing cream (KLENZ-ing KREEM)—a light-textured cream used primarily to dissolve makeup and soil quickly.

cleansing lotion (KLENZ-ing LOH-shun)—a lotion formulated to remove makeup and soil.

cleansing milks (KLENZ-ing MILKS)—non-foaming lotion cleansers designed to cleanse dry and sensitive skin types and to remove makeup.

client base (KLY-ent baze)—customers who are loyal to a particular cosmetologist.

client consultation (KLY-ent KON-sul-tay-shun)—also known as the *needs assessment*; the verbal communication with a client that determines what the client's needs are and how to achieve the desired results.

client consultation form (KLY-ent KON-sul-tay-shun FORM)—a questionnaire used to gather information about a client's needs, history, and preferences; filled out before the client's first service is performed at the salon.

client record keeping (KLY-ent REC-ord KEY-ping)—a method of taking personal notes that helps the professional to remember important data and serve client needs better.

clinic (KLIN-ik)—also known as *student salon*; an establishment where patrons can receive services such as the cosmetology school clinic; a medical clinic is an establishment where patients are received and treated.

clip (KLIP)—a metal or plastic lever-type device used to secure pin curls, waves, or hair rollers.

clipper (KLIP-ur)—electric haircutting tools with a single adjustable blade or detachable blade system; used in freehand or clipper-over-comb cutting to shape, blend, or taper the hair.

clipper oil (KLIP-ur OYL)—a lubricant that reduces friction, heat, and wear when applied to both blades of a hair clipper.

clipper-over-comb (KLIP-ur OVER KOHM)—haircutting technique similar to scissor-over-comb, except that the clippers move side to side across the comb rather than bottom to top.

clipping (KLIP-ing)—the act of cutting split hair ends with shears or scissors; removing hair by using hair clippers.

clockwise (KLOK-wyz)—movement in the same direction as the hands of a clock.

closed-center curls (KLOHZD CEN-ter CURLZ)—pin curls that produce waves that get smaller toward the end.

closed comedo (KLOHZD KAHM-uh-doe)—also known as *whitehead*; hair follicle is closed and not exposed to the environment;

sebum remains a white or cream color and comedone appears as small bump just under the skin surface.

closed end (KLOHZD END)—the rounded (convex) end of a shaping or wave.

close shaving (KLOHS SHAYV-ing)—shaving the beard against the grain of the hair the second time around.

closing consultation (KLOHZ-ing KON-sill-tay-shun)—an opportunity at the end of a treatment session or service to review product recommendations, prepare a home-care program for the client to follow, and provide any additional literature on other treatment options that the client may be interested in.

clot (KLAHT)—a mass or lump of coagulated blood.

clotting (KLAHT-ing)—forming into a mass of coagulated fluid such as blood, caused by exposure of the blood's fibrinogen to oxygen.

cluster (KLUS-tur)—to gather in a mass or group.

coagulant (koh-AG-yuh-lunt)—a substance that produces coagulation or clotting.

coagulate (koh-AG-yuh-layt)—to clot; to convert a fluid into a soft jelly-like solid.

coarse (KORS)—rough or thick in texture; not delicate.

coarse hair (KORS HAYR)—a hair fiber that is relatively large in diameter or circumference having the medulla, cortex, and cuticle.

coated hair (KOHT-ud HAYR)—hair covered with a substance that interferes with, and retards the action of, chemicals on the hair fiber.

coating (KOHT-ing)—in hairdressing, residue left on the hair shaft; coating conditioner that does not penetrate into the hair but coats the hair shaft; in nail technology, coating products, including nail polish, top coats, artificial nail enhancements, and adhesives, that cover the nail plate with a hard film.

cocci (KOK-sye)—round-shaped bacteria that appear singly (alone) or in groups. The three types of cocci are staphylococci, streptococci, and diplococci.

coccygeal plexus (kahk-si-JEE-al PLEX-us)—formed from a portion of the fourth sacral nerve, the fifth sacral nerve, and the coccygeal nerve, supplying the muscles and nerves surrounding the coccyx.

coccyx (KAHK-siks)—the last bone in the vertebral column; tailbone.

coenzyme q10 (KOE-en-zhym KUE TEN)—powerful antioxidant that protects and revitalizes skin cells.

COHNS elements (KONZ ella-mentz)—five elements—carbon, oxygen, hydrogen, nitrogen, and sulfur—that make up human hair, skin, tissue, and nails.

cold sore (KOLD SOR)—also known as *fever blister*; herpes simplex; a recurring viral infection presenting as vesicles with red, swollen, inflamed bases.

cold waving (KOLD WAYV-ing)—a system of permanent waving involving the use of chemicals rather than heating equipment.

collagen (KAHL-uh-jen)—fibrous, connective tissue made from protein; found in the reticular layer of the dermis; gives skin its firmness. Topically, a large, long-chain molecular protein that lies on the top of the skin and binds water; derived from the placentas of cows or other sources.

collarbone (KAHL-ur-BOHN)—the clavicle; the bone connecting the shoulder blade and breastbone.

C

color (KUL-ur)—visual sensation caused by light; any tint or hue distinguished from white; achromatic colors include black, white, and the range of grays in between; chromatic colors are all other colors.

color additive (KUL-ur AD-ih-tiv)—also known as *concentrate*; a concentrated color product that can be added to hair color to intensify or tone down the color.

color base (KUL-ur BAYS)—the combination of dyes that makes up the tonal foundation of a specific hair color.

color blind (KUL-ur BLYND)—partial or total inability to distinguish one or more chromatic colors.

color blocking (KUL-ur BLAH-king)—creating blocks or sections of color on the nail.

color chart (KUL-ur CHART)—a chart of colors produced by manufacturers of haircoloring products to serve as a guide in selecting appropriate colors; the color is shown as it would appear after application to white hair.

color developer (KUL-ur dee-VEL-up-ur)—an oxidizing agent, usually hydrogen peroxide, added to coloring agents before application to develop the color during processing.

color-enhancing shampoo (KUL-ur en-han-sing sham-POO)—a shampoo especially prepared to cleanse the hair and protect the color stability of hair that has been lightened or tinted.

color etching (KUL-ur ECH-ing)—also known as *baliage*; a technique of highlighting the hair by combing a frosting product through the hair.

color fading (KUL-ur FAY-ding)—also known as *color graduation*; when one color fades into the other, and the meeting point is a combination of the two.

colorants (KUL-ur-antz)—substances such as vegetable, pigment, or mineral dyes that give products color.

color fillers (KUL-ur FIL-urz)—equalize porosity and deposit color in one application to provide a uniform contributing pigment on prelightened hair.

color primer (KUL-ur PRY-mer)—applied to the skin before foundation to cancel out and help disguise skin discoloration.

color lift (KUL-ur LIFT)—the amount of change natural or artificial color pigment undergoes when lightened or removed by a substance.

color lifter (KUL-ur LIFT-ur)—a chemical designed to remove artificial color from the hair. Also called a color remover or dye solvent.

color mixing (KUL-ur MIKS-ing)—combining two or more colors together to obtain some in-between shade or tint; creating a custom color.

color palette (KUL-ur PAL-et)—a selection of colors arranged on a kidney-shaped board or in a flat container; used by artists and makeup artists.

color pencil (KUL-ur PEN-sul)—also known as *color stick*; a temporary haircolor in the shape of a pencil used to add color to the scalp where the hair is thin; a pencil with colored lead used as a makeup item.

color pigment (KUL-ur PIG-ment)—the organic coloring matter of the body; substances that impart color to animal or vegetable tissues such as melanin and chlorophyll.

color pigment, hair (KUL-ur PIG-ment, HAYR)—pigment found in the cortex layer of the hair.

color pigment, skin (KUL-ur PIG-ment, SKIN)—coloring matter of the skin such as melanin, hemoglobin (oxygenated and reduced), and carotenes.

color priming (KUL-ur PRYM-ing)—the process of adding pigments to prepare hair for the application of a final color formula.

color refresher (KUL-ur ree-FRESH-ur)—also known as *color wash* or *color enhancer*; color applied to the midshafts and ends of hair to give more uniform color appearance; color applied by a shampoo-in method to enhance the natural color.

color remover (KUL-ur ree-MOOV-ur)—a prepared commercial product designed to remove artificial pigment from the hair; dye solvent color lifter.

color rinse (KUL-ur RINS)—a rinse that gives a temporary tint to the hair.

color shampoo (KUL-ur sham-POO)—a mixture of preparation haircolor and a shampoo product that colors the hair permanently without requiring presoftening treatment.

color swatch (KUL-ur SWAHCH)—a small sample of hair or cloth used to determine matching colors.

color tone (KUL-ur TOHN)—a shade, tint, or degree of a particular color, or a slight modification of a color such as blue with a green undertone or red with an orange tone.

color value (KUL-ur VAL-yoo)—the degree of shading, lightness, or darkness of a color.

color wheel (KUL-ur WHEEL)—a chart, usually circular, used as a tool for selecting and formulating colors for hair, makeup, clothing, and decorating; the arrangement of primary, secondary, and tertiary colors in the order of their relationship to each other; shows harmonizing and contrasting colors.

colorfast (KUL-ur-fast)—resistant to fading or running.

colorist (KUL-ur-ist)—a cosmetologist who specializes in the application of haircolor.

comb (KOHM)—a toothed strip of plastic, metal, bone, or other material used to groom and hold the hair its place; decorative combs are often used to enhance a hairstyle.

comb out (KOHM OWT)—the opening and blending of the hair setting, curls, or waves into the finished style, using a hairbrush and/or comb.

combustion (kum-BUS-chun)—the rapid oxidation of any substance, accompanied by the production of heat and light.

comedone (KAHM-uh-dohn)—also known as *open comedone* or *blackhead*; mass of hardened sebum and skin cells in a hair follicle; an open comedone or blackhead when open and exposed to oxygen. Closed comedones are whiteheads that are blocked and do not have a follicular opening.

comedone extractor (KAHM-uh-dohn eks-TRAK-tur)—an instrument sometimes used as an aid in removing blackheads.

comedogenic (KAHM-uh-doe JEN-ick)—certain cosmetics and skin care products that contain fats, fatty derivatives, or waxes that are known to cause or worsen development of comedones.

comedogenicity (KAHM-uh-doe-jeyn-ih-city)—tendency of any topical substance to cause or to worsen a buildup in the follicle, leading to the development of a comedo.

commission (KAHM-ish-un)—a percentage of the revenue that the salon takes in from services performed by a particular cosmetologist, usually offered to that cosmetologist once the individual has built up a loyal clientele.

common carotid artery (KAHM-un kuh-RAHT-ud ART-uh-ree)—the artery that supplies blood to the face, head, and neck.

common peroneal nerve (KAHM-un per-oh-NEE-al NURV)—a division of the sciatic nerve that extends from behind the knee to wind around the head of the fibula to the front of the leg where it divides into two branches.

communicable (kuh-MYOO-nih-kuh-bul)—able to be communicated; transferable by contact from one person to another as in a communicable disease.

communication (kuh-MYOO-nih-kuh-shun)—the act of sharing information between two people (or groups of people) so that the information is successfully understood.

compact (KAHM-pakt)—closely united; dense; solid; a container, usually having a mirror on one side, and a space for a cosmetic such as powder, eye, or lip makeup on the other.

compact bone (KAHM-pakt BOHN)—hard bone tissue that forms the outer covering of a bone.

compact tissue (KAHM-pakt TISH-oo)—a dense, hard type of bony tissue.

compartmentalization (KOM-part-men-till-iz-ay-shun)—the capacity to keep different aspects of your mental activity separate so you can achieve greater self-control.

competition kit (COMP-uh-tish-on KIT)—a kit you take with you containing all products you will use or might use in a nail competition.

complementary colors (kahm-pluh-MEN-tur-ee KUL-urz)—a primary and secondary color positioned opposite each other on the color wheel. When these two colors are combined, they create a neutral color.

complementary foods (kahm-pluh-MEN-tur-ee KUL-urz)—combinations of two incomplete foods; complementary proteins eaten together provide all the essential amino acids and make a complete protein.

complete electric circuit (kum-PLEET EE-lec-trick SUR-kit)—the path of an electric current from the generating source through conductors and back to its original source.

complexion (kum-PLEK-shun)—hue or general appearance of the skin, especially the face.

complimentary (kahm-plih-MEN-tur-ee)—given free as a favor or courtesy.

component (kahm-POH-nent)—one of the parts of a whole; a constituent part; an ingredient.

composition (kahm-poh-ZISH-un)—the kind and number of atoms constituting the molecule of a substance.

compound (KAHM-pownd)—also known as *compound molecule*; a substance formed by a chemical union of two or more elements in definite proportions by weight and different from any of them.

C

compound dyes (KAHM-pownd DYS)—metallic or mineral dyes combined with a vegetable tint.

compound henna (KAHM-pownd HEN-uh)—Egyptian henna to which one or more metallic preparations has been added.

compound molecules (KAHM-pownd Mahl-eh-cule)—also known as *compounds*; a chemical combination of two or more atoms of different elements in definite (fixed) proportions.

compress (KAHM-pres)—a folded strip of cotton or cloth forming a pad that is pressed on the face or a part of the body; cotton compress as used in facial treatments.

compression (kahm-PRES-shun)—in massage; rhythmic pressing movements directed into muscle tissue by either the hand or fingers.

compressor (kahm-PRES-ur)—a muscle that presses; an instrument for applying pressure on a blood vessel to prevent loss of blood.

compressor nasi (kahm-PRES-ur NAY-zye)—a muscle of facial expression; it is triangular and lies along the side of the nose above the wing.

concave (kahn-KAYV)—hollow and round or curving inward.

concave profile (kahn-KAYV PRO-fyl)—curving inward; prominent forehead and chin, with other features receded inward.

concave rods (kahn-KAYV RAHDZ)—perm rods that have a smaller diameter in the center that increases to a larger diameter on the ends.

concealers (kahn-SEEL-erz)—cosmetics used to cover blemishes and discolorations; may be applied before or after foundation.

concentrated (KAHN-sen-trayt-ud)—condensed; increase of the strength by diminishing the bulk; contains a large quantity of solute in proportion to the quantity of solvent.

concentrator (KAHN-sen-trayt-er)—nozzle attachment of a blowdryer; directs the air stream to any section of the hair more intensely.

concentric (kahn-SEN-trik)—having a common center, such as curls, waves, and other movements of the hair that radiate from a common center.

concentric bits (kahn-SEN-trik BITZ)—balanced bits that do not wobble or vibrate.

concentric contraction (kahn-SEN-trik kahn-TRAK-shun)—a type of isotonic muscle contraction that occurs when the force of a contraction is greater than the resistance and the muscle shortens.

condensation (kahn-den-SAY-shun)—act of changing a gas or vapor into a liquid; reduction to a denser form.

condition (kun-DIH-shun)—to protect or restore the natural strength and body of the hair; the existing state of health of the hair in reference to elasticity, strength, texture, porosity, and evidence of previous treatments.

conditioner (kun-DIH-shun-ur)—special chemical agent applied to the hair to deposit protein or moisturizer to help restore hair strength, give hair body, or to protect hair against possible breakage.

conditioner fillers (kun-DIH-shun FIL-urz)—used to recondition damaged, overly porous hair, and equalize porosity so that the hair accepts the color evenly from strand to strand and scalp to ends.

conditioning (kun- DIH-shun-ing)—the application of special chemical agents to hair to help restore its strength and to give it body to protect it against possible breakage; descriptive of conditioning shampoos and rinses that help to normalize the condition of hair.

conditioning shampoo (kun- DIH-shun-ing SHAM-poo)—also known as *moisturizing shampoo*; shampoo designed to make the hair appear smooth and shiny and to improve the manageability of the hair.

conductivity (kahn-duk-TIV-ut-ee)—the capacity to transmit sound, heat, or electricity.

conductor (kahn-DUK-tur)—any substance, material, or medium that conducts electricity, heat, or sound.

cone-shaped curl (KOHN-SHAYPT KURL)—a curl formed to be smaller at the end of the hair shaft and larger at the scalp.

configuration (kun-fih-gyur-RAY-shun)—the arrangement and spacing of the atoms of a molecule.

congeal (kun-JEEL)—to change from a fluid to a solid condition as in freezing or curdling.

congenital (kahn-JEN-uh-tul)—pertaining to a condition existing at birth.

congestion (kuhn-JES-chun)—excessive or abnormal accumulation of fluid in the vessels of an organ or body part; usually blood, but occasionally bile or mucus; this condition occurs in some diseases, infections, or injuries.

conical hair roller (KAHN-ih-kul HAYR ROHL-ur)—a cone-shaped hair roller.

C

conjunctivitis (kuhn-juhngk-tuh-VAHY-tis)—also known as *pinkeye*; common bacterial infection of the eyes; inflammation of the conjunctiva (the outermost layer of the eye and the inner surface of the eyelids), and extremely contagious.

connecting (kahn-EKT-ing)—in finger waving, the joining of a ridge of wave from one side of the head with the ridge of a wave from the opposite side of the head.

connecting line (kahn-EKT-ing LYN)—a line blending two circular shapes of clockwise and counterclockwise forces; also referred to as a *blending*; connection between two or more shapes; referred to as *blending, dovetailing,* and *dividing.*

connective tissue (Kun-neck-tiv TISH-oo)—fibrous tissue that binds together, protects, and supports the various parts of the body. Examples of connective tissue are bone, cartilage, ligaments, tendons, blood, lymph, and fat.

connective tissue massage (kuh-NEK-tiv TISH-oo muh-SAHZH)—massage directed toward the subcutaneous connective tissue for the treatment of circulatory or visceral disease.

consent form (KUN-sent FORM)—a (customary) written agreement between the client and salon/spa for applying a particular treatment.

consistency (kun-SIS-ten-see)—the degree of density, solidity, or firmness of either a solid or a fluid.

constant base factor (KAHN-stant BAYS FAK-tur)—in haircoloring, the factor that enhances warm tones and adds depth to dark shades; an ingredient in color formulation that neutralizes and balances color and prevents brassy tones.

constrict (kun-STRIKT)—to make narrow; press together.

constructive (kun-STRUK-tiv)—promoting improvement or development.

consultation (kahn-sul-TAY-shun)—verbal communication with a client to determine desired results.

consultative selling (kun-SUL-ta-tive SELL-ing)—a method of advising or consulting to clients and recommending the best treatments and products for their use.

consumer (kun-SOO-mur)—one who uses materials or services; one of the buying public.

consumption supplies (KON-sump-shun sup-LYZ)—supplies used to conduct daily business operations.

contact dermatitis (KAHN-takt dur-mah-TYT-is)—also known as *dermatitis venenata*; inflammatory skin condition caused by contact with a substance or chemical. Occupational disorders from ingredients in cosmetics and chemical solutions can cause contact dermatitis. Allergic contact dermatitis is from exposure to allergens; irritant contact dermatitis is from exposure to irritants.

contagion (kun-TAY-jun)—transmission of specific diseases by direct or indirect contact.

contagious disease (kun-TAY-jus DIZ-eez)—also known as *communicable disease*; disease that is spread from one person to another person. Some of the more contagious diseases are the common cold, ringworm, conjunctivitis (pinkeye), viral infections, and natural nail or toe and foot infections.

contagium animatum (kun-TAY-jee-um AN-ih-may-tum)—any living or animal organism that causes the spread of an infectious disease.

contaminate (kun-TAM-uh-nayt)—to make impure by contact; to taint or pollute.

contamination (kun-tam-uh-NAY-shun)—the presence, or the reasonably anticipated presence, of blood or other potentially infectious materials on an item's surface or visible debris or residues such as dust, hair, and skin.

contour (KAHN-toor)—the outline of a figure or shape, particularly one that curves; to shape the outline or shape something to fit the outline.

contouring (KAHN-toor-ing)—a makeup technique that utilizes the principles of light and shadow to sculpt or contour the face; used in theatrical and corrective makeup.

contour makeup (KAHN-toor MAYK-up)—a cream or powdered makeup used to create optical illusions by the shading and highlighting of facial features.

contract (kun-TRAKT)—to draw together; to acquire a disease by contagion.

contractible (kun-TRAK-tih-bul)—having the ability to contract.

contractile tissues (kun-TRAK-tyl TISH-yoos)—fibrous tissues that have tension placed on them during muscular contractions.

contractility (kahn-trak-TIL-ut-ee)—the property of muscles to contract or shorten, thereby exerting force.

contraction (kun-TRAK-shun)—the act of shrinking or drawing together; the shortening of a functioning muscle.

contracture (kun-TRAK-shur)—occurs when joint mobility is reduced by decreased extensibility of muscle or other tissues crossing the joint.

C

contraindicated (kahn-trah-in-dih-KAYT-ed)—a reason or factor a procedure should be avoided because if performed it may produce undesirable side effects.

contraindication (kahn-trah-in-dih-KAY-shun)—condition that requires avoiding certain treatments, procedures, or products to prevent undesirable side effects.

contrast (KAHN-trast)—a striking difference that appears by comparison.

contrasting lines (KAHN-trast-ing leynz)—horizontal and vertical lines that meet at a 90-degree angle and create a hard edge.

contributing pigment (kun-TRIB-yoot-ing PIG-ment)—also known as *undertone*; the varying degrees of warmth exposed during a permanent color or lightening process.

contusions (kun-TOO-zhunz)—common bruises; common types of hematomas that are generally not serious.

convalesce (kahn-vuh-LES)—to recover health and strength gradually after illness.

conventional straight razor (kun-VEN-shun-ul STRAYT RAY-zor)—a razor made of a hardened steel blade that requires honing and stropping to produce a cutting edge.

converge (kun-VURJ)—to come together at a particular point.

conversion (kun-VUR-zhun)—the act of changing one thing for another thing; conversion of euros into U.S. dollars.

converter (kun-VUR-tur)—an apparatus that changes direct current to alternating current.

convex (kahn-VEKS)—curving outward like an exterior segment of a circle; in a convex profile, the forehead and chin recede.

convex profile (kahn-VEKS pro-fyle)—curving outward; receding forehead and chin.

convolve (kun-VAHLV)—to roll together; to coil, wind, or twist as in braiding the hair.

convulsion (kun-VUL-shun)—an abnormal, violent, involuntary muscular contraction or series of contractions.

cool colors (KOOl KUL-urz)—colors that suggest coolness and are dominated by blues, greens, violets, and blue-reds.

coolant (KOOL-unt)—a substance, usually liquid, used to prevent or control heat buildup.

cooling period (KOOL-ing PIHR-ee-ud)—a waiting period, generally 10 minutes, before removing permanent wave rods from the hair following the neutralizing process.

copper (KAHP-ur)—a metallic element that is a good conductor of heat and electricity.

coracoid (KOR-uh-koyd)—a projecting part of the shoulder blade.

corium (KOH-ree-um)—also known as *dermis, derma, cutis*, or *true skin*; the layer of the skin deeper than the epidermis, consisting of a dense bed of vascular connective tissue.

corkscrew curl (KORK-skroo KURL)—strands of hair having the form of a corkscrew spiral.

corner (KOR-nur)—in haircutting and styling, a point where the direction or outline changes; the point formed where two lines meet.

corneocytes (KOR-nee-ooh-sytz)—another name for a *stratum corneum cell*; hardened, waterproof, protective keratinocytes; these "dead" protein cells are dried out and lack nuclei.

corneum (KOR-nee-um)—also known as *stratum corneum or horny layer of the skin*; the top, outermost layer of the epidermis.

cornrows (KORN ROHS)—also known as *canerows*; narrow rows of visible braids that lie close to the scalp and are created with a three-strand, on-the-scalp braiding technique.

coronal plane (KOR-un-ul PLAYN)—imaginary line that divides body into front and back.

coronal suture (KOR-un-ul SOO-chur)—the line of junction of the frontal bone with the two parietal bones of the skull.

coronary (KOR-uh-nar-ee)—relating to a crown; a term applied to vessels, nerves, or attachments that encircle a part or an organ; pertaining to either of two arteries that supply blood to the heart muscle.

corporation (KOR-pour-aye-shun)—an ownership structure controlled by one or more stockholders.

corpus (KOR-pus)—a body; the human body.

corpuscle (KOR-pus-ul)—a small mass or body; a minute cell; a cell found in the blood.

corpuscles, red (KOR-pus-uls, RED)—cells in blood whose functions are to carry oxygen to the cells.

corpuscles, white (KOR-pus-uls WHYT)—cells in the blood whose functions are to destroy pathogens and harmful bacteria.

corrective coloring (kor-EK-tiv KUL-ur-ing)—the process of altering or correcting an undesirable color.

corrective makeup (kor-EK-tiv MAYK-up)—using light and dark colors to highlight and contour features.

C

corrode (kuh-ROHD)—to eat away or destroy gradually, usually by chemical action.

corrosive (kuh-ROH-siv)—a substance capable of seriously damaging skin, eyes, or other soft tissues on contact. Some corrosives have delayed action (minutes); others affect the skin almost instantly.

corrugated (KOR-uh-gayt-ud)—formed or shaped in wrinkles, folds, or alternate ridges and grooves.

corrugations, nail (kor-uh-GAY-shuns, NAYL)—alternate ridges and furrows; ridges caused by uneven growth of the nail, usually the result of illness or injury; wrinkles.

corrugator muscle (KOR-uh-gayt-or MUS-uhl)—muscle located beneath the frontalis and orbicularis oculi that draws the eyebrow down and wrinkles the forehead vertically.

corrugator supercilii (KOR-uh-gayt-ur SOO-pur-sil-eye)—facial muscle that draws eyebrows down and wrinkles the forehead vertically.

cortex (KOR-teks)—middle layer of the hair; a fibrous protein core formed by elongated cells containing melanin pigment.

cortical (KORT-ih-KUL)—pertaining to or consisting of the outer portion; the bark, rind, or outer layer (cortex) of the hair.

cortical fibers (KORT-ih-KUL FY-burz)—fibers that make up the cortex of the hair.

cortisol (KOR-tih-sawl)—a hormone that acts as an anti-inflammatory and antiallergenic.

cortisone (KOR-tih-sohn)—a powerful hormone extracted from the cortex of the adrenal gland; also made synthetically; used in the treatment of disease and some diseases of the skin.

corynebacterium (kor-uh-nee-bak-TEER-ee-um)—pathogenic bacterium that spreads infection and is usually present in acne lesions along with other bacteria.

coryza (kuh-RY-zuh)—also known as *common cold*; an acute condition affecting the nasal mucous membranes causing a discharge from the nostrils.

cosmeceuticals (KAHZ-muh-SUIT-ick-alz)—a term combining the words *cosmetics* and *pharmaceutical*; products that contain active ingredients that improve the skin's health and appearance.

cosmetic (kahz-MET-ik)—of or pertaining to, or making for beauty, especially of the complexion; any external preparation intended to beautify the skin, hair, or other areas of the body.

cosmetic acne (kahz-MET-ik AK-nee)—acne that becomes activated by improper cleansing and improper use of cosmetics.

cosmetic chemistry (kahz-MET-ik KEM-is-tree)—scientific study of cosmetics.

cosmetic dermatology (kahz-MET-ik der-mah-TAHL-uh-jee)—a branch of dermatology devoted to improving the health and beauty of the skin and its appendages.

cosmetic surgery (kahz-MET-ik SUR-juh-ree)—also known as *esthetic surgery*; elective surgery for improving and altering the appearance.

cosmetician (kahz-muh-TISH-un)—one trained in the use and/or art of selling and demonstrating the application of cosmetics.

cosmetologist (kahz-muh-TAHL-uh-jist)—one skilled in the science and practice of cosmetology.

cosmetology (kahz-muh-TAHL-uh-jee)—the art and science of beautifying and improving the skin, nails, and hair and includes the study of cosmetics and their application.

cosmetics (kahz-met-icks)—as defined by the FDA: articles that are intended to be rubbed, poured, sprinkled, or otherwise applied to the human body or any part thereof for cleansing, beautifying, promoting attractiveness, or altering the appearance.

costal (KAHS-tul)—pertaining to a rib or riblike structure.

cotton compress mask (KAHT-un KAHM-prehs MASK)—strips of cotton moistened in water and applied to the face to aid in the removal of a treatment mask.

cotton mitts (KAHT-un MITZ)—strips of cotton wrapped around the fingers; used to remove cosmetic products following cleansing or other facial treatments.

counterclockwise (kown-tur-KLAHK-wyz)—the movements in the opposite direction to the hands of a clock.

counterirritant (KOWN-tur-IHR-ih-tent)—a substance that produces inflammation of the skin to relieve a more deep-seated inflammation.

couperose (KOO-per-ohs)—redness; distended capillaries from weakening of the capillary walls.

cover letter (KUV-ur LETT-ur)—letter of introduction that highlights your goals, skills, and accomplishments. Usually accompanies a resume or application for employment.

coverage (KUV-ur-ej)—the degree to which gray or white hair has been covered by the coloring process; also references the ability of a color product to conceal gray, white, or other colors of hair; the degree of concealment provided by a cosmetic product, foundation, or coverage stick.

C

cowlick (KOW-lik)—a tuft of hair that stands up straight.

cradle cap (KRAY-dl KAP)—an oily type of dandruff characterized by heavy, greasy crusts on the scalp of an infant.

cranial (KRAY-nee-ul)—of or pertaining to the cranium.

cranial index (KRAY-nee-ul IN-deks)—a method of measuring the skull.

cranial nerves (KRAY-nee-ul NURVZ)—any pair of nerves arising from the lower surface of the brain.

cranium (KRAY-nee-um)—an oval, bony case that protects the brain.

cream (KREEM)—a semisolid cosmetic preparation such as cleansing cream and other skin care creams.

cream masks (KREEM MASQUES)—masks often containing oils and emollients as well as humectants; have a strong moisturizing effect.

crease (KREES)—a line or slight depression in the skin such as grooves across the palms of the hands, at the wrist, or where there are folds of skin.

creatine phosphate (KREE-uh-teen FAHS-fayt)—a compound of creatine with phosphoric acid; a source of energy in the contraction of vertebrate muscle; its breakdown furnishes phosphate for the formation of ATP from ADP.

creme (KREEM)—also known as *cream*; a thick liquid or lotion.

creme bleach (KREEM BLEECH)—also known as *cream bleach*; a chemical preparation of thick consistency used to remove color from hair.

creme rinse (KREEM RINS)—also known as *cream rinse*; a colorless, usually acidic preparation applied to hair to neutralize the effects of a shampoo; it assists in removing tangles from hair and increases its manageability.

creosol (KREE-uh-sawl), cresol (KREE-sul)—a colorless, oily liquid obtained from coal tar and wood tar and used as a disinfectant.

creosote (KREE-uh-soht)—an oily liquid obtained from Beachwood tar and used in antiseptics.

crescent shape (KREHS-ent SHAYP)—in manicuring, a term referring to the small, white area at the base of the nail; a shape like that of the moon when less than half of it is visible.

C

crest (KREST)—also known as *parietal ridge, temporal region, hatband,* or *horseshoe*; the widest area of the head, starting at the temples and ending at the bottom of the crown.

crew cut (KROO KUT)—also known as *brush cut*; a very short men's haircut that leaves a bristle-like surface over the entire head.

crisscross (KRIS-kraws)—to pass back and forth, through or over; to mark with intersecting lines such as the crisscross movement of the fingers while giving a facial.

croquignole Marcel wave (KROH-ken-yohl MAR-sel WAYV)—a wave in the hair produced by the use of a Marcel iron and winding the hair croquignole fashion.

croquignole perm wrap (KROH-ken-yohl PERM RAP)—perms in which the hair strands are wrapped from the ends to the scalp in overlapping concentric layers.

croquignole winding (KROH-ken-yohl WYND-ing)—the process of winding the hair from hair ends toward the scalp.

cross bonds (KRAWS BAHNDZ)—the bonds holding together the long chains of amino acids that compose hair.

cross-checking (KRAWS CHEK-ing)—parting the haircut in the opposite way from which you cut it in order to check for precision of line and shape.

cross-contamination (KRAWS con-tam-in-ay-shun)—contamination that occurs when you touch one object and then transfer the contents of that object to another, such as touching skin, then touching a product without washing your hands.

cross-linker (KRAWS-lynk-ur)—monomer that joins together different polymer chains.

crown (KROWN)—area of the head between the apex and back of the parietal ridge.

crown curls (KROWN KURLZ)—a group of light curls worn on top of the head.

crust (KRUST)—also known as *scab*; dead cells that form over a wound or blemish while it is healing; an accumulation of sebum and pus, sometimes mixed with epidermal material.

cryosurgery (kry-oh-SUR-jur-ee)—the application of extreme cold to destroy abnormal or diseased tissue.

cryotherapy (KRY-oh-theh-rah-pee)—application of cold agents for therapeutic purposes.

cubic (KYOO-bik)—shaped like a cube; having three dimensions.

cubical (KYOO-bih-kul)—any small room or partitioned area such as a facial service cubical.

cuboid bone (KYOO-boyd bohn)—one of the several bones found in the tarsal or ankle region; function of the cuboid is support of the body's movement, weight, and maintain foot stability.

cumulative trauma disorders (CTD) (KYOOM-lah-tiv TRAH-muh dis-OHR-durs)—repetitive motor disorders.

cuneiform bones (kyuh-NEE-uh-form bonez)—three bones in the foot located in front of the navicular bone; they form the arch of the foot.

cure (KYOOR)—to heal or restore to a sound, healthy condition; in nail technology, to harden through exposure to UV light.

curette (KYOOR-et)—a small, scoop-shaped implement used for more efficient removal of debris from the nail folds, eponychium, and hyponychium areas.

curl (KURL)—also known as *circle*; the hair that is wrapped around the roller.

curl, barrel (KURL, BAIR-ul)—a curl made in a similar manner to the standup curl and used where there is insufficient room to place a roller.

curl base (KURL BAYS)—the stationary or immovable foundation of the curl which is attached to the scalp.

curl, cascade (KURL, kahs-KAYD)—also known as *stand-up curls*; pin curls fastened to the head in a standing position to allow the hair to flow upward and then downward.

curl clip (KURL KLIHP)—a pronged device used to secure a curl in place.

curl direction (KURL dih-REK-shun)—the placement of the hair so that it moves or curls toward or away from a certain point.

curl placement (KURL PLAYS-ment)—the positioning of a curl in a predetermined location.

curl, ridge (KURL, RIJ)—a curl placed behind and close to the ridge of a finger wave and pinned across its stem.

curl, roller (KURL, ROHL-ur)—a curl formed over a specially made roller.

curl stem (KURL STEM)—that part of the pin curl between the base and the first arc of the circle.

curl, thermal (KURL, THUR-mul)—a curl formed with thermal irons (electric or stove-heated).

curler (KURL-ur)—that which curls anything.

curling (KURL-ing)—a process of hair waving.

curling iron (KURL-ing EYE-urn)—also known as *thermal iron*; an implement with a long tubelike base over which a top piece can be raised; the hair is placed between the two and curled while it is dry.

curly hair (KUR-lee HAYR)—hair that has a curved or spiral shape; the opposite of straight.

current, alternating (AC) (KUR-ent, AWL-tur-nayt-ing)—rapid and interrupted current, flowing first in one direction and then in the opposite direction; produced by mechanical means and changes directions 60 times per second.

current, direct (DC) (KUR-ent, dih-REKT)—constant, even-flowing current that travels in one direction only and is produced by chemical means.

current, electric (KUR-ent, ih-LEK-trik)—flow of electricity along a conductor.

current, galvanic (KUR-ent gal-VAN-ik)—constant and direct current having a positive and negative pole that produces chemical changes when it passes through the tissues and fluids of the body.

current, high frequency; tesla (KUR-rent, HY FREE-kwen-see; TES-lah)—also known as *violet ray*; thermal or heat-producing current with a high rate of oscillation or vibration, commonly used for scalp and facial treatments.

current strength (KUR-ent STRENGTH)—the relation of the electromotive force to the resistance of the circuit.

C

curvilinear (kur-vuh-LIN-ee-ur)—in hairdressing, formed, bounded, or characterized by curved lines.

curvature (KUR-vuh-chur)—the state of being curved.

curvature lines (KUR-vuh-chur LYNZ)—shaping of the hair and combing out into a series of curved lines running inward and outward.

curvature permanent wrap (KUR-vuh-chur perm-an-ent RAP)—perm wrap in which partings and bases radiate throughout the panels to follow the curvature of the head.

curved lines (KURVD lynz)—lines moving in a circular or semicircular direction; used to soften a design.

cushioning (KOOSH-un-ing)—a form of back combing or back brushing in the scalp area so that the tapered hairs interlock and form a foundation to support the longer lengths of hair.

cut (KUT)—in haircutting, to reduce or shorten by removing the ends with an instrument such as scissors or a razor; a haircut; to style the hair by cutting.

C

cutaneous (kyoo-TAY-nee-us)—pertaining to, involving, or affecting the skin and its appendages.

cutaneous appendage (kyoo-TAY-nee-us uh-PEN-dij)—an organ or structure attached to or embedded in the skin; examples are hair, nails, and sebaceous and sudoriferous glands.

cutaneous colli (kyoo-TAY-nee-us KOH-lih)—a nerve located at the side of the neck affecting the front and side of the neck as far down as the breastbone.

cutaneous diphtheria (kyoo-TAY-nee-us dif-THEER-ee-uh)—a mild form of diphtheria (a contagious disease spread by direct physical contact or breathing the aerosolized secretions of infected individuals) localized on the skin in an ulcer-like formation.

cutaneous gland (kyoo-TAY-nee-us GLAND)—any gland of the skin.

cutaneous horn (kyoo-TAY-nee-us HORN)—a small growth or projection above the skin; commonly found on the face, scalp, or chest.

cutaneous muscle (kyoo-TAY-nee-us MUS-uhl)—a muscle having an insertion into the skin or origin and insertion in the skin.

cutaneous nerves (kyoo-TAY-nee-us NURVZ)—nerves affecting the skin.

cutaneous reaction (kyoo-TAY-nee-us ree-AK-shun)—any reaction of the skin such as a rash or change in appearance as the result of disease, drugs, sunburn, allergy, or the like.

cutaneous reflex (kyoo-TAY-nee-us REE-fleks)—the response of the skin to irritation or sensations, such as goose bumps on the skin as a reaction to cold.

cutaneous sensation (kyoo-TAY-nee-us sen-SAY-shun)—pertaining to the skin's receptors for sensing touch, temperature changes, pain, or irritation.

cutaneous test (kyoo-TAY-nee-us TEST)—a test involving the skin; skin test.

cuticle (KYOO-tih-kul)—in hairdressing, the outermost layer of the hair consisting of a single overlapping layer of transparent, scalelike cells that look like shingles on a roof; in nail technology, the dead, colorless tissue attached to the nail plate.

cuticle nippers (KYOO-tih-kul NIP-urz)—a small cutting tool used in manicuring or pedicuring to nip or cut excess cuticle epidermis; the tool is characterized by its double handle and short clipping blades.

cuticle oil (KYOO-tih-kul OYL)—a special oil used to soften and lubricate the cuticle (epidermis) around fingernails and toenails.

cuticle pusher (KYOO-tih-kul POOSH-ur)—an implement used in manicuring or pedicuring to loosen and push back the cuticle around the fingernails or toenails; the implement is shaped to conform to the shape of the nails.

cuticle remover (KYOO-tih-kul re-MOOV-ur)—a solution of alkali, glycerin, and water used to soften and remove dead cuticle from around the nail.

cuticle scissors (KYOO-tih-kul SIZ-urz)—a small implement designed to trim excess cuticle (epidermis) around the fingernails or toenails. It is distinguished by the long, shank and short, sharp cutting blades.

cuticle softener (KYOO-tih-kul SAW-fuh-nur)—a substance used in manicuring and pedicuring to soften the cuticle (epidermis) around the fingernails and toenails prior to removing the excess cuticle.

cuticularization (kyoo-TIK-uh-lur-ih-zay-shun)—the growth of new skin over a wound or blemish.

cutis (KYOO-tis)—the derma or deeper layer of the skin.

cutis marmorata (KYOO-tis mahr-moh-RAY-tah)—also known as *livedo reticularis*; a common cutaneous finding consisting of a mottled reticulated vascular pattern that appears like a lacelike purplish discoloration of the lower extremities.

cutis rhomboidalis nuchae (KYOO-tis rahm-boy-DAY-lis NOO-kai)—a skin condition characterized by furrows on the back of the neck; usually caused by overexposure to the sun.

cutis verticis gyrata (KYOO-tis VER-tih-sis jy-RAY-tah)—congenital hypertrophy and looseness of the skin or scalp, resulting in folds.

cutting above the fingers (KUT-ing AH-bov THE FING-erz)—in barbering, method of holding the hair section between the fingers so that cutting can be performed on the outside of the fingers; used with horizontal and vertical projections of hair.

cutting below the fingers (KUT-ing BE-low THE FING-erz)—in barbering, method of holding the hair section between the fingers so that cutting can be performed on the inside of the fingers; used in 0- and 45-degree elevation cutting.

cutting line (KUT-ing LYNE)—also known as *finger angle, finger position, cutting position,* or *cutting angle*; angle at which the fingers are held when cutting, and, ultimately, the line that is cut.

C

cutting lotion (KUT-ing LOH-shun)—a wetting agent used to control hair during a haircut.

cutting stroke (KUT-ing STOHK)—correct angle of cutting a beard with a straight razor.

cyanoacrylate (sy-an-oh-AH-cry-late)—also known as *wrap resin*; a specialized acrylic monomer that has excellent adhesion to the natural nail plate and polymerizes in seconds, used to make wraps and nail adhesives.

cyanosis (sy-uh-NOH-sus)—inadequate oxygenation of the blood, causing the skin to take on a bluish cast.

cycle (SY-kul)—a complete wave of an alternating current.

cyclical (SIK-lih-kul)—pertaining to or moving in a circle; having parts arranged in a ring or closed chain structure.

cycloid (SY-kloyd)—arranged in circles; something circular.

cylinder (SIL-in-dur)—a long circular body, solid or hollow, uniform in diameter.

cylindrical (sih-LIN-drih-kul)—pertaining to, or having the form of a cylinder.

cylindrical hair roller (sih-LIN-drih-kul HAYR ROHL-ur)—a roller made of lightweight metal or plastic, in various sizes, lengths, and circumferences, around which strands of hair are wound to create a specific style.

cylindrical-shaped curl (sih-LIN-drih-kul SHAYPT KURL)—a curl that is formed to be about the same circumference along its entire shaft from the ends to the scalp.

cyst (SIST)—closed, abnormally developed sac that contains fluid, pus, semifluid, or dead matter above or below the skin.

cysteic acid (SIS-tee-ik AS-ud)—a chemical substance in the hair fiber produced by the interaction of hydrogen peroxide on the disulfide bond (cysteine).

cysteine (SIS-teen)—an amino acid joined with another cysteine amino acid to create cystine amino acid.

cystic acne (SIS-tik AK-nee)—acne that is distinguished by cysts.

cystine (SIS-teen)—an amino acid that joins together two peptide strands.

cystine links (SIS-teen LINKS)—the crossbonds formed from the amino acid, cystine.

cystoma (sis-TOH-muh)—a tumor containing cysts of pathogenic origin.

cytochemistry (sy-toh-KEM-ih-stree)—the science dealing with the chemistry of cells.

cytocrine theory (SY-toh-krin THEE-uh-ree)—the theory that pigment granules are transferred from melanocytes directly into the cells of the epidermis.

cytogenesis (cy-toh-JEN-uh-sis)—the formation of cells.

cytolysis (sy-TAHL-uh-sus)—the dissolution of cells.

cytoplasm (sy-toh-PLAZ-um)—the protoplasm of a cell, except for the protoplasm in the nucleus, that surrounds the nucleus; the watery fluid that cells need for growth, reproduction, and self-repair.

cytoplasmic organelles (SY-toh-plaz-mik or-guh-NELZ)—structures that perform specific functions necessary for cell survival.

D

damaged hair (DAM-ijd HAYR)—a hair condition characterized by high porosity, brittleness, split ends, dryness, roughness, lifelessness, matting, or sponginess when wet; lacking gloss and elasticity.

D&C colors (DEE and SEE KUL-urz)—colors formulated for and approved by the Food and Drug Administration that are certified to be safe for use in drug and cosmetic products.

dander (DAN-dur)—scales from animal skin, hair, or feathers; may act as an allergen.

dandruff (DAN-druf)—pityriasis; scurf or scales formed in excess on the scalp; greasy or dry keratotic material shed from the scalp.

dandruff conditioner (DAN-druf kun-DIH-shun-ur)—a product containing ingredients formulated to improve or eliminate a dandruff condition of the scalp.

dandruff lotion (DAN-druf LOH-shun)—a lotion applied to the scalp to aid in loosening and removing dandruff scales.

dandruff ointment (DAN-druf OYNT-ment)—a specially formulated salve or unguent applied to the scalp to treat a dandruff condition.

dandruff rinse (DAN-druf RINS)—a liquid applied to the hair and scalp following a treatment or shampoo to control and eliminate a dandruff condition.

dandruff shampoo (DAN-druf sham-POO)—a commercially prepared product designed to control and eliminate dandruff.

dark skin spot (DARK SKIN SPAHT)—also known as *age* or *liver spots*; spots or splotches on the skin indicative of melanosis or melanoderm, a condition in which dark pigment is deposited in the skin and tissues.

day makeup (DAY MAYK-up)—a choice of colors in makeup products to give the face a natural appearance for daylight wear.

day spa (DAY Spah)—a business establishment which people visit for professionally administered personal care treatments such as massages, hair and nail services, and facials. Day spas are visited only for the duration of the client's treatment schedule—usually for a day or part of a day. Conversely, a

Photography by Michael Watson for Salvatore Minardi Salon, Madison, NJ.

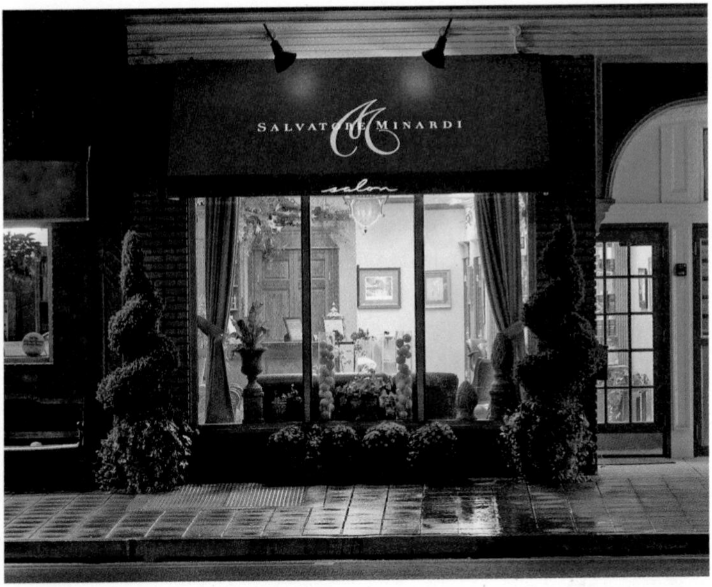

day spa

destination spa offers the same services in a hotel setting where people reside for a day or more.

D

deacidify (dee-uh-SID-uh-fy)—to remove acid from a substance.

decalvant (duh-KAL-vunt)—a substance used to remove or destroy hair.

decimeter (DES-uh-meet-ur)—in the metric system, one-tenth of a meter.

decolorization (dee-KUL-ur-ih-ZAY-shun)—the diffusing of the natural or artificial color from hair.

decolorization process (dee-KUL-ur-ih-ZAY-shun PRAH-ses)—the process of diffusing the natural or artificial color from hair.

decolorize (dee-KUL-ur-yz)—a chemical process involving the lightening of natural pigment or artificial color from the hair.

decompose (dee-kum-POHZ)—to decay or rot; to separate into constituent parts; to bring to dissolution.

decomposition (dee-kahm-poh-ZIH-shun)—to separate or disintegrate into constituent parts or elements.

decontamination (dee-kuhn-tam-ih-NAY-shun)—the removal of blood or other potentially infectious materials on an item's surface and the removal of visible debris or residue such as dust, hair, and skin.

decreasing graduation (dee-KREES-ing GRAJ-oo-ay-shun)—graduation found within two nonparallel lines; it diminishes as it moves back from the face.

deductive reasoning (DEE-duck-tiv REAS-on-ing)—the process of reaching logical conclusions by employing logical reasoning.

deep cervical artery (DEEP SUR-vih-kul ART-uh-ree)—the artery that supplies blood to the deep muscles of the neck.

deep-conditioning treatment (DEEP con-DISH-on-ing TREET-ment)—also known as *hair mask* or *conditioning pack*; chemical mixture of concentrated protein and intensive moisturizer.

deep fascia (DEEP FAYSH-uh)—fibrous tissue that penetrates deep into the body, separating major muscle groups and anchoring them to bone.

deep kneading (DEEP NEED-ing)—a massage movement in which the flesh is lifted and squeezed with the hand.

deep peroneal nerve (DEEP par-uh-NEE-al NURV)—also known as *anterior tibial nerve*; extends down the front of the leg, behind the muscles. It supplies impulses to these muscles and also to the muscles and skin on the top of the foot and adjacent sides of the first and second toes.

D

deep temporal artery (DEEP TEM-puh-rul ART-uh-ree)—the artery that supplies blood to the temporal (temple) muscle and skull.

deep tissue massage (DEEP TISH-shyoo muh-SAHZH)—massage regimens that are directed toward the deeper tissue structures of the muscle and facia using a finger, thumb, several fingers, or entire hand.

deep transverse massage (DEEP TRANZ-vurs muh-SAHZH)—massage that breaks down unwanted fibrous adhesions to restore mobility to the muscles.

defecation (def-ih-cay-shun)—elimination of waste products from digestion.

deficiency disease (dih-FISH-en-see DIZ-eez)—a disease such as pellagra or scurvy caused by the lack of essential vitamins and other nourishment in the body.

defluvium capilorum (duh-FLOO-vee-um kap-ih-LOH-rum)—complete loss of hair.

defluvium unguium (duh-FLOO-vee-um UN-gwee-um)—complete loss of nails.

degenerate (dee-JEN-ur-ayt)—to pass from a higher to a lower type or condition.

degenerative (dee-JEN-ur-uh-tiv)—a biochemical change caused by injury or disease, and leading to loss of vitality or function; prone to deteriorate.

dehydrate (dee-HY-drayt)—to deprive of water or to suffer loss of water; to dry out.

dehydration (dee-HY-dray-shun)—lack of water.

dehydrator (DEE-hy-drayt-ur)—an agent that removes or reduces water in the tissues of the body.

deionized water (DEE-eye-on-ized WAH-ter)—water that has had impurities and other metal ions removed.

delivery systems (DEL-iv-er-ee SIS-tems)—formulations that protect or allow for sustained release of medications or ingredients.

deltoid (DEL-toyd)—a large, triangular muscle covering the shoulder joint that allows the arm to extend outward and to the side of the body.

demarcation (dee-mar-KAY-shun)—a line setting bounds or limits; in makeup, to blend colors to avoid a line of demarcation.

demipermanent haircolor (DEM-ih per-man-ent HARE-kul-ur)—also known as *no-lift deposit-only color*; formulated to deposit but not lift (lighten) natural hair color.

demographics (dem-oh-graf-iks)—information about a specific population, including data on race, age, income, and educational attainment.

denature (dee-NAY-chur)—to change the nature of something by chemical or physical means.

dendrites (DEN-dryts)—tree-like branching of nerve fibers extending from a nerve cell; carry impulses toward the cell and receive impulses from other neurons.

density (DEN-sih-tee)—the quality or condition of being close, thick, or heavy; in hair, refers to how much hair is covering the scalp. Of matter, refers to its weight divided by its volume.

denude (dee-NOOD)—to remove overlying matter or material; to expose to view; to clear the face of makeup.

deodorant soaps (dee-OH-dur-unt SOHPS)—cleansing solutions, including bactericides that remain on the body to kill the bacteria responsible for odors.

deoxyribonucleic acid (DNA) (DEE-ox-ee-RYE-boh-NEW-clay-ic ASUD)—the blueprint material of genetic information;

contains all the information that controls the function of every living cell.

depigment (dee-PIG-ment)—to cause the loss of pigment.

depilate (DEP-uh-layt)—to remove hair from the surface of the skin.

depilation (DEP-uh-lay-shun)—process of removing hair at skin level.

depilatory (dih-PIL-uh-tohr-ee)—substance, usually a caustic alkali preparation, used for temporarily removing superfluous hair by dissolving it at the skin level.

deposit (dee-PAH-zit)—in hairdressing, describes a color product in terms of its ability to add color pigment to the hair. Color added equals deposit.

deposition colors (dep-oh-ZIH-shun KUHL-urs)—color that is deposited in the cortical layer of the hair, as well as coating the shaft.

deposit-only color (dee-PAH-zit-OHN-lee KUL-ur)—a category of haircolor products between permanent and semipermanent colors. Formulated to deposit only color, not lift. They contain oxidation dyes and utilize low-volume developer.

depression (dee-PRESH-un)—a hollow or sunken area; in psychiatry, a state of dejection, sadness, or melancholy.

depressor (dee-PRES-ur)—that which presses or draws down; a muscle that depresses.

D

depressor anguli oris (dee-PRES-ur ANG-yoo-lye OH-ris)—also known as *triangularis muscle*; muscle extending alongside the chin that pulls down the corner of the mouth.

depressor labii inferioris muscle (dee-PRES-ur LAY-bee-eye in-FEER-ee-or-us MUS-uhl)—also known as *quadratus labii inferioris muscle*; muscle surrounding the lower lip; depresses the lower lip and draws it to one side, as in expressing sarcasm.

depressor septi nasi (dee-PRES-ur SEP-tee NAY-zye)—a muscle that widens the nostrils during deep respiration.

depressor supercilii (dee-PRES-ur soo-pur-SIL-eye)—the portion of the orbicularis oculi muscle that draws the eyebrows downward.

depth (DEPTH)—also known as *value* and *level*; distance from top to bottom; in hairdressing: the degree of intensity and saturation of color. The lightness or darkness of a color.

derivative (duh-RIV-uh-tiv)—that which is derived; anything obtained or deduced from another.

derm, derma, dermo (DURM, DURM-uh, DURM-oh)—pertaining to the skin.

dermabrasion (dur-muh-BRAY-zhun)—medical procedure; extreme exfoliation method using a mechanical brush to physically remove tissue down to the dermis.

dermafat (DUR-muh-fat)—the adipose tissue of the skin.

dermal (DUR-mul)—pertaining to the skin.

dermal fillers (DUR-mul FILL-erz)—medical procedure; injectibles used to fill lines, wrinkles, and other facial imperfections.

dermal graft (DUR-mul GRAFT)—a medical procedure in which tissue or organs are transplanted.

dermal papilla (DUR-mul puh-PIL-uh)—small, cone-shaped elevations at the base of the hair follicles that fit into the hair bulb.

dermal papillae (DUR-mul puh-PILL-eye)—membranes of ridges and grooves that attach to the epidermis; contains nerve endings and supplies nourishment through capillaries to skin and follicles.

dermal sense (DUR-mul SENS)—the perception of cold, heat, pain, pressure, or other sensations through the receptors of the skin.

dermatalgia (dur-muh-TAL-jee-uh)—pain accompanied by a burning sensation of the skin when no injury or other changes can be observed.

dermatherm (DUR-muh-thurm)—an apparatus designed to measure skin temperature.

dermatitis (dur-muh-TY-tis)—any inflammatory condition of the skin; various forms of lesions, such as eczema, vesicles, or papules; the three main categories are atopic, contact, and seborrheic dermatitis.

dermatitis combustiones (dur-muh-TY-tis kum-bus-tih-OH-nees)—a type of dermatitis produced by exposure to extreme heat or a burn.

dermatitis, cosmetic (dur-muh-TY-tis, kahz-MET-ik)—an inflammation of the skin caused by contact with some cosmetic product to which the individual may be allergic.

dermatitis medicamentosa (dur-muh-TY-tis med-ih-kuh-men-TOH-suh)—a type of dermatitis caused by the internal use of medicines.

dermatitis, occupational (dur-muh-TY-tis, ohk-yoo-PAY-shun-ul)—an inflammation of the skin caused by the kind of employment in which the individual is engaged and by substances used on the job.

dermatitis seborrheica (dur-muh-TY-tis seb-or-EE-ih-kah)—a type of dermatitis found co-existing with seborrhea.

dermatitis venenata (dur-muh-TY-tis VEN-uh-nah-tuh)—an eruptive skin infection caused by contact with irritating substance such as chemicals or tints.

dermatodysplasia (dur-muh-toh-dis-PLAY-zee-ah)—a condition characterized by abnormal development of the skin.

dermatologist (dur-muh-TAHL-uh-jist)—a physician who specializes in diseases and disorders of the skin, hair, and nails.

dermatology (dur-muh-TAHL-uh-jee)—the medical branch of science that deals with the study of skin and its nature, structure, functions, diseases, and treatment.

dermatomycosis (dur-muh-toh-my-KOH-sis)—a superficial infection of the skin or its appendages caused by pathogenic fungus.

dermatoneurology (dur-muh-toh-noo-RAHL-uh-jee)—the study of the nerves of the skin in health and disease.

dermatopathic (dur-muh-toh-PATH-ik)—pertaining or attributable to disease of the skin.

dermatophyte (DUR-mah-toh-fyt)—a fungus that causes superficial infections of the hair, skin, and nails.

dermatophytosis (dur-muh-toh-fy-TOH-sis)—a condition caused by any of the dermatophytes; characterized by erythema, small vesicles, and scaling; common sites of infection are the feet and scalp.

D

dermatoplasty (DUR-muh-toh-plas-tee)—the science of skin grafting; an operation in which flaps of skin are used from another part of the body to replace lost or damaged skin.

dermatosis (dur-muh-TOH-sis)—any disease of the skin; usually a disease not characterized by inflammation.

dermatotherapy (dur-muh-toh-THAIR-uh-pee)—the treatment of the skin and its diseases.

dermatotrophic (dur-muh-toh-TROHF-ik)—affecting, infesting, or infecting the skin.

dermis (DUR-mis)—also known as *derma, corium, cutis*, or *true skin*; support layer of connective tissue, collagen, and elastin below the epidermis.

dermoid (DUR-moyd)—resembling skin.

desensitize (dee-SEN-sih-tyz)—deprive of sensation; to cause the paralysis of a sensory nerve by blocking.

desiccate (DES-ih-kayt)—to deprive a substance of moisture; to dry.

desiccation (des-ih-KAY-shun)—the process of drying.

design (dee-ZYN)—arrangement of shapes, lines, and ornamental effects that create an artistic unit as in hairstyling, makeup application, and the creation of fashions.

design component (dee-ZYN kahm-POH-nent)—one of four elements (texture, form, structure, and direction) that makes up a hair design.

design line (dee-ZYN LYN)—the artistic concept of a finished hairstyle as expressed in its lines and shapes; a line used as a guide in creating the form of a design. In barbering, usually the perimeter line of the haircut.

design, three-dimensional (dee-ZYN, THREE dih-MEN-shun-ul)—a sculpturing effect with hair, creating volume and/or indentation into a shape.

design, two-dimensional (dee-ZYN, TOO dih-MEN-shun-ul)—a pattern effect on a flat surface.

design sculpture (dee-ZYN sculp-chur)—nail enhancements that have inlaid designs and are produced using either monomer liquid and polymer powder or UV gel products.

design texture (dee-ZYN Teks-chur)—wave patterns that must be taken into consideration when designing a style.

desincrustation (dis-in-krus-TAY-shun)—process used to soften and emulsify sebum deposits (oil) and blackheads in the hair follicles.

desmosine (DES-moh-sin)—a crosslinking amino acid found in elastin.

desmosomes (DEZ-moh-somes)—the structures that assist in holding cells together; intercellular connections made of proteins.

desquamate (DES-kwuh-mayt)—to shed scales; to shed the superficial layer of the skin.

desquamation (DES-kwuh-MAY-shun)—scaling of the cuticle.

detergent (dee-TUR-jent)—a compound or solution used for cleansing; type of surfactant used as cleansers in beauty products; an agent that cleanses the skin and hair.

detoxification (dee-tahk-sih-fih-KAY-shun)—reduction of toxic poisons; ridding the body of toxic substances.

developers (dee-VEL-up-urz)—also known as *oxidizing agents* or *catalysts*; when mixed with an oxidation haircolor, supplies the necessary oxygen gas to develop color molecules and create a change in hair color.

development time (dee-VEL-up-ment TYM)—the oxidation period required for the hair lightener or tint solution to act completely on the hair.

dexterity (deks-TAIR-ih-tee)—skill and ease in using the hands; expertise in manual acts.

diabetes mellitus (dy-uh-BEET-us MEL-uh-tus)—medical term for the condition caused by metabolic disorder or decreased output of insulin by the pancreas.

diagnosis (dy-ag-NOH-sis)—determination of the nature of a disease from its symptoms and/or diagnostic tests. Federal regulations prohibit salon professionals from performing a diagnosis.

diagonal (dy-AG-uh-nul)—a line with a slanting or sloping direction.

diagonal asymmetry (dy-AG-uh-nul Aye-sym-et-ree)—when one side of a design includes a diagonal line while the other does not.

diagonal back design (dy-AG-uh-nul BAK dee-ZYN)—a design resulting in a backward flow of hair from the face.

diagonal forward design (dy-AG-uh-nul FOR-ward dee-ZYN)—a design resulting in a forward movement of hair onto the face.

diagonal left (dy-AG-uh-nul LEFT)—a diagonal line that travels to the left.

diagonal lines (dye-AG-ih-nul LYNES)—lines positioned between horizontal and vertical lines. They are often used to emphasize or minimize facial features.

Used with the permission of the authors, Martin Gannon and Richard Thompson, as featured in their book, Mahogony: Steps to Cutting, Coloring, and Finishing Hair © Martin Gannon and Richard Thompson, 1997.

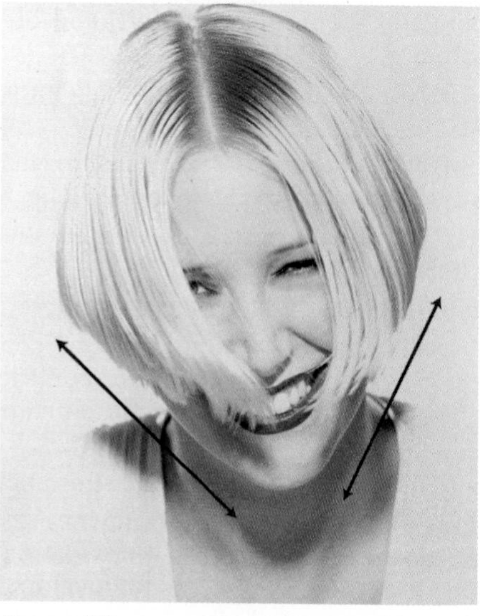

diagonal lines

diagonal right (dy-AG-uh-nul RYT)—a diagonal line that travels to the right.

diagram (DY-uh-gram)—a figure for ascertaining or exhibiting certain relations between objects under discussion; an outline, figure, or scheme of lines, spaces, or points; used in demonstrations.

diameter (dy-AM-ih-tur)—the length from one border to another of a straight line that passes through the center of an object.

diamond shape (DY-uh-mund SHAYP)—a figure bounded by four equal straight lines with two acute angles and two obtuse angles.

diamond-shaped face (DY-uh-mund-SHAYPT FAYS)—a face with a narrow forehead and chin, with the greater width across the cheekbones.

diaphoretic (dy-uh-fuh-RET-ik)—cool, clammy skin; producing perspiration.

diaphragm (DY-uh-fram)—a muscular wall that separates the thorax from the abdominal region and helps to control breathing.

diarthrotic joints (dy-ar-THRAH-tik JOYNTS)—freely movable joints.

diathermy (DY-uh-thur-mee)—the method of raising the temperature in the deep tissues by using high-frequency current; the application of oscillating electromagnetic fields to the tissues.

dichromatic (dy-kroh-MAT-ik)—having two colors.

diencephalon (DY-en-sef-ah-lon)—located in the uppermost part of the midbrain; consists of two main parts, the thalamus and the hypothalamus.

diet (DY-it)—a selection of foods in a regulated course of eating and drinking, especially for health reasons; to regulate kinds and amounts of food and drink for specific reasons.

dietetics (dy-uh-TET-iks)—the science of regulating the diet for hygienic or therapeutic purposes.

differentiation (dif-ur-en-chee-AY-shun)—repeated division of the ovum during early developmental stages, resulting in specialized cells that differ from one another and have specialized functions.

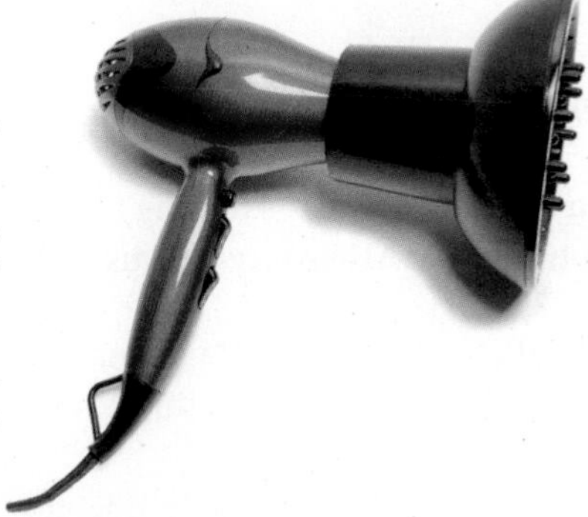

© Milady, a part of Cengage Learning

blowdryer and diffuser

diffuse (dih-FYOOZ)—to pour out; to break down and spread in every way; scattered; not limited to one spot.

diffuser (dih-FYOOZ-er)—blowdryer attachment that causes the air to flow more softly and helps to accentuate or keep textural definition.

diffusion (dih-FYOO-zhun)—spreading out; the process

D

by which substances move from areas of higher concentration to lower concentration.

digest (dy-JEST)—to prepare for absorption; to change food chemically in the alimentary canal for assimilation by the body.

digestion (dy-JES-chun)—the process of converting food into a form that can be readily absorbed; the breaking down of substances into simple forms, such as food into simpler chemical compounds.

digestive enzymes (dy-JES-tiv EN-zymz)—chemicals that change certain types of food into a soluble (capable of being dissolved) form that can be used by the body.

digestive system (dy-JES-tiv SIS-tum)—also known as *gastrointestinal system*; responsible for breaking down foods into nutrients and wastes; consists of the mouth, stomach, intestines, salivary and gastric glands, and other organs.

digit (DIJ-ut)—a finger or toe.

digital artery (DIJ-ut-ul ART-uh-ree)—the artery that supplies blood to the fingers and toes.

digital function (DIJ-ut-ul FUNK-shun)—a massage technique using fingertips in a rotating motion; pressing and rotating the fingers on the skin.

digital nerves (DIJ-ut-ul NURVZ)—sensory-motor nerve that, with its branches, supplies impulses to the fingers.

digital stroking (DIJ-ut-ul STROHK-ing)—a massage movement in which the fingertips are used to lightly glide over the face and neck.

digital tapotement (DIJ-ut-ul tah-POT-ment)—a massage movement to promote stimulation of blood to the skin surface; consists of light, tapping movements with the tips of the fingers.

digital vibration (DIJ-ut-ul vy-BRA-shun)—a massage movement using the tips of the fingers pressed on a pressure point such as the temples, then using a rapid shaking movement for a few seconds.

digiti manus (DIJ-ih-ty MAN-us)—the digits of the hand.

digiti pedis (DIJ-ih-ty PED-us)—the digits of the foot.

digitus (DIJ-ih-tus)—finger.

digitus annularis (DIJ-ih-tus an-yuh-LAHR-is)—the ring finger.

digitus demonstrativus (DIJ-ih-tus duh-MAHN-stray-tee-vus)—the index finger.

digitus medius (DIJ-ih-tus MEE-dee-us)—the middle finger.

digitus minimus (DIJ-ih-tus MIN-ih-mus)—the little finger.

dilate (DY-layt)—to enlarge; expand; distend.

dilator (dy-LAYT-ur)—that which expands or enlarges; an instrument for stretching or enlarging a cavity or opening.

dilute (dy-LOOT)—to make less concentrated, thinner, or more liquid by mixing with another substance, especially water.

dimension (dih-MEN-shun)—any measurable extent such as length, breadth, or thickness.

dimensional coloring (dih-MEN-shun-ul KUL-ur-ing)—two or three different shades of the same color on the same head of hair.

dimensional design (dih-MEN-shun-ul dee-ZYN)—three-dimensional sculpturing effect with hair, creating volume or indentation into a shape and silhouette.

dimensional styling (dih-MEN-shun-ul STYL-ing)—hairstyling achieved by creating volume or indentation.

dimethicone—(DYE-meth-ih-kone) cosmetic ingredient that is derived from silicon polymers; creates slip and seals in hydration.

dimethyl urea hardeners (DMU) (DY-meth-il YUR-ee-ah HAR-den-urs)—a hardener that adds cross-links to the natural nail plate. Unlike hardeners containing formaldehyde, DMU does not cause adverse skin reactions.

dimethylaminoethanol (DMAE) (dy-meth-il-uh-MEEN-noh-eth-uh-nol)—antioxidant that stabilizes cell membranes and boosts the effect of other antioxidants.

dimple (DIM-pul)—a slight depression or indentation on the body, usually the cheeks or chin.

dioxide (dy-AHK-syd)—a molecule containing two atoms of oxygen.

diphtheria (dif-THEER-ee-uh)—an infectious disease in which the air passages, and especially the throat, become coated with a false membrane caused by a specific bacillus.

diplococci (dip-loh-KOK-sy)—spherical bacteria that grow in pairs and cause diseases such as pneumonia.

diplomacy (dih-PLOH-muh-see)—the practice of negotiations; skill and tact when dealing with others, the art of being tactful.

direct current (DC) (dy-REKT KUR-ent)—constant, even-flowing current that travels in one direction only and is produced by chemical means.

direct dye (dy-REKT DYE)—a preformed color that dyes the fiber directly without the need for oxidation.

direct marketing (dy-REKT MAR-ket-ing)—any attempt to reach the consumer directly with an offer such as direct mail post-cards, coupons, newsletters, sales letters, telemarketing, electronic mail, and text messages.

directional massage (dy-REK-shun-ul ma-SAHZH)—technique using a short "J" stroke on a specified body area or muscle.

directional roller (dy-REK-shun-ul ROHL-ur)—a roller used to direct the hair forward or backward to create a specific style.

direct surface application (dy-REKT SUR-fas APP-li-cay-shun)—high-frequency current performed with the mushroom- or rake-shaped electrodes for its calming and germicidal effect on the skin.

direct transmission (dy-REKT trans-MISH-uhn)—transmission of blood or body fluids through touching (including shaking hands), kissing, coughing, sneezing, and talking.

directional lines (dr-REKT-shun-uhl LYNZ)—lines with a definite forward or backward movement.

disaccharides (DYE-sack-uh-ridz)—sugars made up of two simple sugars, such as lactose and sucrose.

discharge (dis-CHARJ)—to set free; to remove the contents or load; to relieve of responsibility; the escape or flowing away of the contents of a cavity.

discolor (dis-KUL-ur)—to change or destroy the color.

discoloration (dis-kul-ur-AY-shun)—the development of an undesired color shade through chemical reaction.

discolored nails (dis-KUL-urd NAILZ)—a condition in which the nails turn a variety of colors; may indicate surface staining, a systemic disorder, or poor blood circulation.

D

disease (DIZ-eez)—an abnormal condition of all or part of the body, or its systems or organs, that makes the body incapable of carrying on normal function.

disease carrier (DIZ-eez KAIR-ee-ur)—a healthy person, who may be affected by or not affected by a disease, who carries and may transmit disease to another person.

disentangle (dis-en-TANG-ul)—to free from clumping together; to straighten out snarls in hair.

disfigure (dis-FIG-yur)—to impair or destroy the beauty of a person or object.

disinfectants (dis-in-FEK-tents)—EPA-registered products used on nonporous surfaces that destroy organisms such as bacteria, viruses, and fungi, when used according to the disinfectant label instructions.

disinfection (disinfecting) (dis-in-FEK-shun)—a chemical process that uses specific products to destroy organisms on nonporous surfaces.

disintegrate (dis-IN-tuh-GRAYT)—to separate or decompose a substance into its component parts; to reduce to fragments or powder.

dislocation (dis-loh-KAY-shun)—a bone displaced within a joint.

dispensary (dis-PEN-suh-ree)—room or area used for mixing products and storing supplies.

dispersion (dis-PUR-zhun)—the act of scattering or separating; the incorporation of the particles of one substance into the body of another comprising solutions, suspensions, and colloid solutions.

disposable implements (dis-POH-zuh-bul IMP-luh-ments)—also known as *single-use implements*; implements that cannot be reused and must be thrown away after a single use.

dissipate (DIS-ih-payt)—to dissolve.

dissociation (dih-soh-see-AY-shun)—the process by which combined chemicals are changed into simpler constituents.

dissoluble (dis-AHL-yuh-bul)—capable of being dissolved or decomposed.

dissolve (dih-ZAHLV)—to cause to become a solution; to break into parts; to disintegrate.

distal (DIS-tul)—farthest from the center or median line.

distend (dis-TEND)—to expand; to swell.

distill (dis-TIL)—to extract the essence or active principle of a substance.

distillation (dis-tuh-LAY-shun)—the process of distilling.

distilled water (dis-TILD WAH-tur)—purified or refined water.

distribute (dis-TRIB-yoot)—to disperse through space or over an area; to arrange; in hairdressing and design, distribution refers to the direction hair is combed in relation to its base parting.

disulfide (dy-SUL-fyd)—a chemical compound in which two sulfur atoms are united with a single atom of an element; for example, carbon, an amino acid found in hair.

disulfide bonds (dy-SUL-fyed BAHNDS)—also known as *sulfur bonds*; strong chemical side bond that joins the sulfur atoms of two neighboring cysteine amino acids to create one cystine, which joins together two polypeptide strands like rungs on a ladder.

disulfide links (dy-SUL-fyd LINKS)—bonds or cross-linkages between the polypeptide chains of the hair cortex.

dominant (DAHM-ih-nent)—the prominent part or position; large or more impressive as in a dominant facial feature.

dorsal (DOR-sul)—pertaining to the back of a part.

dorsal nasal artery (DOR-sul NAY-zul ART-uh-ree)—artery that supplies blood to the side of the nose.

dorsal nerve (DOR-sul NURV)—also known as *dorsal cutaneous nerve*; a nerve that extends up from the toes and foot, just under the skin, supplying impulses to toes and foot, as well as the muscles and skin of the leg, where it becomes the superficial peroneal nerve or the musculocutaneous nerve.

dorsal vertebrae (DOR-sul VURT-uh-bray)—the bones of the vertebral or spinal column located in the midsection of the back.

dorsalis pedis artery (DOR-sul-is PEED-us ART-uh-ree)—supplies blood to the foot.

dorso, dorsi (DOR-soh, DOR-see)—pertaining to the back of the body; denoting relationship to a dorsum or to the posterior aspect of the body.

double application tint (DUB-ul ap-lih-KAY-shun TINT)—also known as *two-process tint, double-process tint,* and *double-process application*; a product requiring two separate applications to the hair, a softener or lightener followed by a penetrating tint.

D

double bond (DUB-ul BAHND)—a chemical bond consisting of two bonds between two atoms of a molecule, each bond formed by shared electrons.

double chin (DUB-ul CHIN)—a fleshy fold under the chin giving the appearance of two chins.

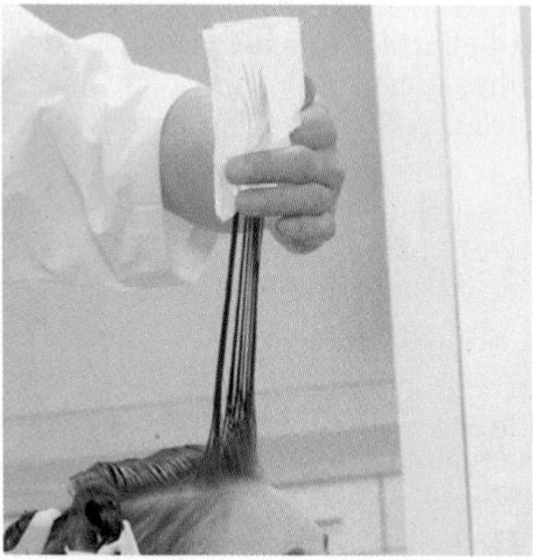

© Milady, a part of Cengage Learning. Photography by Paul Castle, Castle Photography.

double flat wrap

double flat wrap (DUB-ul FLAT RAP)—perm wrap in which one end paper is placed under and another is placed over the strand of hair being wrapped.

double-process application (DUB-ul PRAH-ses APP-lih-cay-shun)—also known as *two-step coloring*; a coloring technique requiring two separate procedures in which the hair is prelightened before the depositing color is applied to the hair.

double-press (DUB-ul PRESS)—a technique of passing a hot curling iron though the hair before performing a hard press.

double-prong clips (DUB-ul-PRAWNG KLIPS)—small clips with short prongs used to hold pin curls flat; also used in other shaping, rolling, and setting of hair.

double-rod wrap (DUB-ul ROHD RAP)—also known as *piggyback wrap*; a wrap technique whereby extra-long hair is wrapped on one rod from the scalp to midway down the hair shaft, and another rod is used to wrap the remaining hair strand in the same direction.

dovetail (DUV-tayl)—a connecting line in a style between two or more shapes.

down stroke (DOWN STROHK)—a stroke made with a razor while shaving; in facials, stroking lightly upward and downward with the tips of fingers.

downy hair (DOWN-ee HAYR)—soft, lightweight hair growth; fine hair.

drab (DRAB)—also known as *ash*, or *dull*; a shade that has no red or gold tones; usually a dull brown or gray color.

drab color (DRAB KUL-ur)—a hair color lacking red and gold tones; colors such as ash, gray, silver, white, platinum, smoky, or steel gray.

drabber (DRAB-ur)—a concentrated coloring agent designed to reduce the presence of red or gold tones.

drabbing agent (DRAB-ing AY-jent)—a chemical used to eliminate red or gold tones from the hair color.

drafting (DRAFF-ting)—putting thoughts and information into cohesive sentences and paragraphs.

drag (DRAG)—a term to describe a feeling of resistance when a product is applied; the opposite of slip or ease of application.

drape (DRAYP)—to arrange or cover with cloth; a cape or covering placed on a client to protect clothing while receiving salon services; a coverlet placed over a client during a facial or massage treatment.

draw (DRAW)—in haircutting, to bring the section of hair through the fingers to hold it taut while cutting and shaping.

dressing (DRES-ing)—arranging hair in a style; a substance applied to the hair; a salve or pomade.

dropping a wave (DRAHP-ing UH WAYV)—the act of discontinuing a wave rather than carrying it around the entire head.

drug (DRUG)—a substance other than food intended to affect the structure or function of the body; a chemical compound or substance used in some medications.

Dr. Jacquet Movement (DAHK-tur Jah-ket MOOV-ment)—a kneading movement beneficial for oily skin; it helps move sebum out of the follicles and up to the skin's surface.

Dr. Vodder's Manual Lymph Drainage (DAHK-tur VAHD-urz MAN-yooul LIMF DRAYN-ij)—a method of gentle, rhythmical massage along the surface lymphatics to accelerate functioning of the lymphatic system that treats chronic lymphedema.

dry cut (DRY KUT)—a technique for cutting hair while it is dry; to cut hair before it is shampooed, or after it has been shampooed and dried.

dry hair (DRY HAYR)—hair lacking sufficient or normal oils; a condition that may be temporary or chronic in nature; hair that is free from moisture.

dry heat (DRY HEET)—used to sterilize sheets, towels, gauze, cotton, and similar materials.

dry nail polish (DRY-NAYL-POL-ish)—powder or paste used with the chamois buffer to add shine to the nails.

dry shampoo (DRY sham-POO)—also known as *powder shampoo*; shampoo that cleanses the hair without the use of soap and water.

D

dryer chair (DRY-ur CHAYR)—a chair to which a hair dryer is attached.

drying lamp (DRY-ing LAMP)—an infrared lamp used to dry wet hair during a haircutting procedure.

dry (cabinet) sanitizer (DRY SAN-ih-tyz-ur)—an airtight cabinet containing an active fumigant used to store cleaned and disinfected tools and implements until needed.

dry skin (DRY SKIN)—skin that is deficient in oil and/or moisture.

duct (DUKT)—a passage or canal for fluids.

duct gland (DUKT GLAND)—gland that produces a substance that travels through small tube-like ducts; examples are the sudoriferous (sweat) glands and sebaceous (oil) glands.

ductless gland (DUKT-lis GLAND)—a gland that has no excretory duct but releases secretions directly into the blood or lymph.

dull (DUL)—also known as *drab*; used to describe hair or hair color without sheen.

duodenum (doo-uh-DEE-num)—the part of the small intestines just below the stomach.

dye (DYE)—to stain or color; a chemical compound or mixture formulated to penetrate the hair and effect a change in hair color; made from plants, metals, or synthetic compounds; artificial pigment.

dye brush (DYE BRUSH)—also known as *color brush*; a small, flat, long-handled brush designed for the application of haircoloring or hair treatment products.

© Milady, a part of Cengage Learning. Photography by Yanik Chauvin.

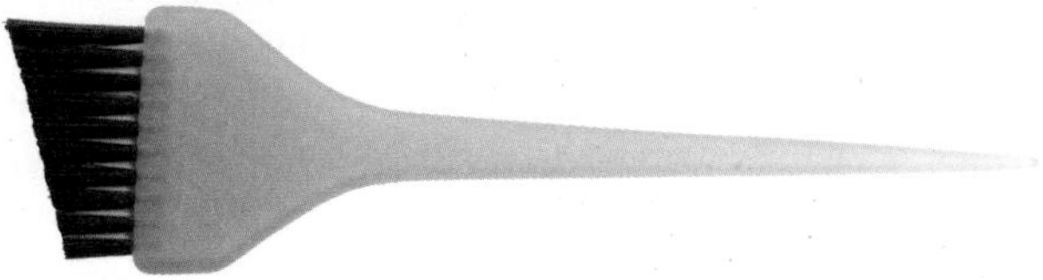

dye or color brush

dye intermediate (DYE in-tur-MEE-dee-it)—a material that develops into color only after reaction with developer (hydrogen peroxide); also known as *oxidation dyes*.

dye remover (DYE ree-MOOV-ur)—also known as *color remover*, a prepared commercial product that removes tint from the hair.

dye solvent (DYE SAHL-vunt)—a chemical solution that is employed to remove artificial color from the hair.

dye stain remover (DYE STAYN ree-MOOV-ur)—a chemical substance used to remove tint stains from the skin following a hair tinting procedure.

dyschromias (diz-KRO-me-ahz)—abnormal colorations of the skin that accompany many skin disorders and systemic disorders.

dyskeratoma (dis-kair-uh-TOH-muh)—a skin tumor; warty growth; a brownish-red nodule with a soft, yellowish keratotic plug appearing on the face or scalp.

dyskeratosis (dis-kair-uh-TOH-sis)—imperfect keratinization of individual epidermal cells.

ear lobe (EER lohb)—the soft, fleshy lower part of the external ear.

ear protector (EER proh-TEK-tur)—a plastic ear-shaped shell used over the ears as a protection during the hair-drying procedure.

earlap (EER-lap)—the external ear, especially the ear lobes.

earwax (EER-waks)—also known as *cerumen*; a yellowish-brown substance secreted by the glands lining the passages of the external ear.

ecchymosis (ek-ih-MOH-sus)—also known as *bruise*; a discoloration such as a bluish spot caused by the rupture of a small blood vessel beneath the surface of the skin.

eccrine glands (EK-run GLANZ)—sweat glands found all over the body with openings on the skin's surface through pores; not attached to hair follicles, secretions do not produce an offensive odor.

ecderon (EK-dur-ahn)—the epithelial, outermost layer of the skin and mucous membrane.

ecology (ee-KAHL-uh-jee)—the study of the environmental relationship of organisms.

ecthyma (ek-THY-muh)—a viral disease that forms ulcerating pustules on the skin.

ectoderm (EK-tuh-durm)—the outermost layer of the cells in an embryo that develops into skin after the establishment of the three primary germ layers.

ectodermic (ek-tuh-DUR-mik)—pertaining to the outer layer of cells formed from the inner cell mass in the embryonic cell.

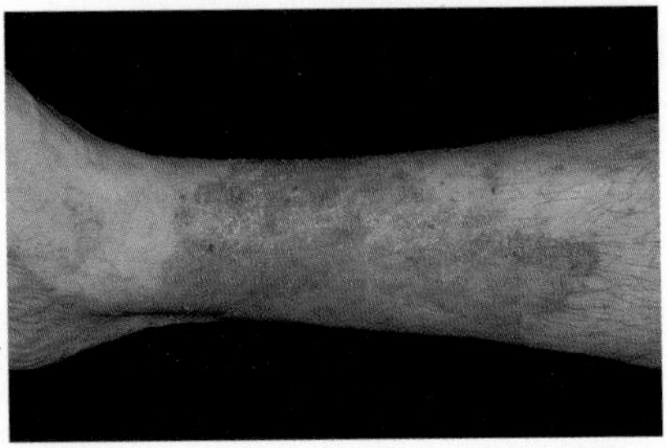

Courtesy of www.dermnet.com

eczema

ectomorph (EK-tuh-morf)—a person who is characterized by a lean, lanky body structure.

ectothrix (EK-toh-thriks)—a fungal parasite that affects the hair shaft.

eczema (EG-zuh-muh)—inflammatory, painful itching disease of the skin, acute or chronic in nature, with dry or moist lesions. This condition should be referred to a physician.

eczematoid reaction (ek-ZEE-muh-toyd ree-AK-shun)—a dermal and epidermal condition of the skin resembling eczema.

eczematosis (ek-zee-muh-TOH-sus)—any eczematous skin disease.

eczematous (ek-ZEE-muh-tus)—having the characteristics of eczema.

edema (ih-DEE-muh)—swelling caused by a fluid imbalance in cells or a response to injury or infection.

edge (EJ)—the cutting side of a blade.

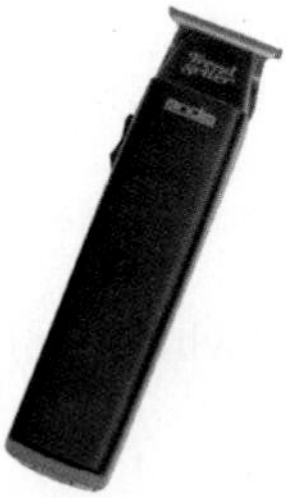
© Milady, a part of Cengage Learning. Photography by Paul Castle, Castle Photography.
edgers

edgers (EJ-urs)—also known as *outliners,* or *trimmers*; small, electric clippers used to remove superfluous hair from the hairline and create straight or creative lines in short taper cuts.

edging (EJ-ing)—the process of cutting the sideburn and nape area.

effective communication (uh-FEK-tive COM-yun-ik-ay-shun)—the act of sharing information between two people (or main groups of people) so that the information is successfully understood.

efferent (EF-uh-rent)—conveying outward, as efferent nerves conveying impulses away from the central nervous system from the brain to muscles.

efferent lymphatic (EF-uh-rent lim-FAT-ik)—a vessel conveying lymph away from a lymph node.

efferent neuron (EF-uh-ent NOO-rahn)—a neuron conducting impulses away from a nerve center.

efficacy (ef-ih-KUH-see)—the ability to produce an effect.

efficiency (ih-FISH-un-see)—usefulness; quality or degree of being able to produce results; economic productivity.

efficient (ih-FISH-unt)—characterized by energetic and useful activity.

effilate (EF-ih-layt)—to cut the hair strand by a sliding movement of the scissors while keeping blades partially opened.

effilating (EF-ih-layt-ing)—a method of thinning hair with scissors.

E

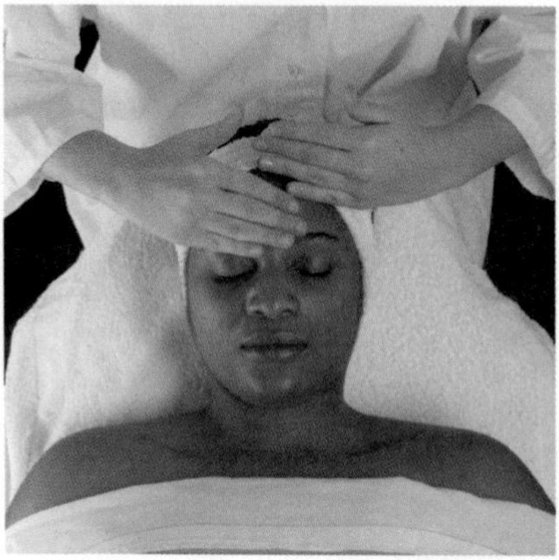

© Milady, a part of Cengage Learning. Photography by Paul Castle, Castle Photography.

effleurage

effleurage (EF-loo-rahzh)—light, continuous stroking movement applied with the fingers (digital) or the palms (palmar) in a slow, rhythmic manner.

efflorescence (ef-luh-RES-uns)—a rash or eruption of the skin.

effusion (eh-FYOO-zhun)—the act of pouring out; the escape of fluid from the blood vessels or lymphatics into tissue or cavity.

egg (EG)—ovum; a round or oval reproductive body produced by female birds, fish, and the like; used primarily as a food and in some products such as shampoos and facial masks.

eggshell nails (EG-shell NAYLZ)—noticeably thin, white nail plates that are more flexible than normal.

elastic (ee-LAS-tik)—capable of returning to the original form after being stretched; having the ability to stretch and return to the original form.

elastic cartilage (ee-LAS-tik KART-ul-ij)—a resistant cartilage found in the external ear and larynx.

elasticity (ee-las-TIS-ih-tee)—of hair, the ability of the hair to stretch and return to normal; important in the ability of hair to retain curl or withstand chemical treatments; of skin, the tissue's ability to return to normal resting length when a stress that was placed on it is removed; of muscles, the ability of muscles to return to their original shape after being stretched.

E

elastin (ee-LAS-tin)—protein fiber found in the dermis; gives skin its elasticity and firmness.

elastoma (ee-las-TOH-muh)—a tumor formed by an excess of elastic tissue fibers or abnormal collagen fibers of the skin.

elastosis senilis (ee-las-TOH-sis seh-NIL-is)—degeneration of the elastic connective tissues in advanced age.

electric clippers (ee-LEK-trik KLIP-urz)—an electrically powered implement used to cut and trim hair.

electric current (ee-LEK-trik KUR-unt)—the movement of electricity along a conductor.

electric facial mask (ee-LEK-trik FAY-shul MASK)—a contoured pad heated electrically and placed over the face to soften oil/sebum deposits and induce deep penetration of beneficial products into the skin.

electric hair roller (ee-LEK-trik HAYR ROHL-ur)—a cylindrical roller designed to retain heat and used to style dry hair.

electric massager (ee-LEK-trik muh-SAJH-ur)—massaging unit that attaches to a barber's hand to impart vibrating massage movements to the skin surface.

electric pressing iron (ee-LEK-trik PRES-ing EYE-urn)—a curling iron designed with a larger barrel for straightening curly hair.

electric shaver (ee-LEK-trik SHAYV-ur)—also known as *electric razor*; an electrically powered device used to remove facial and body hair.

electric straightening comb (ee-LEK-trik STRAYT-un-ing KOHM)—a comb with a wooden handle and metal teeth that contains a heating element and is used to straighten curly hair.

electricity (ee-lek-TRIS-ih-tee)—the movement of particles around an atom that creates pure energy.

electricity, chemical (ee-lek-TRIS-ih-tee, KEM-ih-kul)—electricity generated, by chemical action in a galvanic cell.

electricity, galvanic (ee-lek-TRIS-ih-tee, gal-VAN-ik)—electricity generated by chemical action in a galvanic cell.

electricity, induced or inductive (ee-lek-TRIS-ih-tee, in-DOOST OR in-DUK-tiv)—electricity produced by proximity to an electrified body.

electricity, magnetic (ee-lek-TRIS-ih-tee, mag-NET-ik)—electricity developed by bringing a conductor near the poles of a magnet.

electricity, static (ee-lek-TRIS-ih-tee, STAT-ik)—frictional electricity.

electricity, voltaic (ee-lek-TRIS-ih-tee, vohl-TAY-ik)—galvanic or chemical electricity.

electrification (ee-lek-trih-fih-KAY-shun)—the process of applying electricity to the body by holding an electrode in the hand and charging the body with electricity.

electrocoagulation (ee-lek-troh-koh-ag-yoo-LAY-shun)—the single-needle shortwave method of electrolysis; the use of high-frequency current to remove superfluous hair.

electrocution (ee-lek-troh-KYOO-shun)—occurs from either low- or high-voltage currents when a person makes contact with an electric outlet or pathway and simultaneously touches a metal object that extends to the ground, is standing on a wet surface, or has damp skin.

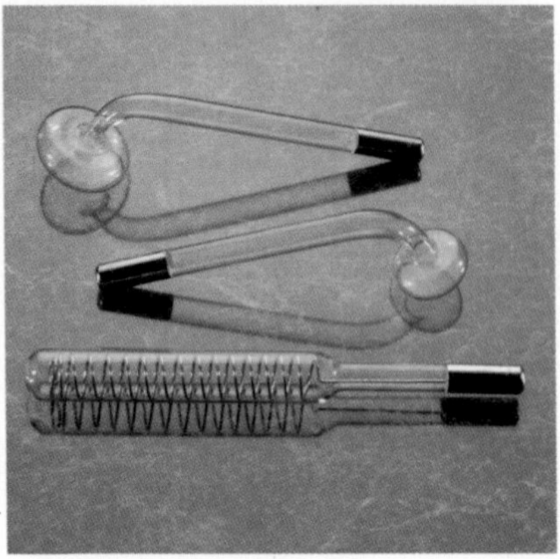
© Milady, a part of Cengage Learning. Photography by Larry Hamill.
electrodes

electrode (ee-LEK-trohd)—also known as *probe*; applicator for directing electric current from an electrotherapy device to the client's skin.

electrode gel (ee-LEK-trohd JEL)—a gel used to improve contact between the electrode and the skin when the electrode is used in a specific treatment.

electrologist (ee-lek-TRAHL-uh-just)—one who removes hair by means of an electric current applied to the body with a needle-shaped electrode.

electrolysis (ee-lek-TRAHL-ih-sis)—removal of hair by means of an electric current that destroys the root of the hair.

electromagnetic spectrum (ee-LEK-troh-MAG-net-ik SPECK-trum)—also known as *electromagnetic spectrum of radiation*; name given to all of the forms of energy (or radiation) that exist.

electron (ee-LEK-trahn)—a basic negatively charged particle found outside the nucleus of an atom, arranged in orbits or shells.

electronic tweezing (ee-lek-TRAHN-ik TWEEZ-ing)—the use of high-frequency current in removal of superfluous hair.

electropositive (ee-lek-troh-PAHZ-ih-tiv)—relating to or charged with positive electricity.

E

electrostatic (ee-lek-troh-STAT-ik)—pertaining to static electricity.

electrotherapeutics (ee-lek-troh-thair-uh-PYOO-tiks)—the application of electricity for therapeutic purposes.

electrotherapy (ee-lek-troh-thair-uh-py)—the use of electrical currents to treat the skin.

element (EL-uh-ment)—the simplest form of chemical matter; an element cannot be broken down into a simpler substance without a loss of identity.

elemental molecule (EL-uh-ment-uhl mahl-ick-yule)—molecule containing two or more atoms of the same element in definite (fixed) proportions.

elements in hair (EL-uh-ments IN HAYR)—elements commonly found in hair are nitrogen, oxygen, carbon, sulfur, hydrogen, and phosphorus.

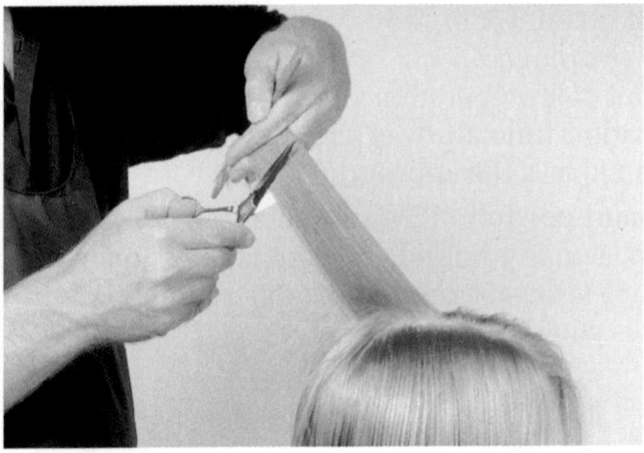

© Milady, a part of Cengage Learning. Photography by Yanik Chauvin.

elevation

elevation (el-uh-VAY-shun)—also known as *projection* or *lifting*; angle or degree at which a subsection of hair is held, or lifted, from the head when cutting.

eleventh cranial nerve (ee-LEV-unth CRAY-nee-ul NURV)—also known as *accessory nerve*; a motor nerve that controls the motion of the neck and shoulder muscles.

elimination (ee-lim-ih-NAY-shun)—act of expelling or excreting.

ellipse (ee-LIPS)—a wide oval curve.

emaciation (ee-MAY-shee-AY-shun)—the state of being wasted away; physically, loss of body fat; extreme leanness.

embed (em-BED)—to fix firmly in surrounding matter.

emery board (EM-ur-ee BORD)—a disposable manicuring instrument having rough cutting ridges; used for shaping nails with the coarse side, and for smoothing them with the finer side.

emit (ee-MIT)—to send out; to give off light, heat, sound.

emollient (ee-MAHL-yunt)—oil or fatty ingredients that prevent moisture from leaving the skin.

emollient cream (ee-MAHL-yunt KREEM)—a cream used in facial and body massage.

emphasize (EM-fuh-syz)—also known as *focus*; the place in a hairstyle where the eye is drawn first before traveling to the rest of the design.

employee (EM-ploy-ee)—employment classification in which the employer withholds certain taxes and has a high level of control.

employee evaluation (EM-ploy-ee EE-val-you-aye-shun)—a periodic assessment of an employee's skills, attitudes, and behaviors and how they are used and perceived in the work setting.

employee manual (EM-ploy-ee MAN-yu-ehl)—handbook or guide for employees; contains important general information about salon operations, such as the number of sick days or vacation time allowed, holiday closings, how to call in late or sick, and the appropriate dress code for technicians.

employment portfolio (EM-ploy-ment PORT-fo-lee-oh)—a collection, usually bound, of photos and documents that reflect your skills, accomplishments, and abilities in your chosen career field.

© Milady, a part of Cengage Learning. Photography by Yanik Chauvin.

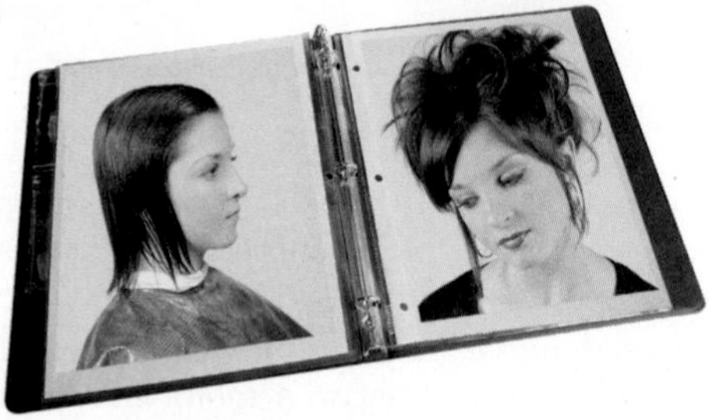

employment portfolio

emulsified (ee-MUL-suh-fyd)—made into an emulsion.

emulsifier (ee-MUL-suh-fy-ur)—an ingredient that brings two normally incompatible materials together and binds them into a uniform and fairly stable blend.

emulsion (ee-MUL-shun)—an unstable physical mixture of two or more immiscible substances (substances that normally will not stay blended) plus a special ingredient called an emulsifier.

E

enamel (ee-NAM-ul)—in nail technology; gloss; nail polish.

encephalitis (en-SEF-uh-ly-tus)—a viral disease causing inflammation of the brain.

end bonds (END BAHNDZ)—also known as *peptide bonds*; the chemical bonds that join amino acids to form the long chains characteristic of all proteins.

end curls (END curlz)—used to give a finished appearance to hair ends either turned under or over.

end organ (END OR-gun)—the termination of nerve fiber in the skin, muscle, mucous membranes, and the like.

end papers (END PAY-perz)—also known as *end wraps*; absorbent papers used to control the ends of the hair when wrapping and winding hair on perm rods.

endepidermis (end-ep-ih-DUR-mus)—the inner layer of the epidermis.

endermic (en-DUR-mik)—acting through the skin by absorption such as a product applied to the skin.

endermology (ENDER-mol-oh-gee)—treatment for cellulite.

endermosis (en-dur-MOH-sus)—the application of a product to the skin by rubbing; any eruptive disease of the mucous membrane.

endocardium (EN-doh-kar-dee-um)—innermost layer of the heart.

endocrine gland (EN-duh-krin GLAND)—also known as *ductless glands*; ductless glands that release hormonal secretions directly into the bloodstream. They are a group of specialized glands that affect the growth, development, sexual activities, and health of the entire body.

endocrine system (EN-duh-krin SIS-tum)—a group of specialized glands that affect the growth, development, sexual activity, and health of the entire body.

endocrinology (EN-duh-krin-ahl-uh-jee)—the study of the endocrine glands and their function.

endoderm (EN-doh-derm)—the innermost layer of cells of the skin; a layer of cells developing in a human fetus to produce tissue for specialized function.

endomysium (en-do-MY-see-um)—delicate connective tissue covering muscle fibers.

endosteum (en-DAHS-tee-um)—a layer of cells covering the inner surface of bone in the medullary cavity.

endothelium (en-duh-THEE-lee-yum)—a thin lining of the interior of the heart, blood vessels, lymphatics, and the like.

endothermic method (en-duh-THUR-mik METH-ud)—perm activation by an outside heat source, usually a conventional hood-type hair dryer.

endothermic waves (en-duh-THUR-mik wayvz)—perm activated by an outside heat source, usually a conventional hood-type hair dryer.

endotoxin (en-doh-TAHK-sun)—a toxic substance found in some forms of bacteria.

energy (EN-ur-jee)—internal or inherent power or capacity for performing work.

enlarged pores (en-LARJD PORZ)—follicles (pores) that have been stretched due to accumulation of sebum and dead surface cells.

entangle (en-TANG-gul)—to intertwine the hair in a confused manner.

environment (en-VY-run-ment)—the surrounding conditions; influences or forces that influence or modify.

Environmental Protection Agency (EPA) (en-VY-ron-men-tal PROTECK-shun AGE-en-see)—a governmental agency whose purpose is to ensure that all Americans are protected from significant risks to human health and the environment where they live, learn, and work.

envisioning (EN-vijg-ohn-ing)—the process of visualizing a procedure or finished haircut style.

enzyme (EN-zym)—catalysts that induce chemical changes in the body, such as breaking down complex food molecules to utilize extracted energy.

enzyme peels (EN-zym PEELZ)—also known as *keratolytic enzymes* or *protein-dissolving agents*; a type of chemical exfoliant that works by dissolving keratin protein in the surface cells of the skin.

EPA-registered disinfectant (EE-PEE-AYE REJ-ih-stired dis-in-FECT-ant)—a product that has been approved by the Environmental Protection Agency as an effective disinfectant against certain disease-producing organisms.

epicardium (ep-ih-KARD-ee-um)—a protective layer of the heart.

epicranial aponeurosis (ep-ih-KRAY-nee-al ap-uh-noo-ROH-sus)—also known as *galea aponeurotica*; a tough layer of dense fibrous tissue which covers the upper part of the cranium; and connects the occipitalis and frontalis muscles.

epicranium (ep-ih-KRAY-nee-um)—a broad band of muscles covering the cranium.

E

epicranius (ep-ih-KRAY-nee-us)—also known as *occipitofrontalis*; the broad muscle that covers the top of the skull and consists of the occipitalis and frontalis.

epidermal (ep-ih-DUR-mul)—pertaining to or arising from the outer layer of the skin.

epidermal-dermal junction (ep-ih-DUR-mul DUR-mul JUNK-shun)—the top of the papillary layer of the dermis where it joins the epidermis.

epidermal growth factor (EGF) (ep-ih-DUR-mul GROWTH FAK-tor)—a protein involved in the skin repair process.

epidermin (ep-ih-DUR-min)—a regenerating substance; an extract of animal tissues that has been used in the renewal of destroyed skin such as in wounds and burns.

epidermis (ep-uh-DUR-mis)—outermost and thinnest layer of the skin; it is made up of five layers: stratum corneum, stratum lucidum, stratum granulosum, stratum spinosum, and stratum germinativum.

epilate (EP-ih-layt)—to remove hair from below the skin surface; to uproot hair.

epilation (ep-uh-LAY-shun)—the removal of hair by the roots. Examples are waxing or tweezing.

epilator (eh-PIL-ayt-or)—substance used to remove hair by pulling it out of the follicle.

epilatory (eh-PIL-uh-toh-ree)—a device used to remove hair by pulling it out of the follicle.

epimysium (ep-i-MI-see-um)—layer of connective tissue that closely covers a skeletal muscle.

epinephrine (ep-ih-NEF-run)—a hormone and a neurotransmitter. It increases heart rate, constricts blood vessels, dilates air passages, and participates in the fight-or-flight response of the sympathetic nervous system. Used as an injection for the relief of some allergic reactions.

epiphysis (eh-PIF-uh-sis)—the enlarged area on the end of the long bones that articulates with other bones.

epithelial cell (ep-ih-THEE-lee-ul SEL)—one of various kinds of cells that form the epidermis; lines hollow organs such as the stomach and all passages.

epithelial tissue (ep-ih-THEE-lee-ul TISH-oo)—a protective covering on body surfaces, such as the skin, mucous membranes, lining of the heart, digestive and respiratory organs, and glands. It is capable of constant reproduction.

epithelioma (ep-ih-thee-lee-OH-muh)—an abnormal growth consisting of epithelial cells.

epithelium (ep-ih-THEE-lee-um)—a cellular tissue covering a free surface (internal and external) or lining a tube or cavity; it consists of cells joined by small amounts of cementing substances. Epithelial tissue is classified into types based on how many layers deep it is and the shape of the superficial cells.

eponychium (ep-oh-NIK-ee-um)—living skin at the base of the natural nail plate that covers the matrix area.

equation (ee-KWAY-zhun)—a method of expressing a chemical reaction by using chemical or mathematical formulas and symbols.

equilibrium (ee-kwoh-LIB-ree-um)—the state of balance between two or more forces acting within or on a body in such a way that stability is maintained.

equipment (ee-KWIP-ment)—supplies and tools required to perform a particular service.

equivalent (ee-KWIV-uh-lent)—a state of being or having equal values; equal in volume, area, or force.

erector (ih-REK-tur)—an elevating muscle.

erector pilae (ih-REK-tur PEE-lye)—minute muscles located at the base of each hair that contract when the skin becomes cold, causing the hair to stand erect; compression of skin glands. The muscle contractions are commonly known as *gooseflesh*, or *goose bumps*.

erector muscle (ih-REK-tur MUS-uhl)—a muscle that produces erection; for example, the erector pili, fanlike muscles attached to hair follicles, which contract, especially when cold, causing the hair to stand up.

ergonomics (UR-go-nom-icks)—the scientific discipline of designing the workplace as well as its equipment and tools to make specific body movements more comfortable, efficient, and safe.

erosion (ih-ROH-zhun)—the eating away of tissue.

eructation (ee-ruk-TAY-shun)—belching; that which is forced out.

eruption (ih-RUP-shun)—a visible lesion of the skin due to disease; marked by redness or papular condition, or both.

erysipelas (er-uh-SIP-uh-lus)—an acute infectious disease accompanied by a diffused inflammation of the skin and mucous membrane.

E

erythema (er-uh-THEE-muh)—a superficial blush or redness of the skin.

erythematous (er-uh-THEM-ut-us)—pertaining to or characterized by abnormal redness of the skin caused by a congestion of capillaries.

erythrasma (er-ih-THRAZ-muh)—eruption of reddish brown patches in the axillae and groin, especially due to the presence of a fungus.

erythrism (ER-uh-thrizm)—exceptional redness of the hair, beard, and skin.

erythrocyte (ih-RITH-ruh-syt)—a red blood cell; red corpuscle; carries oxygen from the lungs to body cells and carbon dioxide from cells back to the lungs.

eschar (ES-kar)—a dry crust of dead tissue or a scab caused by heat or a corrosive substance.

esophagus (eh-SOF-uh-gus)—the canal leading from the pharynx to the stomach.

essential fatty acid (ih-SEN-shul FAT-ee AS-ud)—any of the polyunsaturated fatty acids that are required in the diet, including linoleic, linolenic, and arachidonic acids.

essential oils (ih-SEN-shul OYLZ)—oils extracted using various forms of distillation from the seeds, bark, roots, leaves, wood, and/or resin of plants.

ester (ES-tur)—an organic compound formed by the reaction of an acid and an alcohol.

esthetic (es-THET-ik)—of or relating to beauty; describing beauty in art and nature; appreciation of beauty.

esthetician (es-thuh-TISH-un)—also known as *aesthetician*; a specialist in the cleaning, beautification, and preservation of the health of the skin on the entire body, including the face and neck.

esthetics (es-THET-iks)—also known as *aesthetics*; from the Greek word *aesthetikos* (meaning "perceptible to the senses"); a branch of anatomical science that deals with the overall health and well-being of the skin, the largest organ of the human body.

estrogen (ES-truh-jin)—any of various substances that influence estrus (the phase when a female is sexually receptive) or produce changes in the sexual characteristics of female mammals.

ethics (ETH-iks)—the moral principles by which we live and work.

ethmoid (ETH-moyd)—resembling a sieve; a bone forming part of the walls of the nasal cavity.

ethmoid bone (ETH-moyd BOHN)—a light, spongy bone between the eye sockets; forming part of the nasal cavity.

ethmonasal (eth-moh-NAY-zul)—pertaining to the ethmoid and nasal bones.

ethyl acetate (ETH-ul AS-uh-tayt)—a colorless liquid with a fruity odor that occurs in fruits and some berries; used as a solvent in nail polish and polish remover.

ethyl alcohol (ETH-ul AL-kuh-hawl)—the basis of some alcoholic beverages; used in cosmetic products such as astringents, antiseptics, and fragrances.

ethyl methacrylate (ETH-ul meth-AK-ry-layt)—a compound of ethyl alcohol and methacrylic acid used in the chemical formulation of many nail enhancements.

etiology (eet-ee-AHL-uh-jee)—the study of the causes of disease and their mode of operation.

eukeratin (yoo-KAIR-uh-tin)—a hard keratin found in hair, nails, feathers, hooves, horns, and the like.

eumelanin (yoo-MEL-uh-nin)—a type of melanin that is dark brown to black in color. People with dark-colored skin mostly produce eumelanin. There are two types of melanin; the other type is pheomelanin, which is red to yellow in color.

evaporate (ee-VAP-uh-rayt)—change from liquid to vapor form.

evascularization (eh-vas-kyoo-lar-ih-ZAY-shun)—the destruction of a vessel or a duct that conveys blood to a part of the body.

excitation (ek-sy-TAY-shun)—the act of stimulating or irritating.

excoriate (ek-SKOR-ee-ayt)—to wear away, scrape, or strip off the skin.

excoriation (ek-skor-ee-AY-shun)—skin sore or abrasion produced by scratching or scraping.

excrement (EKS-kruh-ment)—also known as *feces*; waste material expelled from the body.

excrescence (ik-SKRES-uns)—a disfiguring outgrowth.

excrete (eks-KREET)—to eliminate from the blood or tissue from the body as through the kidneys or sweat glands.

excretion (eks-KREE-shun)—that which is thrown off or eliminated from the body; a substance that is produced by some cells, but is of no further use to the body; the act or process of excreting.

excretory system (EKS-kruh-toh-ree SIS-tum)—group of organs including the kidneys, liver, skin, large intestine, and lungs, that are responsible for purifying the body by eliminating waste matter.

exfoliants (EKS-foh-LEE-entz)—mechanical and chemical products or processes used to exfoliate the skin.

exfoliating scrubs (eks-FOH-LEE-ate-ing SCRUBZ)—water-based lotions that contain a mild gritty-like abrasive and moisturizers to help in removing dry, flaky skin and reducing calluses.

exfoliation (eks-FOH-lee-AY-shun)—the removal of excess dead cells from the skin surface.

exfoliative dermatitis (eks-FOH-lee-ay-tiv dur-MUH-TY-tus)—any dermatitis where there is excessive hair loss and denudation of the skin.

exhalation (eks-huh-LAY-shun)—the act of breathing outward, expelling carbon dioxide from the lungs.

exhaustion (ek-ZAWS-chun)—loss of vital and nervous power from fatigue or protracted disease.

exocrine gland (EK-suh-krin GLAND)—also known as *duct glands*; produces a substance that travels through small tubelike ducts; sweat glands and oil glands of the skin belong to this group.

exothermic (ek-soh-THUR-mik)—characterized by or formed with the giving off of heat. In permanent waving, activation by heat created chemically within the product.

exothermic waves (ek-soh-THUR-mik WAYVZ)—permanent wave solutions that create an exothermic chemical reaction that heats up the waving solution and speeds up processing.

expansion (eks-PAN-shun)—distention, dilation, or swelling; the distance a completed sculptured form extends into space.

expel (eks-PEL)—to force out; to eject or dislodge; to remove a blackhead from a follicle.

expert (EKS-purt)—an experienced person; one who has special knowledge in a particular subject.

expertise (ek-spur-TEES)—knowledge or skill in a particular field.

expiration (ek-spih-RAY-shun)—the act of breathing out; expelling air from the lungs.

expire (ek-SPYR)—to breathe out air from the lungs; to exhale; to die.

exposure (eks-POH-zhoor)—state of being open to view or unprotected, as from the weather.

exposure incident (eks-POH-zhoor in-SI-dent)—contact with nonintact (broken) skin, blood, body fluid, or other potentially infectious materials that is the result of the performance of an employee's duties.

extend (ek-STEND)—to open or stretch more, or to full length.

extensibility (eks-ten-sih-BIL-ih-tee)—capable of being extended or stretched.

extensor (ik-STEN-sur)—muscle that straightens the wrist, hand, and fingers to form a straight line.

extensor carpi radialis (ik-STEN-sur KAR-pih ray-DEE-ay-lis)—a strong muscle in the wrist that operates with other muscles to bend the hand backward.

extensor digitorum brevis (ik-STEN-sur giji-TORE-ee-um brev-IS)—muscle of the foot that moves the toes and helps maintain balance while walking and standing.

extensor digitorum longus (ik-STEN-sur dij-ih-TOR-um LONG-us)—muscle that bends the foot up and extends the toes.

extensor hallucis longus (ik-STEN-surha-LU-sis LONG-us)—muscle that extends the big toe and flexes the foot.

extensors (ik-STEN-surz)—muscles that straighten the wrist, hand, and fingers to form a straight line.

external carotid arteries (eks-TUR-nul kuh-RAHT-ud ART-uh-rees)—supplies blood to the anterior (front) parts of the scalp, ear, face, neck, and sides of the head.

external jugular veins (eks-TUR-nul JUG-yuh-lur VAYNS)—the veins located on the sides of the neck that carry blood returning to the heart from the head, face, and neck.

external maxillary artery (eks-TUR-nul MAK-sah-lair-ee ART-uh-ree)—the artery that supplies blood to the nose, mouth, and the lower region of the face.

external respiration (eks-TUR-nul res-pih-RAY-shun)—the exchange of oxygen and carbon dioxide during normal respiration.

external vertebral plexus (eks-TUR-nul VURT-uh-brul PLEK-sus)—vein located anterior and posterior to the vertebral column.

E

externus (eks-TUR-nus)—external; pertaining to the outside.

exteroceptors (ek-STUH-ro-sep-tuhrs)—group of sensory nerves that record conscious sensations such as heat, cold, pain, and pressure throughout the body.

extracellular (eks-truh-SEL-yuh-lur)—outside of a cell or cells.

extraction (EKS-trakt-shun)—manual removal of impurities and comedones from follicles.

extraocular muscle (ek-struh-AI-IK-yah-lur MUS-uhl)—the six small voluntary muscles that control the movement of the eyeball within its orbit.

extreme (eks-TREEM)—to a very great or to the greatest degree; to the farthest point.

extremity (ek-STREM-ih-tee)—the distant end or part of any structure.

extrinsic factors (EKS-trinz-ik FAC-torz)—primarily environmental factors that contribute to aging and the appearance of aging.

exudation (eks-yoo-DAY-shun)—act of discharging sweat, moisture, or other liquid from a body through pores or incisions; oozing out.

exudative eczema (EK-suh-day-tiv EG-zuh-muh)—an acute form of dermatitis in which serum is exuded; also called "weeping eczema."

exude (EKS-ood, eks-OOD)—to discharge slowly from a body through pores or incisions such as sweat.

eye (EYE)—organs through which we see.

eye color (EYE KUL-ur)—the color of the iris of the eye; color in eye makeup products.

eye cream (EYE KREEM)—a cream or emollient formulated for the delicate skin around the eyes; some of the ingredients used in eye creams are beeswax, cholesterol, lanolin, sodium benzoate, boric acid, mineral oil, almond oil, ascorbyle palmitate, and lecithin.

eye cup (EYE KUP)—a small cup with a curved rim to fit the eye; used when washing or applying lotion or liquid to the eye.

eye makeup (EYE MEYK-up)—cosmetics created especially for the enhancement of brows, lashes, and eyelids.

eye makeup removers (EYE MEYK-uhp RE-moverz)—special preparations for removing eye makeup.

eye pads (EYE PADZ)—cotton pads shaped to fit over the eyelids during a facial treatment.

eye shadows (EYE shad-oh)—cosmetics applied on the eyelids to color, accentuate, or contour.

eye shadow primer (EYE shad-oh PRIH-mur)—a product applied beneath eye shadow to create a smooth application base and extend wearability.

eye tabbing (EYE tab-ing)—procedure in which individual synthetic eyelashes are attached directly to a client's own lashes at their base.

eyeball (EYE-bawl)—the ball-shaped part of the eye; the globe of the eye.

eyebrow (EYE-brow)—the bony ridge on which hair grows in an arch above the eye.

eyebrow arching (EYE-brow ARCH-ing)—the tweezing, trimming, or waxing of the brow hair to create a neat arched effect.

eyebrow brush (EYE-brow BRUSH)—a small, short-handled brush used to groom the eyebrows.

eyebrow comb (EYE-brow KOHM)—a small comb with a short handle used for grooming the eyebrows.

eyebrow pencil (EYE-brow PEN-sul)—also known as *eyebrow shadow*; pencil used to add color and shape to the eyebrows.

eyebrow tint (EYE-brow TINT)—a metallic salt dye formulated to be used in tinting eyebrows and eyelashes.

eyehole (EYE-hohl)—an opening for the eyes as in a gauze mask.

eyelash adhesive (EYE-lash ad-HEE-siv)—a product used to make artificial eyelashes adhere, or stick, to the natural lash line.

eyelash brush (EYE-lash BRUSH)—a small, long-handled brush with short bristles used to groom the eyelashes and to apply mascara.

eyelash comb (EYE-lash KOHM)—a small comb with a long handle designed to comb and curl the eyelashes.

eyelash curler (EYE-lash KUR-lur)—an implement designed to fit the curve of the eyelid so when lashes are pressed between two parts, they will be curled upward.

eyelash remover (EYE-lash ree-MOOV-ur)—a liquid used to remove artificial eyelashes by dissolving the adhesive that fastens the lashes to the natural lash line.

eyelash tint (EYE-lash TINT)—a metallic salt dye formulated to be used in dyeing eyelashes and eyebrows.

eyelashes (EYE-lash-iz)—the hair of the eyelids.

eyelashes, artificial (EYE-lash-iz, ar-tih-FISH-ul)—individual lash hair on a strip, applied with adhesive to the natural lash line.

eyelid (EYE-lid)—the movable fold of skin over the eye; the protective covering of the eyeball.

eyeliner (EYE-lyn-ur)—cosmetic used to outline and emphasize the eyes.

eyewash (EYE-wash)—a soothing lotion to alleviate fatigue and to cleanse the eyes.

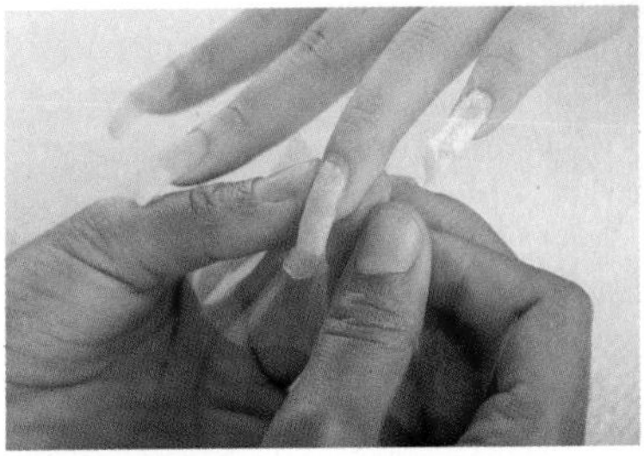
© Milady, a part of Cengage Learning. Photography by Dino Petrocelli.
fabric wrap

fabric wrap (FAB-rick rap)—nail wrap made of silk, linen, or fiberglass.

face framing (FAYS FRAYM-ing)—a frame formed by lightening (one or two shades) or by haircutting a narrow section of hair around the face.

face lift (FAYS LIFT)—also known as *rhytidectomy*; the removal of excess skin to correct sagging areas of the face.

face powder (FAYS POW-dur)—cosmetic powder, sometimes tinted and scented, that is used to add a matte or nonshiny finish to the face.

facial (FAY-shul)—pertaining to the face; also, the seventh cranial nerve, a sensory-motor nerve that controls the motion of the face, scalp, neck, ear, and sections of the palate and tongue; professional service designed to improve and rejuvenate the skin.

facial artery (FAY-shul ART-uh-ree)—also known as *external maxillary artery*; supplies blood to the lower region of the face, mouth, and nose.

facial bones (FAY-shul bonez)—two nasal bones; two lacrimal bones; two zygomatic or malar bones; two maxillae; the mandible; two turbinal bones; two palatine bones; and the vomer.

facial chair (FAY-shul CHAYR)—a reclining chair with a headrest.

facial cream (FAY-shul KREEM)—a product in cream form used during a facial treatment for specific purposes such as cleansing and hydrating.

facial hair (FAY-shul HAYR)—any hair on the face; whiskers, beard, mustache, eyebrows; superfluous facial hair, usually found on upper lip and between the eyebrows.

facial index (FAY-shul IN-deks)—a number that expresses the ratio of the breadth of the face to the length multiplied by 100.

facial machines (FAY-shul muh-SHEENZ)—specially constructed apparatus, appliances, and equipment used to give facial treatments.

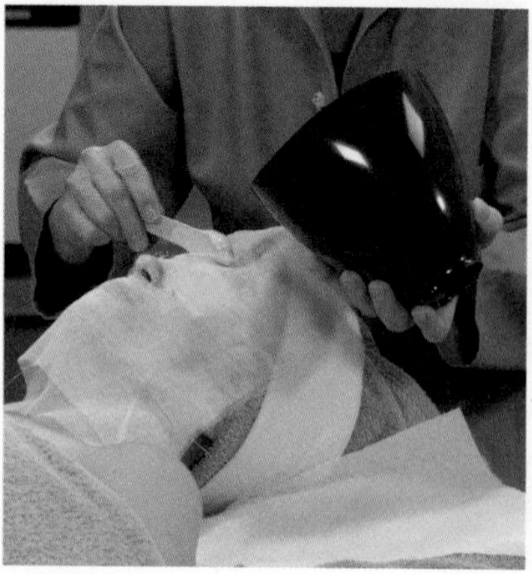

© Milady, a part of Cengage Learning. Photography by Larry Hamill.

facial mask

facial mask (FAY-shul MASK)—also known as *pack* or *masques*; concentrated treatment products often composed of herbs, vitamins, mineral clays, moisturizing agents, skin softeners, aromatherapy oils, beneficial extracts, and other beneficial ingredients to cleanse, exfoliate, tighten, tone, hydrate, and nourish and treat the skin.

facial massage (FAY-shul muh-SAHZH)—a series of movements designed to benefit the facial muscles, skin, and tissues; a procedure given by a trained esthetician to stimulate, tone, cleanse, and beautify the skin.

facial movements (FAY-shul MOOV-ments)—a massage procedure where certain manipulation and movements are used in facial treatments to benefit the skin.

facial nerve (FAY-shul NURV)—also known as the *seventh cranial nerve*; one of a pair that serves to activate the muscles that control facial expressions.

facial proportions (FAY-shul proh-POR-shunz)—the dimensional relationship of one facial feature to another, to be considered in makeup artistry and hairstyling.

facial skeleton (FAY-shul skell-uh-tin)—framework of the face composed of 14 bones.

facial steamer (FAY-shul STEEM-ur)—an apparatus used to apply steam at a comfortable temperature to the face during a facial treatment.

facial towel (FAY-shul TOW-ul)—a small towel, usually of white cotton terry cloth about 16 x 24 inches (40.64 cm x 60.96 cm); used to apply warm, moist steam to the face during a facial treatment or a shaving procedure.

facial treatment (FAY-shul TREET-munt)—a cosmetic treatment applied to the face and neck generally for preventive or corrective purposes, and for the general enhancement of skin and muscle tone.

facial veins (FAY-shul VAYNZ)—veins located on the anterior side of the head.

F

facioplasty (FAH-shee-oh-plas-tee)—plastic surgery of the face.

Fahrenheit (FAYR-un-hyt)—pertaining to the Fahrenheit thermometer or scale; water freezes at 32°F and boils at 212°F.

fallen hair (FAWL-en HAYR)—hair that has been shed from the head or gathered from a hairbrush, as opposed to hair that has been cut; the cuticles of the strands will move in different directions (opposite of turned or Remi hair).

fallopian tube (fu-LO-pee-an TOOB)—egg-carrying tube of the female reproductive system.

fall point (FAWL POYNT)—point at the crown of the head from which hair grows in a circular direction.

fan brush (FAN BRUSH)—flat brush where the bristles or hairs are spread out like a fan. This brush is most commonly used for blending and special effects.

fantail comb (FAN-tayl KOHM)—also known as *tail comb, rattail comb, sectioning comb*; a comb with a tapering tail used for sectioning and parting hair, and for use in wrapping and smoothing.

fantasy (FAN-tuh-see)—a type of hairpiece, makeup application, or nail enhancement that is intended only as a form of art and not for practical usage.

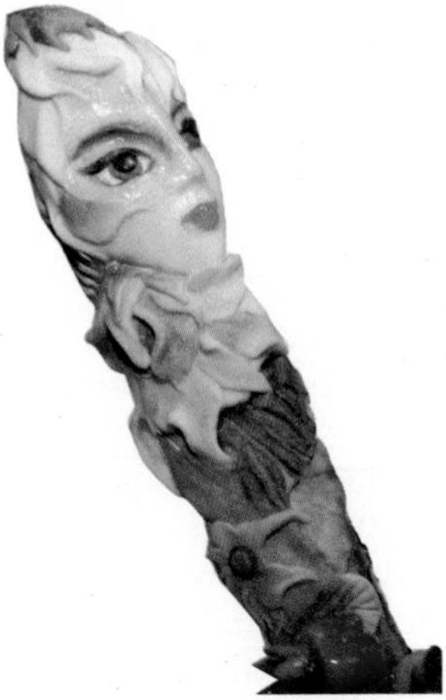

Courtesy of Catherine Wong, Ecsalonce.

fantasy art

fantasy art (FAN-tuh-see ART)—nail art category or competition where all art mediums are allowed and the only limitation is the imagination.

faradic current (fuh-RAD-ik KUR-unt)—alternating current that produces a mechanical reaction without chemical effect.

faradism (FAR-ah-diz-um)—a form of electrical treatment used for stimulating activity of the tissues.

fascia (FAYSH-ah)—a sheet of fibrous tissue that encloses bundles of muscles and separates their layers and groups.

fats (FATS)— also known as *lipids*; macronutrients used to produce energy in the body; the materials in the sebaceous glands that lubricate the skin.

fatty acid (FAT-ee AS-ud)—emollients; lubricant ingredients derived from plant oils or animal fats.

F

fatty alcohols (FAT-ee AL-kuh-hawlz)—emollients; fatty acids that have been exposed to hydrogen.

fatty esters (FAT-ee ES-terz)—emollients produced from fatty acids and alcohols.

favus (FAY-vus)—a contagious parasitic disease of the skin or scalp; chronic ringworm, characterized by dry, sulfur-yellow, cuplike crusts called scutula.

feather stroking (FEH-thur STROK-ing)—massage movement using very light pressure of the fingertips or hands with long, flowing strokes.

feathering (FEH-thur-ing)—also known as *tapering*; shortening the hair in a graduated effect.

female reproductive system (FE-mail ree-pro-DUK-tiv SIS-tum)—functions to produce the ovum and female hormones, to receive the sperm during the sex act, and to carry the fetus during pregnancy.

feminine (FEM-uh-nin)—pertaining to the female sex; womanly.

femur (FEE-mur)—heavy, long bone that forms the leg above the knee.

ferrous sulfate (FAIR-us SUL-fayt)—a salt of sulfuric acid derived from iron.

ferrule (FAIR-uhl)—the metal band around the brush that helps to hold the bristles in place.

fertilization (fur-tih-lih-ZAY-shun)—the union of the male and female reproductive cells.

fester (FES-tur)—to develop inflammation and pus.

fetid (FET-ud)—having a foul smell.

fetus (FEE-tus)—the developing child from the third month of pregnancy until birth.

fever blister (FEE-vur BLIS-tur)—also known as *cold sore*; herpes simplex; a recurring viral infection presenting as vesicles with red, swollen, inflamed bases.

fiber (FY-bur)—a slender, thread-like structure that combines with others to form animal or vegetable tissue.

F

fiberglass (FYB-bur-glas)—a thin synthetic mesh with a loose weave, used as a nail enhancement wrap.

fibroblasts (fy-BROH-blasts)—the most common type of cell found in connective tissue. Fibroblasts secrete collagen proteins that are used to maintain a structural framework for many tissues. They also play an important role in healing wounds.

fibrocartilage (fy-broh-KART-ul-ij)—cartilage found between tendons or ligaments or bones.

fibroma (fy-BROH-muh)—a tumor composed mainly of fibrous or fully developed connective tissue.

fibromyalgia (fy-broh-my-ALG-uh)—a medical disorder characterized by chronic widespread pain and pain from stimuli which are not normally painful such as a heightened and painful response to pressure.

fibrosis (fy-BROH-sus)—the formation of fibrous tissue.

fibrous connective tissue (FY-brus kuh-NEK-tiv TISH-oo)—composed of collagen and elastic fibers, closely arranged, forming tendons and ligaments.

fibrous joints (FY-brus JOYNTS)—held together by fibrous connective tissue.

fibula (FIB-yuh-luh)—smaller of the two bones that form the leg below the knee. The fibula may be visualized as a bump on the little-toe side of the ankle.

fifth cranial nerve (FIFTH KRAY-nee-ul NURV)—also known as *trifacial* or *trigeminal nerve*; it is the chief sensory nerve of the face, and it serves as the motor nerve of the muscles that control chewing. It consists of three branches.

filament (FIL-uh-ment)—a thread-like structure.

file (FYL)—a hardened steel instrument with cutting ridges for the removal of portions of anything; nail file: used to remove portions of the free edge of the nail.

filler (FIL-ur)—a dual-purpose haircoloring product that is able to create a color base and to equalize porosity. Any liquid-like substance to help fill a void.

fill-in curl (FIL-in KURL)—a pin curl used between roller shapings for continuous style.

film (FILM)—a membranous covering causing opacity; thin skin.

filterable virus (FIL-tuh-ruh-bal VY-rus)—living organisms so small they can pass through the pores of a porcelain filter; causes the common cold, and other respiratory and gastrointestinal infections.

filtration (fil-TRAY-shun)—process in which blood pressure pushes fluids and substances through the capillary wall into the tissue spaces.

Finasteride (fin-ASTER-eyed)—also known as *Propecia®*; an oral medication prescribed for men only to stimulate hair growth.

fine-grit abrasives (FYN GRIT uh-BRAS-ives)—240-grit and higher abrasives designed for buffing, polishing, and removing very fine scratches from the natural nail or nail enhancement.

fine hair (FYN HAYR)—a hair fiber that is relatively small in diameter or circumference.

finger bowl (FING-gur BOHL)—a small bowl used to hold water for soaking the fingers during a manicure procedure; a small bowl used to cleanse the fingers following the serving of food.

finger breadth (FING-gur BREDTH)—the width of a finger, about three-quarters to one inch.

finger curls (FING-gur KURLZ)—elongated, spiral wound curls resembling the fingers; long curls.

finger dexterity (FING-gur deks-TAIR-ih-tee)—skill and ease in using the fingers.

finger shield (FING-gur SHEELD)—a small metal cap worn to protect the finger.

finger test (FING-gur TEST)—also known as *porosity test*; a test given to determine the degree of porosity in the hair. Strands of hair are held away from the head by one hand, while the fingers of the other hand slide down the hair shaft and feel the texture of the strand. Smooth texture indicates low porosity; rough texture indicates high porosity.

finger wave comb (FING-gur WAYV KOHM)—a small tapered comb used to sculpture finger waves in the hair.

finger waving (FING-gur WAYV-ing)—process of shaping and directing the hair into an S pattern through the use of the fingers, combs, and waving lotion.

fingernail (FING-gur-nayl)—the horny protective substance (hard keratin) on the upper surface of the fingers and thumb; the nail.

fingernail brush (FING-gur-nayl BRUSH)—a small brush with semi-hard bristles; used to cleanse the fingers and nails during the manicure procedure.

F

fingernail buffer (FING-gur-nayl BUF-ur)—a padded implement used for polishing the nails without nail enamel; used to stimulate blood flow to the nail bed.

fingernail composition (FING-gur-nayl kahm-poh-ZIH-shun)—the material that composes the nail, mainly keratin, a protein substance that forms the base of all horny tissue.

fingernail file (FING-gur-nayl FYL)—a steel instrument with fine filing edges designed for filing and shaping the fingernails; an emery board with sandpaper surfaces; used to smooth and shape the nails.

fingernail polish (FING-gur-nayl PAHL-ish)—a clear or colored enamel used to beautify and protect the nails.

fingernail polish remover (FING-gur-nayl PAHL-ish ree-MOOV-ur)—a product containing acetone, usually formulated with some water, lanolin fragrance, and coloring agents; used to remove nail enamel.

fingernail repair (FING-gur-nayl ree-PAYR)—the art of restoring and mending damaged nails by replacing the natural nail with a nail extension or nail enhancement.

fingernail sculpturing (FING-gur-nayl SKULP-chur-ing)—a technique that uses a product to build and form realistic nail enhancements.

fingernail shapes (FING-gur-nayl SHAYPS)—the general classification of nail shapes such as square, rounded, oval, and pointed.

fingers-and-shear (FING-ers and SHEER)—technique used to cut hair by holding the hair into a position to be cut.

fingertip (FING-gur-tip)—the extreme end of a finger.

finishing knot (FIN-ish-ing NAHT)—the technique used in securing the final strand of hair, on a wig or hairpiece, to make certain that the hair does not come loose.

finishing rinse (FIN-ish-ing RINS)—a conditioning rinse used as the final step of a shampoo or chemical service to close the cuticle and normalize the pH of the hair.

first-degree burn (FIRST-duh-GREE BURN)—a mild burn characterized by some pain and reddening of the skin; less severe than a second- or third-degree burn.

first-time-over shave (FIRST-tyme-OVER-shayv)—first part of the standard shave consisting of shaving areas of the face; followed by the second-time-over shave to remove residual missed or rough spots.

fishhook (FISH-hook)—a flaw in the curling of hair that results in the tip of the hair bending in a direction opposite to that of the rest of the curl.

fishtail braid (FISH-tayl BRAID)—simple two-strand braid in which hair is picked up from the sides and added to the strands as they are crossed over each other.

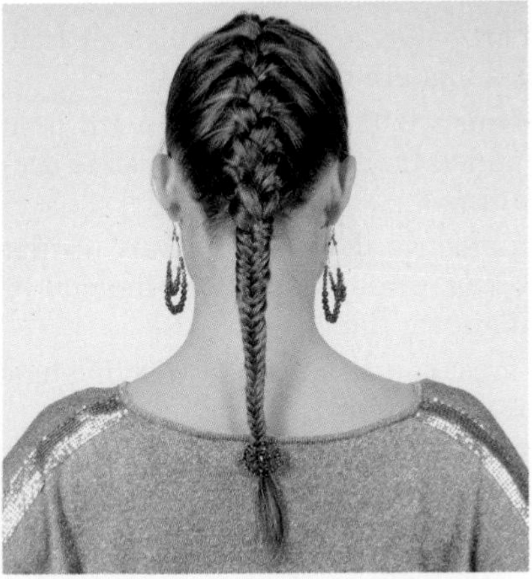

© Milady, a part of Cengage Learning. Photography by Yanik Chauvin.

fishtail braid

F

fission (FISH-un)—reproduction of bacteria by cellular division; the splitting of an atomic nucleus.

fissure (FISH-ur)—a crack in the skin that penetrates the dermis. Examples are severely cracked and/or chapped hands or lips.

Fitzpatrick scale (FITS-pat-rick scayl)—scale used to measure the skin type's ability to tolerate sun exposure.

fixative (FIK-suh-tiv)—a hairstyling product used to keep hair in place; in cold waving, an agent that stops the chemical action of the cold waving solution and sets or hardens the hair by reforming most of the disulfide bonds; a chemical agent capable of stopping the processing of the chemical hair relaxer and hardening the hair in its new form.

fixed costs (fixed COSTS)—operating costs that are constant, for example, rent and loan payments.

flagella (fluh-JEL-uh) (singular: flagellum)—also known as *cilia*; slender, hairlike extensions used by bacilli and spirilla for locomotion (moving about).

flake (FLAYK)—a small particle of a substance; to scale or chip as shedding of the skin in a dandruff condition; sloughing off of the epidermis due to dryness.

flammable (FLAM-uh-bul)—capable of being easily ignited and burning with great rapidity.

flap surgery (flap SIR-jer-ee)—a surgical technique that involves the removal of a bald scalp area and the attachment of a flap of hair-bearing skin.

flare curl (FLAYR KURL)—a pin curl that is rolled and placed so that it stands slightly away from the scalp; semi-standup curl.

flash cure (FLASH cyoor)—placing wet UV gel product under the UV light for five to ten seconds.

flat art (FLAT ART)—a nail art category that includes all free-hand painting techniques that are flat, not raised.

flat brush (FLAT brush)—a brush with a square tip with long bristles, which gives it added flexibility. This brush is useful for blending and shading.

F

flat iron (FLAT EYE-urn)—a electric device that heats up flat metal plates and, once run through the hair, flattens or smoothes hair making it appear flat.

flat weft (FLAT WEFT)—the most common type of weaving hair on silks; woven on three silks.

flattop hairstyle (FLAT-top HAYR-styl)—a hairstyle for men in which the hair is cut short on top so that the ends create a horizontal line.

flex (FLEKS)—to bend, especially repeatedly; as to exercise a muscle.

flexible (FLEK-sih-bul)—capable of being bent; pliable; not stiff; able to adjust to change.

flexor (FLEK-sur)—extensor muscles of the wrist involved in flexing the wrist.

flexor carpi ulnaris (FLEK-sur KAR-pih ul-NAIR-is)—the extensor muscles of the wrist, which are involved in bending the hand backward.

flexor digiti minimi (FLEK-sur di-JEE-tee min-EH-me)—muscle that moves the little toe.

flexor digitorum brevis (FLEK-sur di-jee-TORE-ee-uhm BREV-us)—muscle that moves the toes and helps maintain balance while walking and standing.

florid (FLOR-id)—flushed; tinged with red; ruddy.

fluctuate (FLUK-choo-ayt)—to shift back and forth; to move like a wave.

fluid movement (FLOO-id MOOV-ment)—the appearance of a finished hairstyle achieved from a predetermined change of direction in the setting pattern.

fluidity (floo-ID-uh-tee)—the state of being fluid; the physical property of a substance that enables it to flow; the ability of the hair to flow and move easily.

fluorescent (flur-ES-ent)—an ability to emit light after exposure to light; the wavelength of the emitted light being longer than that of the light absorbed.

flush (FLUSH)—to become red in the face due to emotion, fever, or a skin condition that causes blood to rush to the undersurface of the skin; to blush.

flute (FLOOT)—in nail technology, long, slender cut or groove found on carbide bits.

flyaway (FLY-uh-way)—of or pertaining to an excessive electrostatic condition of hair that causes individual strands to repel one another and stand away from the head.

foam (FOHM)—also known as *mousse*; a light, airy, whipped styling product that resembles shaving foam and builds moderate body and volume into the hair.

foaming cleansers (FOHM-ing KLEN-surz)—cleansers containing surfactants (detergents) which cause the product to foam and rinse off easily.

foil (FOYL)—a very thin sheet of metal used in coloring and highlighting techniques when hair is sliced or weaved out in thin sections or strands.

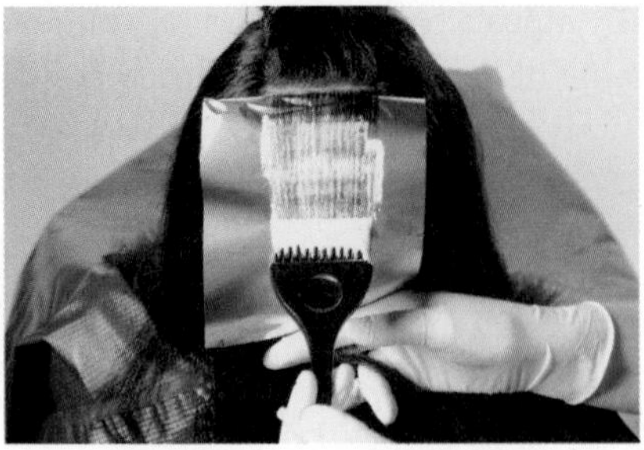

© Milady, a part of Cengage Learning. Photography by Yanik Chauvin.

foil technique

foil technique (FOYL tek-NEEK)—highlighting technique that involves coloring selected strands of hair by slicing or weaving out sections, placing them on foil or plastic wrap, applying lightener or permanent haircolor, and then sealing them in the foil or plastic wrap.

folic acid (FOH-lik AS-ud)—vitamin B complex, found in green, leafy vegetables and some animal products.

follicle (FAWL-ih-kul)—hair follicles and sebaceous follicles are tube-like openings in the epidermis.

follicular (fah-LIK-yuh-lar)—affecting or arising from the follicles.

folliculitis (fah-lik-yuh-LY-tis)—also known as *folliculitis barbae, sycosis barbae,* or *barber's itch.* Inflammation of the hair follicles caused by a bacterial infection from ingrown hairs. The cause is typically from ingrown hairs from shaving or other epilation methods. Folliculitis is generally classified as both infectious and non-infectious depending on the cause of the inflammation.

folliculosis (fah-lik-yuh-LOH-sis)—the presence of an excessive number of lymph follicles.

fomentation (foh-men-TAY-shun)—application of warm moisture in treating a disease.

Food and Drug Administration (FDA) (FOOD AND DRUG ad-mi-nih-STRAY-shun)—an agency of the United States government responsible for ensuring that cosmetics, drugs, and foods are safe, correctly packaged, and truthfully labeled.

foot file (FOOT FEYE-uhl)—also known as *paddle*; large, abrasive file used to smooth and reduce thicker areas of callus.

F

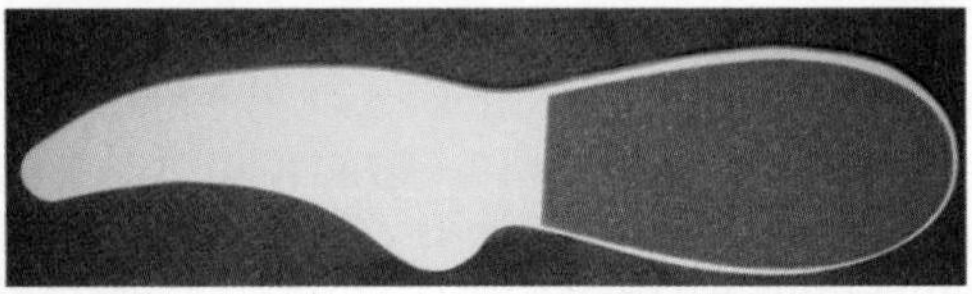

© Milady, a part of Cengage Learning. Photography by Dino Petrocelli.

foot file

foot reflexology (FOOT reflex-OL-oo-jee)—technique of applying pressure to the feet based on a system of zones and areas on the feet that directly correspond to the anatomy of the body. Reflexology is also performed on the hands and ears.

foot soaks (FOOT SOHKS)—products containing gentle soaps, moisturizers, and other additives that are used in a pedicure bath to cleanse and soften the skin.

footrest (FOOT-rest)—a small stool or platform on which to place the feet; the extension of the service chair used in a salon on which the client may place his or her feet.

foramen (fuh-RAY-mun)—a passage or opening through a bone or membrane.

foreign matter (FOR-un MAT-ur)—undesirable substance or particles from outside the body found on or in the skin, hair, nails, or body, occurring where they are not normally found.

forelock (FOR-lok)—a small section of hair growing over the forehead.

forged (FORJed)—process of working metal to a finished shape by hammering or pressing.

form (FORM)—the mass or general outline of a hairstyle. It is three-dimensional and has length, width, and depth.

formaldehyde (for-MAL-duh-hyd)—a pungent gas manufactured by an oxidation process of methyl alcohol, powerful disinfectant; used as a preservative in soap, cosmetics, nail hardeners, and polishes. Suspected cancer-causing agent. Prolonged exposure can cause symptoms similar to chronic bronchitis or asthma.

formalin (FOR-muh-lin)—a 37% to 40% disinfectant solution of formaldehyde in water.

formation (for-MAY-shun)—the manner in which a thing is formed or shaped.

formula (FOR-myuh-luh)—a prescribed method or rule; a recipe or prescription mixture of two or more ingredients; abbreviation for a chemical compound containing the elements used and their proportions.

formulate (FOR-myoo-layt)—to put into a systematized statement or expression; the art of mixing to create a blend or balance of two or more ingredients.

forward curls (FOR-word KURLZ)—curls directed toward the face; curls wound in a clockwise direction on the left side of the head and counterclockwise on the right side of the head.

forward wave (FOR-word WAYV)—a wave shaped toward the face.

fortified (FOUR-ti-fiyd)—indicating that a vitamin has been added to a food product.

fossa (FAHS-uh); pl., fossae (FAHS-ee)—a depression, furrow, or sinus below the level of the surface of a part.

foundation (fown-DAY-shun)—also known as *base makeup*; a tinted cosmetic used to cover or even out the coloring of the skin.

foundation cream (fown-DAY-shun KREEM)—a cream sometimes used in place of a colored makeup base or as a protective film applied before the makeup base and/or powder.

four corners (FOR COR-nerz)—points on the head that signal a change in the shape of the head, from flat to round or vice versa.

fracture (FRAK-chur)—the breaking or cracking of a bone or cartilage.

fragile hair (FRAJ-il HAYR)—hair that is lacking in normal flexibility, tensile strength, and resilience; is usually brittle and easily broken.

fragilitas (fruh-JIL-ih-tus)—brittleness.

fragilitas crinium (fruh-JIL-ih-tus KRY-nee-um)—technical term for brittle hair.

frail (FRAYL)—easily broken or damaged; delicate.

frame (FRAYM)—in hairstyling, hair arranged to create a pleasing outline for the face.

franchise (FRAN-chyz)—a right granted to an individual or group to market a company's goods or services within a certain territory or location.

franchised salon or spa (FRAN-chyz-ed salon or spah)—a salon or spa owned by an individual(s) who pays a certain fee to use the company name and is part of a larger organization or chain of salons. The franchise operates according to a specified business plan and set protocols.

frayed (FRAYD)—worn away by friction or use, especially an edge of cloth.

freckle (FREK-ul)—also known as *freckle*; a small yellow- to brown-colored spots on skin exposed to sunlight and air.

F

free amino-acids (FREE uh-MEE-no A-suds)—located between the chains of keratin in the cortex, holding the moisture within the cortex at a desirable level.

free edge (FREE EJ)—part of the nail plate that extends over the tip of the finger or toe.

free radicals (FREE RAD-ih-culs)—unstable molecules that can cause inflammation and disease, especially wrinkling and sagging of the skin.

free styling (FREE STYL-ing)—a technique using the fingers of one hand with a hand-held dryer in the other; to direct and style the hair.

free-form haircoloring technique (FREE form hayr-CULUR-ing tek-NEEK)—also known as *baliage*; the painting of a lightener on clean, styled hair.

free-hand (FREE-HAND)—a hand position and kind of stroke used when shaving the face.

free-hand clipper cutting (FREE-hand CLIP-uhr CUT-ing)—generally interpreted to mean that guards are not used in the cutting process.

free-hand notching (FREE-hand NOCH-ing)—haircutting technique in which pieces of hair are snipped out at random intervals.

free-hand shear cutting (FREE-hand SHEER CUT-ing)—cutting with shears without the use of fingers or a comb to control the hair.

free-hand slicing (FREE-hand sly-SING)—technique used to release weight from the subsection, allowing the hair to move more freely.

French braiding (FRENCH BRAYD-ing)—also known as *invisible braid*, or *inverted braid*; a technique using strands of hair interlaced close to the head to form a pattern.

French knot (FRENCH NAHT)—also known as *classic knot, chignon*; in hairstyling, a hairstyle where the hair is smoothed off the face and gathered into a twisted roll at the nape of the neck.

French lacing (FRENCH LAYS-ing)—also known as *teasing, backcombing, backbrushing*; the technique of combing small sections of hair from the ends toward the scalp, causing it to form a cushion on which the hair is combed into the desired style.

French manicure (FRENCH MAN-eh-cyoor)—nail art technique where the nail bed is one color, usually pink, peach, or beige (depending upon the client's skin tone), and the free edge of the nail is another color, usually white.

French twist (FRENCH TWIST)—in hairdressing, a vertical seam-like arrangement at the back of the head. In nail technology, a competition where you may use pink, white, clear, and glittered products to produce a unique twist on the French manicure look.

frequency (FREE-kwen-see)—the number of complete cycles per second of current produced by an alternating current generator; standard frequencies are 25 and 60 cycles per second.

freshener (FRESH-un-ur)—also known as *skin-freshening lotion*; skin-freshening lotions with a low alcohol content.

friction (FRIK-shun)—deep rubbing movement requiring pressure on the skin with the fingers or palm while moving them under a underlying structure. Chucking, rolling, and wringing are variations of friction. Created using fingers or palms while moving them over an underlying structure.

fringe (FRINJ)—hair that partially or completely covers the facial area near the hairline; a small hairpiece.

frizzy (FRIZ-ee)—hair formed into small, tight curls or narrow waves.

frontal (FRUNT-ul)—in front; relating to the forehead; the bone of the forehead.

frontal artery (FRUNT-ul ART-uh-ree)—supplies blood to the forehead and upper eyelids.

frontal bone (FRUNT-ul BOHN)—bone that forms the forehead.

frontal nerve (FRUNT-ul NURV)—a somatic sensory nerve that innervates the skin of the upper eyelids, the forehead, and the scalp.

frontal vein (FRUNT-ul VAYN)—the diploic vein (veins located between the bony tissue between the external and internal layers of the skull) of the cranial bones.

frontalis (frun-TAY-lus)—front (anterior) portion of the epicranius; muscle of the scalp that raises the eyebrows, draws the scalp forward, and causes wrinkles across the forehead.

frostbite (FRAWST-byt)— localized damage is caused to skin and other tissues due to extreme cold. Frostbite is most likely to happen in body parts farthest from the heart and those with large exposed areas.

F

frosting (FRAWST-ing)—also known as *highlighting*, *streaking*, or *low-lighting*; to lighten or darken small selected strands of hair over the entire head to blend with the rest of the hair.

frosting cap (FRAWST-ing KAP)—a plastic cap-like head covering with small holes through which strands of hair are pulled to the surface to be tinted, lightened, or darkened as desired.

fulcrum finger (FULL-crum fing-UHR)—also known as *balance point*; balancing the tip of one pinky finger with the tip of the pinky finger on the other hand as you work.

full-base curls (FUL BAYS CURLZ)—thermal curls that sit in the center of their base; strong curls with full volume.

full head bonding (FUL head BAHND-ing)—the process of attaching a hair replacement system to all areas of the head with an adhesive bonding agent.

full stem (FUL STEM)—a curl or curling device such as a roller that is rolled up to the base part.

full stem curl (FUL STEM KURL)—curl placed completely off the base; allows for the greatest mobility.

full twist (FUL TWIST)—a ropelike winding of the hair on the rod in spiral permanent waving.

fulling (FUL-ing)—form of pétrissage in which the tissue is grasped, gently lifted, and spread out; used mainly for massaging the arms.

fumigant (FYOO-mih-gant)—a gaseous substance capable of destroying pathogenic bacteria.

fumigate (FYOO-mih-gayt)—disinfect by the action of smoke or fumes.

function (FUNK-shun)—the normal or special action for which a part is especially suited or used.

functional ingredients (FUNBK-shun-al in-GREED-ee-antz)—ingredients in cosmetic products that allow the products to spread, give them body and texture, and give them a specific form such as a lotion, cream, or gel.

fundus (FUN-dus)—the bottom or lowest part of a sac or hollow organ.

fungicidal (FUN-gih-side-uhl)—capable of destroying fungi.

fungus (FUN-gus), pl. fungi (FUN-ji)—microscopic plant parasites, which include molds, mildews, and yeasts; can produce contagious diseases such as ringworm and that live on dead or decaying things.

furrow (FUR-oh)—corrugation (lengthwise or across) in nails; a groove; wrinkle.

furuncle (FYOO-rung-kul)—also known as *boil*; acute, localized bacterial infection of the hair follicle that produces constant pain.

fuse (FYOOZ)—device that prevents excessive current from passing through a circuit.

fusion (FYOO-zhun)—the act of uniting, blending, or melting together; something formed by fusing.

fusion bonding (FYOO-zhun BAHND-ing)—method of attaching extensions in which extension hair is bonded to the client's own hair with a bonding material that is activated by heat from a special tool.

fuzz (FUZ)—fine, lightweight hair.

G

galea aponeurotica (GAY-lee-uh ap-uh-noo-RAHT-ih-kuh)—the intermediate tendon joining the frontal and occipital muscles in the scalp.

galvanic current (gal-VAN-ik KUR-unt)—a constant and direct current having a positive and negative pole that produces chemical changes when it passes through the tissues and fluids of the body; named for Galvani (1737–1798).

galvanic machine (gal-VAN-ik muh-SHEEN)—an apparatus with attachments designed to produce galvanic current; used primarily to introduce water-soluble products into the skin during a facial treatment.

galvanism (GAL-vuh-niz-um)—a constant current of electricity, the action of which is chemical.

game plan (GAYM PLAN)—the conscious act of planning your life, instead of just letting things happen.

gamete (GA-meet)—reproductive cell that can unite with another gamete to form the cell that develops into a new individual.

gamma globulin (GAM-uh GLAHB-yuh-lin)—a globulin in the blood plasma that contains antibodies effective against pathogenic microorganisms.

gamma rays (GAM-uh RAYZ)—powerful electromagnetic radiation having a frequency greater than X-rays.

ganglion (GANG-glee-un); pl., **ganglia** (GANG-glee-ah)—subcutaneous tumors; bundles of nerve cells in the brain, in organs of special sense of forming units of the sympathetic nervous system.

gangrene (gang-GREEN)—the death of tissue due to lack of blood supply, allowing bacteria to proliferate. The primary cause of gangrene is reduced blood supply to the affected tissues, which results in cell death.

gas (GAS)—matter without a definite shape or size; no fixed volume or shape; takes the shape of its container.

gastric juice (GAS-trik JOOS)—the digestive fluid secreted by the glands of the stomach.

gastrocnemius (gas-trok-NEEM-e-us)—muscle attached to the lower rear surface of the heel and pulls the foot down.

gastrointestinal (gas-troh-in-TES-tun-ul)—pertaining to the stomach and intestines.

gauge (GAYJ)—to estimate; appraise; judge.

gauze (GAWZ)—a thin, open-meshed cloth used for dressings and for facial masks in some types of facial treatments.

gauze mask (GAWZ MASK)—a mask made by cutting a piece of thin, open mesh cloth (cheesecloth) to fit over the client's face and neck; the material is moistened with warm water, applied to the face, and then mask ingredients or other thin substances are applied over the cloth. The purpose of the gauze is to keep the mask from running or crumbling.

gel (JEL)—a substance comprised of a solid and a liquid that exists as a solid or semisolid mass (jelly-like); a thickened styling preparation that comes in a tube or bottle and creates a strong hold.

gene (JEEN)—a unit of heredity in a living organism. It normally resides on a stretch of DNA that codes for a type of protein or for an RNA chain that has a function in the organism.

general circulation (JEN-ur-ul sir-kyoo-LAY-shun)—also known as *systemic circulation*; blood circulation from the left side of the heart throughout the body and back to the heart.

general infection (JEN-ur-ul in-FEK-shun)—when bacteria enters the bloodstream and is carried throughout an infection results in all parts of the body.

generic product (juh-NAIR-ik PRAHD-ukt)—a product, especially a drug, not protected by a trademark and not registered.

genetics (juh-NET-iks)—the science that deals with the heredity and variation of organisms.

genitalia (jen-uh-TAY-li-ya)—the organs of the reproductive system, especially the external organs.

geriatrics (jeer-ee-AH-triks)—the branch of medicine that deals with the physical and psychological changes that affect humans during the aging process.

germ (JURM)—a minute, one-celled vegetable microorganism that causes disease; a microbe; a bacillus; an embryo in its early stages.

germ layer (JURM LAY-ur)—any of three primary layers of cells from which the various organs of most embryos develop by further differentiation.

germicidal (jer-muh-SYD-ul)—destructive to germs.

germicide (JER-muh-syd)—a solution that destroys germs.

germination (jer-muh-NAY-shun)—the formation of an embryo from an impregnated ovum; the first act of growth in a germ, seed, or bud.

germinative (JER-muh-na-tiv)—having the power to grow or develop.

germinative layer (JER-muh-na-tiv LAY-ur)—also known as *stratum germinativum* or *basal layer*; the deepest layer of the epidermis from which new tissue is constantly formed.

glabrous (GLAY-brus)—smooth; without hair.

gland (GLAND)—specialized organs that remove certain elements from the blood to convert them into new compounds.

glandular (GLAN-juh-lur)—pertaining to a gland.

glaze (GLAYZ)—a nonammonia color that adds shine and tone to the hair.

gliding (GLYD-ing)—moving the hand over some portion of the client's body with varying amounts of pressure.

globule (GLAHB-yool)—a small, spherical droplet of fluid or semifluid material.

glomus tumor (GLOH-mus TOO-mur)—a tumor affecting the digits; usually painful, bluish, and benign.

glossal (GLAWS-ul)—pertaining to the tongue.

glossing (GLAWS-ing)—also known as *glazing*; a technique in haircoloring designed to add shine to the hair.

glossopharyngeal (glahs-oh-fa-rehn-JEE-ul)—also known as *ninth cranial nerve*; pertaining to the pharynx and tongue; controls the sense of taste.

glucose (GLOO-kohs)—a monosaccharide (dextrose) found in fruit and other foods, and in the blood; the chief source of energy for living organisms.

glutamate (GLOOT-uh-mayt)—a salt or ester of glutamic acid used to enhance the flavor of foods; used as an antioxidant in cosmetics to prevent spoilage.

glutamic acid (gloo-TAM-ik AS-ud)—an amino acid from vegetable or grain protein; used in cosmetics as an antioxidant and as a softener in permanent wave solutions.

gluteus muscle (GLOOT-ee-us MUS-uhl)—any of three muscles of the buttocks.

glycation (GLIE-kay-shun)—caused by an elevation in blood sugar, glycation is the binding of a protein molecule to a glucose molecule resulting in the formation of damaged, nonfunctioning structures, known as *advanced glycation end products* (AGES). Glycation alters protein structures and decreases biological activity.

glycerin (GLIS-ur-in)—sweet, colorless, slippery substance used as a solvent and as a moisturizer in skin and body creams.

glycerol monothioglycolate (GMTG) (GLIS-ur-awl mon-oh-thy-oh-GLY-co-layt)—main active ingredient in true acid and acid-balanced waving lotions.

glycine (GLY-seen)—amino acetic acid.

glycolic acid (gly-KAHL-ik AS-ud)—the strongest alpha hydroxy acid (AHA) and is derived from sugar cane. One of many acids are used in different percentages and pH factors to dissolve the desmosomes between cells to keep skin cells exfoliated.

glycoproteins (GLY-co-pro-teenz)—skin-conditioning agents derived from carbohydrates and proteins that enhance cellular metabolism and wound healing.

glycosaminoglycans (gly-kose-ah-mee-no-GLY-cans)—a water-binding substance between the fibers of the dermis.

goal setting (GOHL SET-ing)—the identification of long-term and short-term goals that helps you decide what you want out of life.

goals (GOHLZ)—a set of benchmarks that, once achieved, help you to realize your mission and your vision.

gold bands (GOHLD BANDZ)—uneven effect and brassy areas occurring in some hair-lightening procedures.

golgi tendon organ (GTO) (GOHL-jee TEN-dun OHR-gun)—multi branched sensory nerve ending embedded among the fibers of a tendon.

gommages (goh-MAJ-ez)—also known as *roll-off masks*; exfoliating creams that are rubbed off of the skin.

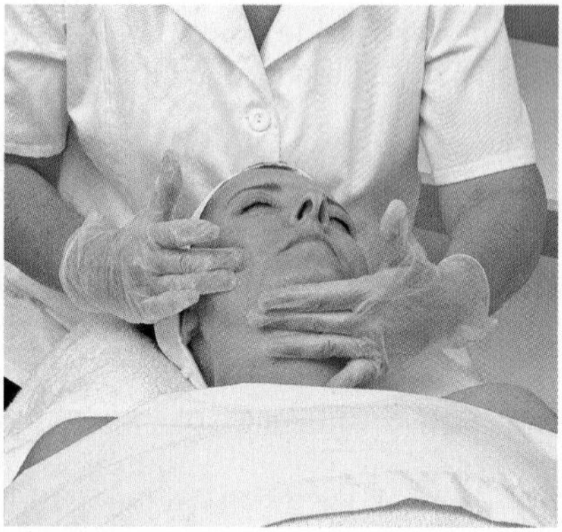

© Milady, a part of Cengage Learning. Photography by Rob Werfel.

gommages

G

gonads **(GOH-nadz)**—primary sex glands that produce reproductive cells; ovaries and testes.

gonorrhea **(gahn-uh-REE-uh)**—a contagious sexually transmitted disease caused by the presence of the gonococci bacteria in the genital tract, characterized by discharge and burning sensation when urinating.

grab **(GRAB)**—to react very rapidly to some stimulus; in haircoloring, pertaining to color that takes quickly.

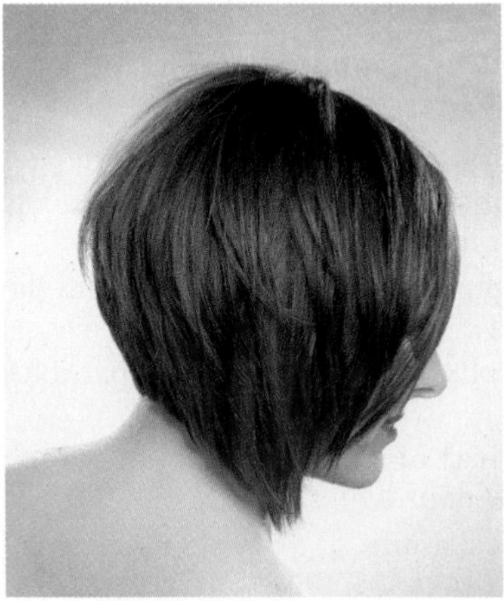

Photography by Tom Carson. Hair by Antonio Morosi, hairstylist for Above and Beyond Salon, Vermillion, Ohio, Laura Hall, color, for Above and Beyond Salon, Vermillion, Ohio. Makeup by Laura Hall.

graduated haircut

graduated haircut **(GRAJ-oo-ayt-ud HAYR-kut)**—graduated shape or wedge; an effect or haircut that results from cutting the hair with tension, low-to-medium elevation, or overdirection.

graduation **(GRAJ-oo-ay-shun)**—elevation occurs when a section is lifted above 0 degrees.

gram **(GRAM)**—the basic unit of mass or weight in the metric system.

granular layer **(GRAN-yuh-lur LAY-ur)**—a layer of granular, nondividing cells lying immediately above the stratum basale in most parts of the epidermis.

granules **(GRAN-yoo-ulz)**—small grains or particles; in haircoloring, granules contain melanin pigment.

granulosum **(gran-yoo-LOH-sum)**—granular layer of the epidermis.

grattage **(grah-TAHZH)**—the scrubbing, scrapping, or brushing of a part during treatment.

gravity **(GRAV-ih-tee)**—the effect of the attraction of the earth on matter; the quality of having weight.

gravity-fed **(GRAV-ih-tee FED)**—airbrush system designed to pull the paint into the airbrush using gravity.

gray hair **(GRAY HAYR)**—hair with decreasing amounts of natural pigment; hair with no natural pigment is actually white; white hair looks gray when mingled with the still-pigmented hair.

grayed **(GRAYD)**—in coloring, dulled or diluted by the addition of gray.

greasepaint (GREES paint)—heavy makeup used for theatrical purposes.

greater auricular nerve (GRAYT-ur aw-RIK-yuh-lur NURV)—located at the side of the neck; affects the face, ears, neck, and parotid gland.

greater multangular (GRAY-tur mul-TANG-yuh-lur)—also known as *trapezium*; bone of the wrist.

greater occipital nerve (GRAY-tur ahk-SIP-ut-ul NURV)—located in the back of the head; affects the scalp as far up as the top of the head.

great saphenous vein (GRAYT sah-FEE-nus VAYN)—a large superficial vein in the leg.

great toe (GRAYT TOH)—the first inner digit of the foot.

green light (GREEN lyte)—a light-emitting diode for use on clients with hyperpigmentation or for detoxifying the skin.

gristle (GRIS-ul)—cartilage; tough, elastic, connective tissue in the body.

grit (GRIT)—in nail technology; the number of abrasive particles per square inch.

groove (GROOV)—the hollow part of a curling iron into which the rod fits; a long, narrow depression.

gross (GROHS)—in mathematics, a unit of quantity comprising 12 dozen.

gross anatomy (GROHS an-AT-o-mee)—the study of large and easily observable structures on an organism as seen through inspection with the naked eye.

ground (GROWND)—in electricity, the connection of an electrical current with the earth through some form of conductor such as a ground wire that connects an electrical apparatus with the ground object.

ground fault circuit interrupter (GFCI) (GROWND FAWLT sir-CUT in-ter-UP-ter)—a device that senses imbalances in an electric current.

ground wire (GROWND WYR)—a wire that connects an electric current to a ground.

grounding (GROWND-ing)—completes an electric circuit and carries the current safely away.

growth (GROHTH)—lengthening of hair, nails, and the like; the process of growing larger or longer; increase in size or maturity; abnormal formation of tissue such as a tumor.

growth direction (GROHTH dih-REK-shun)—the direction in which the hair grows from the scalp.

growth pattern (GROHTH PAT-urn)—also known as *natural fall* or *natural falling position*; direction in which the hair grows from the scalp.

guards (GARDZ)—plastic or hard rubber comb attachments that fit over clipper blades to minimize the amount of hair being cut with the clippers; metal shields applied over a haircutting razor for protection.

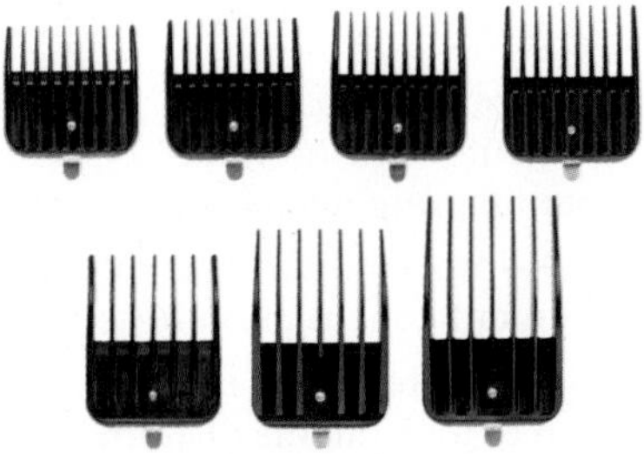

Courtesy of The Andis Company

guards

guide (GYDE)—something that serves as a model to follow or provides information; a rule to follow.

guideline (GYDE-lyn)—also known as *guide*; section of hair, located either at the perimeter or the interior of the cut, that determines the length the hair will be cut; usually the first section that is cut to create a shape.

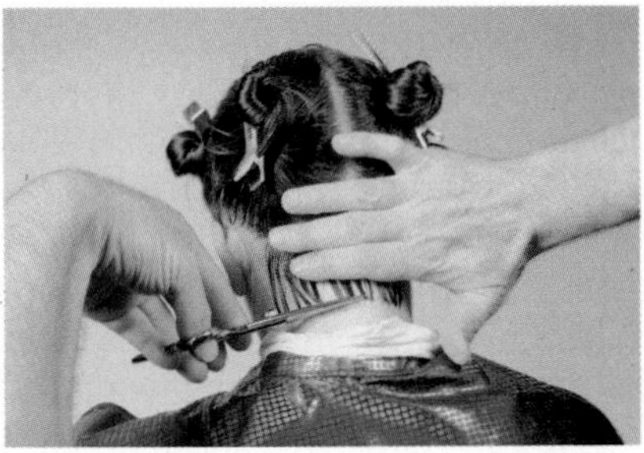

© Milady, a part of Cengage Learning. Photography by Yanik Chauvin.

guideline

guttate (GUT-ayt)—drop-like form characterizing certain cutaneous lesions.

gynecology (gy-nuh-KAHL-uh-jee)—the science and branch of medicine dealing with women's health and diseases of the reproductive organs.

G

H

H (AYCH)—in chemistry, the symbol for hydrogen.

hacking (HAK-ing)—a chopping movement done with the edge(s) of the hand(s) in massage.

hackle (HAK-ul)—an oblong board designed with metal upright teeth through which hair or other fiber is pulled to remove tangles; a disentangling device used in wig making.

hackling (HAK-ling)—process used to comb through hair strands in hair replacement construction to separate them.

hair (HAYR)—a slender thread-like filament of protein. The protein is made up of long chains of amino acids which in turn are made up of elements. The major elements that make up human hair are carbon, oxygen, hydrogen, nitrogen, and sulfur. Hair is an appendage or outgrowth of the skin of the head and body, and once it protrudes from the scalp it is completely keratinized and is a nonliving fiber composed of keratin protein.

hair analysis (HAYR uh-NAL-ih-sis)—the examination of the hair to determine its condition such as strength, elasticity, porosity, and moisture content; the study of the mineral and chemical content of hair.

hair bleaching (HAYR BLEECH-ing)—also known as *lightening* or *decolorizing*; chemical process involving the diffusion of the natural hair color pigment or artificial haircolor from the hair; the partial or total removal of natural pigment or artificial color from the hair.

hair bulb (HAYR BULB)—swelling at the base of the follicle that provides the hair with nourishment; the thickened, club-shaped structure that forms the lower part of the hair root.

hair canal (HAYR kuh-NAL)—the space in the hair follicle occupied by the hair root.

hair care products (HAYR KAYR PRAHD-ukts)—products formulated especially for the hair to condition, cleanse, and beautify.

hair clip (HAYR KLIP)—a metal or plastic device with prongs that open and close to secure a curl, curler, or subsection of hair in place.

hair clipper (HAYR KLIP-ur)—also known as *clipper, edger,* or, *trimmer*; an implement designed to cut and trim hair.

hair, coarse (HAYR, KORS)—hair that is extremely large in circumference.

hair color (HAYR-kul-ur)—this spelling is used to indicate the hair's natural color.

haircolor (HAYR-kul-ur)—professional, salon industry term referring to artificial haircolor products and services.

H

haircolor filler (HAYR KUL-ur FIL-ur)—a product used to fill porous spots in the hair and deposit base color during the lightening, tinting, or perming process.

haircoloring (HAYR-KUL-ur-ing)—the science and art of changing the color of the hair.

haircoloring brush (HAYR-KUL-ur-ing BRUSH)—also known as *dye brush*; a flat, short-bristled brush with a long, pointed handle, designed to be used when applying a coloring product to the hair.

haircoloring classification (HAYR-KUL-ur-ing klas-ih-fih-KAY-shun)—the four main categories of haircoloring are: temporary, semipermanent, demipermanent, and permanent.

haircolor glaze (HAYR-KUL-ur GLAYZ)—common way to describe a haircolor service that adds shine and color to the hair.

haircolor mousse (HAYR-KUL-ur MOOS)—foam that adds temporary color or highlights, and aids with styling in one process.

haircolor remover (HAYR-KUL-ur ree-MOOV-ur)—a product formulated to remove tint from the hair.

haircolor rinse (HAYR-KUL-ur RINS)—a temporary rinse used to color and highlight the hair.

haircolor spray (HAYR-KUL-ur SPRAY)—a spray, available in an array of colors, applied from an aerosol container; generally used for shows and special effects.

hair composition (HAYR kahm-poh-ZIH-shun)—hair is chiefly composed of protein keratin; the primary elements in average hair are carbon (50.65%), hydrogen (6.36%), nitrogen (17.14%), sulfur (5.0%), and oxygen (20.85%); hair also contains phosphorus in measurable amounts; the exact composition varies with the type of hair, depending to a large extent on age, race, sex, and color.

hair condition (HAYR kun-DIH-shun)—the state of health of the hair.

hair conditioner (HAYR kun-DIH-shun-ur)—a product formulated to be used in the hair to improve its health and appearance.

hair cortex (HAYR KOR-teks)—the middle layer of hair between the cuticle and the medulla. It is a fibrous protein core formed by elongated cells containing melanin pigment. The elasticity of the hair and its natural color are the result of unique protein structures located within the cortex.

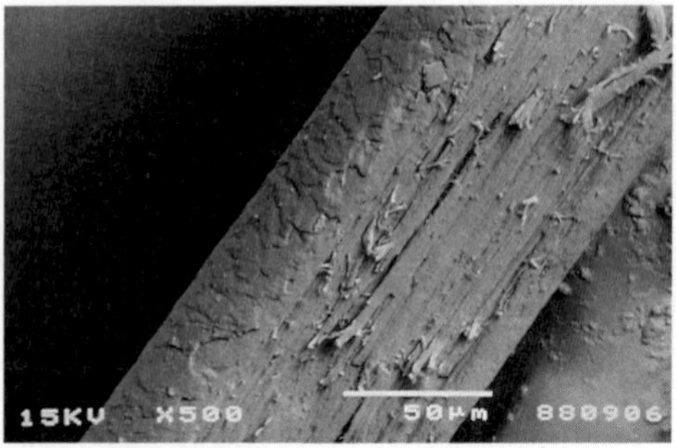

Courtesy of P & G's Beauty from John Grey's The World of Hair Care

hair cortex

hair cowlick (HAYR KOW-lik)—a tuft of hair that stands up.

hair crayons (HAYR KRAY-uns)—sticks of coloring material compounded with soaps or synthetic waxes; used to retouch the hair growth between coloring.

hair cuticle (HAYR KYOO-tih-kul)—outermost layer of hair; consisting of a single, overlapping layer of transparent, scale-like cells that look like shingles on a roof.

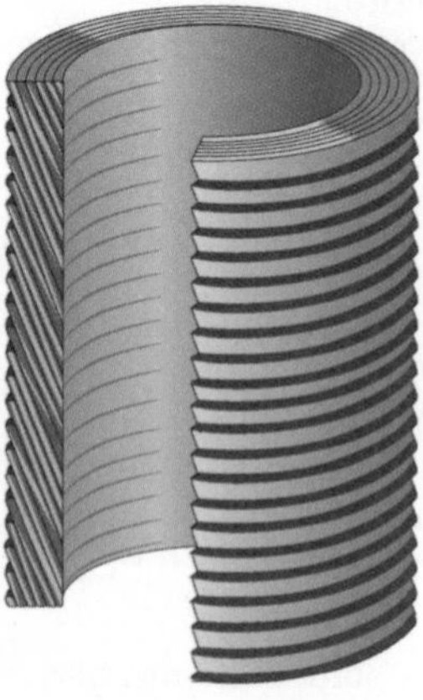
© Milady, a part of Cengage Learning

hair cuticle

haircutting implements (HAYR-kut-ing IM-pluh-ments)—the tools used to cut, trim, and shape the hair such as scissors or shears, thinning shears, straight razors, combs, hair clippers, and safety guards.

haircutting lotion (HAYR-kut-ing LOH-shun)—also known as *cutting lotion*; a liquid applied to wet hair before cutting to aid the cutting process.

haircutting shears (HAYR-kut-ing SHEERZ)—also known as *shears* or *scissors*; implement used to cut hair.

Haircutting shears are composed of two blades, one movable and the other stationary, fastened with a screw that acts as a pivot.

hair density (HAYR DEN-sih-tee)—the number of individual hair strands on 1 square inch (2.5 square centimeters) of scalp.

hair design (HAYR dee-ZYN)—the art of styling the hair; a specific style or trend.

hair dryer (HAYR DRY-ur)—a machine used to dry the hair; chair with drying hood; handheld hair dryer.

hair-drying lamp (HAYR DRY-ing LAMP)—an infrared lamp with a reflector designed to dry wet hair.

hair elasticity (HAYR ee-las-TIS-ut-ee)—the ability of hair to stretch and return to its original form without breaking.

hair ends (HAYR ENDZ)—the last one- to one-half inch (2.54–3.81 cm) of hair growth furthest from the scalp.

hair extensions (HAYR ex-TEN-shunz)—hair additions that are secured to the base of the client's natural hair in order to add length, volume, texture, or color.

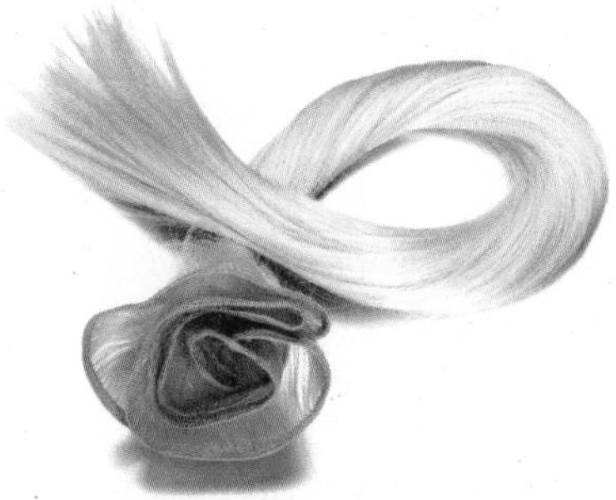

© Camilla Wisbauer/iStockphoto.com

hair extension or weft

hair, fine (HAYR, FYN)—hair that is extremely small in circumference.

hair follicle (HAYR FAHL-ih-kul)—the tubelike depression or pocket in the skin or scalp that contains the hair root.

hair goods (HAYR GOODS)—wigs, hairpieces, and decorative items for the hair.

hair lacquer (HAYR LAK-ur)—also known as *hairspray, finishing spray,* or *designing spray*; a product used to hold a hairstyle in place; usually used in spray form.

hair-locking (HAYR lock-ing)—the process that occurs when curly/coily hair is allowed to develop in its natural state without the use of combs, heat, or chemicals.

hair lightening (HAYR LY-ten-ing)—also known as *bleaching* or *decolorizing*; chemical process involving the diffusion of the natural hair color pigment or artificial haircolor from the hair.

hair loss (HAYR LAWS)—also known as *alopecia*; unnatural loss of hair or premature baldness.

H

hair net (HAYR NET)—a cap-shaped, open mesh head covering made of nylon or rayon; used to hold the hair in place while drying; also made in a three-cornered scarf style which is tied over the head.

hair oil (HAYR OYL)—also known as *shiner* or *smoother*; an oil used to lubricate dry hair and scalp.

hair ornament (HAYR OR-nuh-ment)—a decorative object added to the finished hairstyle (comb, ribbon, feathers, bow, or clasp).

hair papilla (HAYR pah-PIL-uh)—a small cone-shaped elevation at the bottom of the hair follicle.

hair parting (HAYR PART-ing)—separating the hair by a line to comb or create a set, or as an aid in styling the hair; the sectioning of hair to apply tint or bleach to the scalp.

hair pilus (HAYR Pil-us)—a slender threadlike outgrowth on the body.

hair porosity (HAYR puh-RAHS-ut-ee)—the ability of hair to absorb moisture.

hair pressing (HAYR PRES-ing)—method of temporarily straightening extremely curly or unruly hair by means of a heated iron or comb.

hair-pressing cream (HAYR PRES-ing KREEM)—a cream used in hair pressing as a protective lubricant.

hair-pressing oil (HAYR PRES-ing OYL)—an oily or waxy mixture used in hair pressing.

hair relaxer (HAYR ree-LAKS-ur)—a chemical product used to soften or remove natural curl from the hair.

hair relaxing (HAYR ree-LAKS-ing)—a method used to chemically straighten extremely curly or unruly hair so that it can be styled in less curly arrangements.

hair roll (HAYR ROHL)—a sausage-like shape in various lengths; used to fill under hair to create special effects.

hair roller (HAYR ROHL-ur)—a tube-shaped device made of metal, plastic, or other material of various lengths and diameters; used to set wet or dry hair.

hair roller pick (HAYR ROHL-ur PIK)—a toothpick-shaped plastic pick used to hold a hair roller in place.

hair roller pin (HAYR ROHL-ur PIN)—a flat, long, closed "U" shaped pin; used to secure hair rollers.

hair root (HAYR ROOT)—the part of the hair located below the surface of the epidermis. Anchors hair to the skin cells and is part of the hair located at the bottom of the follicle below the surface of the skin; part of the hair that lies within the follicle at its base, where the hair grows.

hair sample (HAYR SAM-pul)—a swatch of hair taken from a client's head for purposes of testing or matching.

hair set (HAYR SET)—the technique of placing the hair into roller or pin curl patterns, finger waving, or other manipulations, and then combing and brushing it into a finished style.

hair set tape (HAYR SET TAYP)—a type of tape that is used to assist in the foundation of hairlines and curves when the hair is too short to set on rollers or in pin curls.

hair-setting product (HAYR SET-ing PRAHD-ukt)—a lotion, spray, or gel used to make the hair easier to set and to hold the finished style in place.

hair shaft (HAYR SHAFT)—the portion of hair that projects above the epidermis.

hair shaping (HAYR SHAYP-ing)—the art of haircutting; molding the hair into a style.

hair shingling (HAYR SHING-gling)—the technique of cutting the hair close to the nape, with the hair becoming gradually longer toward the crown.

hair slithering (HAYR SLITH-ur-ing)—the process used in thinning and tapering the hair at the same time using scissors.

hair spray (HAYR SPRAY)—also known as *finishing spray*; a styling product applied in the form of a mist to hold a style in position; available in a variety of holding strengths.

hair straightener (HAYR STRAYT-en-ur)—a chemical agent or a heated mechanical device (iron) used to straighten extremely curly or unruly hair.

hair straightening (HAYR STRAYT-en-ing)—straightening extremely curly or unruly hair by use of chemical agents or a heated mechanical device (iron).

hair stream (HAYR STREEM)—hair flowing in the same direction, resulting from follicles sloping in the same direction.

hair, superfluous (HAYR, soo-PUR-floo-us)—unwanted or excess hair on the face or body.

hair texture (HAYR TEKS-chur)—the thickness or diameter of the individual hair strand.

hair thinning (HAYR THIN-ing)—a procedure to reduce the bulk and density of hair.

hair tint (HAYR TINT)—also known as *haircoloring* or *tinting*; changing the color of the hair in whole or in part.

hair tint test (HAYR TINT TEST)—also known as *patch test*, or *predisposition test*; the testing of a product on the client's skin to determine predisposition to the ingredients in the product to be used; a test to determine the reaction of a tint on a sample strand of hair.

hair transplantation (HAYR TRANZ-plant-ay-shun)—any form of hair restoration that involves the surgical removal and relocation of hair, including scalp reduction and flap surgery.

hair treatment (HAYR TREET-munt)—a procedure using appropriate products to improve the condition of the hair and scalp.

hair trim (HAYR TRIM)—trimming; cutting the hair slightly; following the existing lines.

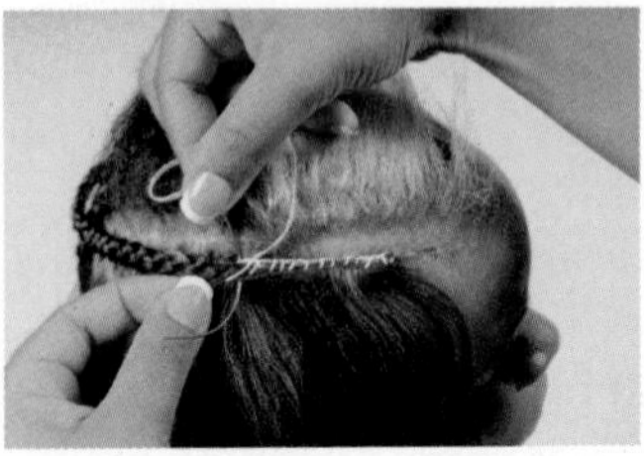

© Milady, a part of Cengage Learning. Photography by Yanik Chauvin.

hair weaving

hair weaving (HAYR WEEV-ing)—the practice of sewing a foundation or weft into the remaining hair on the head in an effort to eliminate the appearance of thinning or baldness, or to add length to natural hair.

hair weft (HAYR WEFT)—a section of woven hair.

hair wrapping (HAYR RAP-ing)—a technique used to keep curly hair smooth and straight.

hairband (HAYR-band)—also known as *head band*; an elasticized band used to hold the hair in place during a facial treatment; a decorative ribbon or material worn to hold the hair back from the face.

hairbrush (HAYR-brush)—an implement designed with bristles on one end and a handle on the other; used for grooming and styling the hair.

haircut (HAYR-kut)—the act of cutting the hair; the result of cutting the hair.

haircut, blunt (HAYR-kut, BLUNT)—refers to a haircut in which there is no elevation; hair is cut off squarely, without taper, so all hairs are the same length at the ends.

haircut, graduated (HAYR-kut, GRAD-yoo-ate-ed)—graduated shape or wedge; an effect or haircut that results from cutting the hair with tension, low-to-medium elevation, or overdirection.

haircut, reverse elevation (HAYR-kut, ree-VURS el-uh-VAY-shun)—the longest length of hair is at the lower hairline, with the haircut progressively shorter toward the crown and front hairline.

haircut, shag (HAYR-kut, SHAG)—a haircut combining high and low elevation with fringed effect around the hairline.

haircut, tailored neckline (HAYR-kut, TAYL-urd NEK-lyn)—a hairline length with low elevation in the nape section; haircut with fitted nape line.

haircut, tapering (HAYR-kut TAY-pur-ing)—cutting the hair at various lengths within the strands.

haircut, thinning (HAYR-kut THIN-ing)—cutting off small strands of hair at the scalp to reduce bulk.

haircutting (HAYR-kut-ing)—shortening and thinning of the hair and molding the hair into a becoming style; hair shaping.

haircutting comb (HAYR-kut-ing KOHM)—a comb specifically designed to be used in haircutting; usually it is narrow with short, fine teeth.

hairdresser (HAYR-dres-ur)—also known as *cosmetologist, stylist, beautician,* or *technician*; one who is skilled in the art and science of beautifying and improving the skin, nails, and hair and includes the study of cosmetics and their application.

hairdressing (HAYR-dres-ing)—art of arranging the hair into various becoming shapes or styles.

hairdressing adhesive (HAYR-dres-ing ad-HEE-siv)—also known as *hairdressing tape*; a substance used to hold small curls in place.

hairless (HAYR-les)—without hair; bald.

hairline (HAYR-lyn)—hair that grows at the outermost perimeter along the face, around the ears, and on the neck.

hairpiece (HAYR-pees)—also known as *toupee, hair solution,* or *hair replacement system*; small wig used to cover the top or crown of the head, or a hair attachment of some sort.

hairpin (HAYR-pin)—a slender, elongated "U"-shaped pin of plastic or metal, used to secure the hair in place; a pin shaped like a clasp with ridges or plain sides.

hairstyle (HAYR-styl)—also known as *style, design, hairdo, coif,* or *coiffure*; a way of wearing the hair.

hairstyling (HAYR-styl-ing)—the art of dressing the hair.

hairstylist (HAYR-styl-ist)—a specialist in the creation and design of hair fashions.

hairy (HAYR-ee)—also known as *hirsute*; having excessive hair growth.

hairy nevus (HAYR-ee NEE-vus)—a mole; a pigmented, brownish growth covered with hair.

H

H

half base (HAF-BAYS)—position of a curl or a roller half off its base, giving medium volume and movement.

half-base curls (HAF-BAYS kurlz)—curls placed half off their base; strong curls with moderate lift or volume.

half moon (HAF MOON)—also known as *lunula*; in manicuring, a term pertaining to the light, crescent shape at the base of each nail where the matrix and the connective tissue of the nail bed join. May be polished or left unpolished.

half off-base placement (HAF-OFF-BAYS PLAYSZ-ment)—base control in which the hair is wrapped at an angle of 90 degrees or perpendicular to its base section, and the rod is positioned half off its base section.

half-stem curl (HAF-stem KURLZ)—curl placed half off the base; permits medium movement and gives good control to the hair.

half tone (HAF TOHN)—a semitone, halfway between a highlight and a shadow.

half wig (HAF WIG)—a hair piece formed on one-half of a wig base to blend with the natural hair on the head.

halitosis (hal-uh-TOH-sus)—also known as *bad breath*; offensive odor from the mouth.

hallux (HAL-uks)—the first and innermost digit of the foot; the great toe.

hamstring (HAM-string)—in human anatomy, one of the tendons at the back of the knee.

hand care (HAND KAYR)—pertaining to beneficial exercises and grooming of the hands and nails.

hand care products (HAND KAYR PRAHD-ukts)—any cream, lotion, or other preparation used to soften and smooth the skin of the hands, and to aid in care of the nails.

hand massage (HAND muh-SAHZH)—a series of massage movements for the hands, included with a manicure.

hand mirror (HAND MEER-ur)—a small mirror with a handle used in the salon to enable the client to view the back and sides of the finished hairstyle.

handheld implement (HAND-HELD IM-pluh-ment)—any item such as a blow-dryer, clippers, cutting shears, and facial apparatus held in the hand and used to perform a service.

hand-tied wigs (HAND-tyd WHIGZ)—also known as *hand-knotted wigs*; wigs made by inserting individual strands of hair into mesh foundations and knotting them with a needle.

hanging curls (HANG-ing KURLZ)—curls hanging downward from the head.

hangnail (HANG-nayl)—also known as *agnail*; a condition in which the living tissue surrounding the nail plate splits or tears.

hardener, nail (HARD-un-ur NAYL)—a substance used to strengthen the fingernails.

hard press (HARD PRES)—technique that removes 100 percent of the curl by applying the pressing comb twice on each side of the hair.

hard rubber (HARD RUB-ur)—a substance used in the manufacture of combs for the cosmetology and barbering industry.

hard UV gels (HARD yoo-vee JELZ)—also known as *traditional UV gels*; gels that cannot be removed with a solvent and must be filed off the natural nail.

hard water (HARD WAW-tur)—water that contains minerals that reduce the ability of soap or shampoo to lather.

harmony (HAR-muh-nee)—the creation of unity in a design; the most important of the art principles; holds all the elements of the design together.

haversian canals (huh-VUR-zhun kuh-NALZ)—small channels through which the blood vessels travel in the bone.

Hazard Communication Rule (HAZ-ard comm-YOON-eh-cay-shun ROOL)—requires that chemical manufacturers and importers evaluate and identify possible health hazards associated with their products.

H-bond (AYCH-BAHND)—a hydrogen bond; physical cross bond in the cortical layer.

head form (HED-form)—also known as *head shape*; shape of the head, which greatly affects the way the hair falls and behaves.

health screening form (HELTH SCREEN-ing FORM)—a questionnaire that discloses all medications, both topical (applied to the skin) and oral (taken by mouth), along with any known skin disorders or allergies that might affect treatment.

heart (HART)—muscular cone-shaped organ that keeps the blood moving within the circulatory system.

heart-shaped face (HART-SHAYPT FAYS)—a face with a wide forehead and a narrow, pointed chin.

heel (HEEL)—point at which the bristles of the brush meet the ferrule.

H

helical winding (HEEL-ih-kul WYND-ing)—also known as *spiral winding*; winding the hair from the scalp to the ends.

heliotherapy (hee-lee-oh-THAIR-uh-pee)—the therapeutic use of solar energy; use of the sun's rays as a beneficial treatment.

helix (HEE-liks)—spiral shape of a coiled protein created by polypeptide chains that intertwine with each other.

hematidrosis, hemidrosis (hem-ah-tih-DROH-sus, hem-ih-DROH-sus)—the excretion of sweat stained with blood or blood pigment.

hematocyst (heh-MAT-uh-sist)—a cyst containing blood.

hematocyte (heh-MAY-uh-syt)—a blood corpuscle.

hematology (hee-muh-TAHL-oh-jee)—the science of the blood, its functions, composition, and diseases.

hematoma (hee-muh-TOH-muh)—mass of blood trapped in tissue or in a cavity as a result of internal bleeding.

hemifacial (hee-mih-FAY-shul)—pertaining to one side of the face.

hemiplegia (hee-mi-PLEE-jeea)—unilateral paralysis caused by a stroke.

hemoglobin (HEE-muh-gloh-bun)—complex iron protein in red blood cells that binds to oxygen; gives blood color.

hemophilia (hee-moh-FEE-lee-uh)—disease characterized by slow blood clotting and excessive bleeding.

hemopoietic tissue (hee-muh-poy-ET-ik TISH-oo)—tissue found in bone marrow and the vascular system.

hemorrhage (HEM-uh-rij)—heavy or uncontrollable bleeding.

hemostatic (hee-muh-STAT-ik)—also known as *styptic*; a substance used to control bleeding.

henna (HEN-uh)—the leaves of an Egyptian plant, *Lawsonia inermis*; used as a dye, imparting bright shades of red; also used as a cosmetic.

henna, compound (HEN-uh KAHM-pownd)—also known as *progressive dye*; Egyptian henna to which has been added one or more metallic preparations to alter color and adhere like a coating to the hair.

henna shampoo (HEN-uh sham-POO)—a shampoo to which henna has been added to add color and luster to the hair.

hepatitis (HEP-uh-tight-is)—the inflammation of the liver caused by viruses or toxic agents and characterized by the presence of inflammatory cells in the tissue of the organ.

herbal shampoo (URB-ul sham-POO)—shampoo containing substances extracted from bark, roots, and herbs known to aid in cleansing the hair and scalp; shampoo to which saponin products have been added.

herbal therapy (URB-ul THAIR-uh-pee)—the use of etheric oils of plants and natural oils, applied to the skin as a stimulant, and to impart a sense of physical well-being.

herbs (URBS)—a plant with leaves, stems, or parts used in cookery, and in medicinal and cosmetic preparation. Hundreds of different herbs that contain phytohormones are used in skin care products and cosmetics; they heal, stimulate, soothe, and moisturize.

hereditary (huh-RED-ih-teh-ree)—descending from ancestor to heir; genetically transmitted from parent to offspring.

heredity (huh-RED-ih-tee)—the genetic capacity of the organism to develop ancestral characteristics; the transfer of qualities or disease from parent to offspring.

herpes (HER-peez)—an inflammatory disease of the skin caused by a viral infection and characterized by small vesicles in clusters.

herpes simplex virus 1 (HER-peez SIM-pleks VY-rus ONE)—strain of the herpes virus that causes fever blisters or cold sores; it is a recurring, contagious viral infection consisting of a vesicle or group of vesicles on a red, swollen base. The blisters usually appear on the lips or nostrils.

herpes simplex virus 2 (HER-peez SIM-pleks VY-rus TOO)—strain of the herpes virus that infects the genitals.

herpes zoster (HER-peez ZOS-ter)—also known as *shingles*; a painful viral infection skin condition from the chicken pox virus; characterized by groups of blisters that form a rash in a ring or line.

hidrosis (hid-ROH-sus)—the production and excretion of sweat; abnormally profuse sweating.

high elevation (HY el-uh-VAY-shun)—haircutting term indicating that hair is held 90 degrees or more from the head and then cut, causing it to fall in a layered effect.

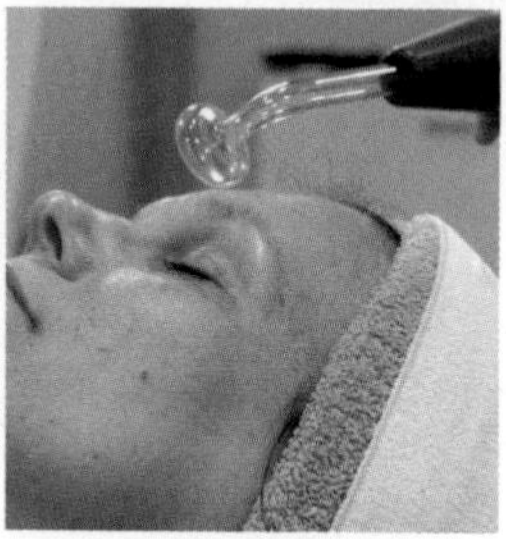

© Milady, a part of Cengage Learning. Photography by Larry Hamill.

high-frequency machine

high-frequency current (HY-FREE-kwen-see KUR-ent)—current with a high oscillation or vibration.

high-frequency machine (HY-FREE-kwen-see muh-SHEEN)—also known as *tesla high-frequency* or *violet ray*; apparatus that utilizes alternating, or sinusoidal, current to produce a mild-to-strong heat effect.

H

high frequency, tesla (HY FREE-kwen-see TES-luh)—violet ray; an electric current of medium voltage and medium amperage producing a slight thermal response, and that has a bactericidal effect on the skin.

high-lift tinting (HY-LIFT TINT-ing)—a single-process color with a higher degree of lightening action and a minimum amount of color deposit.

high molecular weight (HY muh-LEK-yuh-lur WAYT)—large size and density of a specific molecular construction.

highlight (HY-lyt)—brightness or luster added to the skin or hair by some artificial means; a lighter cosmetic applied to a facial feature to improve its contours.

highlighting (HY-lyt-ing)—also known as *foiling*, *baliage*, or *lightening*; coloring some of the hair strands lighter than the natural color to add a variety of lighter shades and the illusion of depth.

highlighting shampoo (HY-lyt-ing sham-POO)—colors prepared by combining permanent haircolor, hydrogen peroxide, and shampoo.

hinge joints (HINJ JOYNTS)—joints in the elbow and knee; two or more bones that connect like a door.

hirsute (HUR-soot, hur-SOOT)—hairy; having coarse, long hair; shaggy.

hirsuties (hur-SOO-teez)—also known as *hypertrichosis*; growth of an unusual amount of hair on parts of the body normally bearing only downy hair, such as the faces of women or the backs of men.

hirsutism (HUR-soo-tiz-um)—condition pertaining to an excessive growth or cover of hair.

histology (his-TAHL-uh-jee)—also known as *microscopic anatomy*; the study of tiny structures found in living tissues.

hold (HOLD)—pertaining to the ability of a hair spray to keep a hairstyle in place.

holding angle (HOLD-ing ANG-gul)—also known as *cutting angle*; angle at which the hand is held while cutting hair from the head form.

homeostasis (hoh-mee-oh-STAY-sus)—the maintenance of normal, internal stability in an organism.

homogeneous (hoh-moh-jeen-ee-us)—having the same nature or quality; a uniform character in all parts.

homogenizer (huh-MAHJ-uh-nyz-ur)—a substance that produces a uniform suspension of emulsions from two or more normally immiscible substances.

hone (HOHN)—a fine grit stone used to sharpen a cutting tool such as a razor; used for haircutting or for shaving the beard.

horizontal lines (hor-ih-ZAHN-tul LYNZ)—lines parallel to the floor or horizon; create width in design.

hormone (HOR-mohn)—chemicals released by cells or tissues that influence other cells or tissues, such as secretions of insulin, adrenaline, and estrogen, that stimulate functional activity or other secretions in the body. Hormones influence the welfare of the entire body.

hospital disinfectants (HOS-pih-tal dis-in-FEKT-ants)—disinfectants that are effective for cleaning blood and body fluids.

hot iron (HAHT EYE-urn)—another term for curling iron.

hot oil (HAHT OYL)—a warmed oil used in facial and manicure treatments.

hot rollers (HAHT ROHL-urz)—rollers that are preheated before being placed in the hair.

hue (HYOO)—pertaining to a particular color, tint, or shade; gradation of color.

human disease carrier (HYOO-mun DIZ-eez KAIR-ih-ur)—person who is immune to a disease, but harbors germs that can infect other people.

human hair (HYOO-mun HAYR)—hair that grows on a human being; the facial, head, or body hair of a person.

human hair wig (HYOO-mun HAYR WIG)—a wig made with human hair, considered to be of excellent quality.

human immunodeficiency virus (HIV) (HYOO-mun ih-MYOO-noh-di-FISH-en-see VY-rus)—a pathogen that is most often the precursor to acquired immune deficiency syndrome (AIDS). By impairing or killing the immune system affected with it, HIV progressively destroys the body's ability to fight infections or certain cancers.

human papilloma virus (HPV) (HYOO-mun pap-uh-LOW-ma VY-rus)—also known as *plantar warts*; a virus that can infect the bottom of the foot and resembles small black dots, usually in clustered groups. It is also a cutaneous viral infection commonly caused by sexual transmission and exhibited by genital warts.

H

humectant (hyoo-MEK-tent)—also known as *hydrators* or *water-binding agents*; ingredients that attract water, absorb moisture, or promote the retention of moisture.

humerus (HYOO-muh-rus)—the uppermost and largest bone in the arm extending from the elbow to the shoulder.

humidity (hyoo-MID-ih-tee)—dampness; a moderate amount of wetness, especially in the atmosphere.

hyaline (HY-uh-lin)—cartilage found in the nose, trachea, and on the ends of bones and in movable joints.

hydrate (HY-drayt)—a compound formed by the union of water with some other substance; to combine a substance with water; to add moisture to the skin.

hydrating agent (HY-drayt-ing AY-jent)—a substance used in facial treatments to restore moisture to dry (dehydrated) skin.

hydration (hy-DRAY-shun)—the chemical union of a substance with water.

hydrocarbon (hy-droh-KAR-bun)—any compound composed only of hydrogen and carbon.

hydrochloric acid (hy-droh-KLOR-ik AS-ud)—an aqueous solution of hydrogen chloride (HCl) that is a strong, corrosive, irritating acid.

hydrocyst (HY-droh-sist)—a cyst containing a watery fluid.

hydrocystoma (hid-roh-sis-TOH-muh)—an eruption of deeply seated vesicles due to water retention in the sweat follicles.

hydrogen (HY-druh-jun)—in chemistry, the symbol H; the lightest element; it is an odorless, tasteless, colorless gas found in water and all organic compounds.

hydrogen bond (HY-druh-jun BAHND)—a weak, physical, cross-link side bond that is easily broken by water or heat.

hydrogen peroxide developer (HY-druh-jun puh-RAHK-syd devel-UP-uhr)—oxidizing agent that, when mixed with an oxidation hair color, supplies the necessary oxygen gas to develop the color molecules and create a change in natural hair color.

hydrogenate (hy-DRAHJ-uh-nayt)—to combine or treat with hydrogen.

hydrogenated lanolin (HY-druh-jen-ayt-ud LAN-ul-un)—lanolin treated with hydrogen so that it retains its emollient qualities while losing unwanted odor, color, and tackiness; used in cosmetic preparations such as creams, lotions, powders, sprays, suntan products, hair and nail preparations, and perfumes.

hydrolysis (hy-DRAHL-uh-sus)—chemical process of decomposition involving splitting of a bond with the addition of the elements of water (hydrogen and oxygen).

hydrolyze (HY-droh-lyz)—to decompose as a result of the incorporation and splitting of water; the two resulting products divide the water: the hydroxyl group is attached to one and the hydrogen atom to the other.

hydrolyzed elastin (HY-druh-lyzd ih-LAS-tun)—the product (hydrolysate) of animal ligaments and other connective tissue used in creams formulated to help retain the skin's elasticity.

hydromassage (hy-druh-muh-SAHZH)—massage by means of moving water.

hydrometer (hy-DRAHM-ut-ur)—an instrument used to measure the strength (volume) of peroxide and other liquids.

hydrophilic (hy-drah-FIL-ik)—easily absorbs moisture; in chemistry terms, capable of combining with or attracting water (water-loving).

hydrophobia (hy-druh-FOH-bee-uh)—an abnormal fear of water.

hydrophobic (hy-druh-FOH-bik)—naturally resistant to being penetrated by moisture.

hydroquinone (hy-droh-kwin-OHN)—a topical medication that is used for bleaching or reducing excessive melanin lesions in the epidermis.

hydrosis (hy-DROH-sis)—excretion of perspiration.

hydrotherapy (hy-druh-THAIR-uh-pee)—the therapeutic use of water in the treatment of injuries, diseases, or for mental well-being; physical therapy using water.

hydroxide (hy-DRAHKS-yd)—any compound formed by the union of one oxygen atom and one hydrogen atom with a group of atoms known as a radical.

hydroxide neutralization (hy-DRAHKS-yd new-trull-eye-ZAY-shun)—an acid-alkali neutralization reaction that neutralizes (deactivates) the alkaline residues left in the hair by a hydroxide relaxer and lowers the pH of the hair and scalp; hydroxide relaxer neutralization does not involve oxidation or rebuild disulfide bonds.

hydroxide relaxers (hy-DRAHKS-yd re-LAX-ors)—very strong alkalis with a pH over 13; the hydroxide ion is the active ingredient in all hydroxide relaxers.

hygiene (HY-jeen)—a set of practices that help to preserve health.

hygienic (hy-JIEN-ik)—having to do with preserving health.

H

H

hygroscopic (hy-gruh-SKAHP-ik)—readily absorbing and retaining moisture.

hyoid bone (HY-oyd bohn)—U-shaped bone at the base of the tongue that supports the tongue and its muscles.

hyper (HY-pur)—a prefix denoting excessive; above normal; above; beyond.

hyperacidity (hy-pur-uh-SID-ih-tee)—an excess of acidity.

hyperadrenalism (hy-pur-uh-DREN-al-is-um)—excessive release of adrenal hormones into the bloodstream.

hyperhidrosis, hyperidrosis (hy-per-hy-DROH-sus, hy-pur-ih-DROH-sis)—excessive sweating, caused by heat or general body weakness.

hyperkeratosis (hy-pur-kair-uh-TOH-sis)—thickening of the skin caused by a mass of keratinized cells (keratinocytes).

hyperkeratosis subungualis (hy-pur-kair-uh-TOH-sis sub-un-GWAY-lis)—hypertrophy affecting the nail bed.

hyperostosis (hy-puh-rahs-TOH-sus)—excessive growth or thickening of bone tissue.

hyperpigmentation (hy-pur-pig-men-TAY-shun)—darker-than-normal pigmentation, appearing as dark splotches.

hyperplasia (hy-pur-PLAY-zhuh)—excessive formation of tissue; an increase in the number of cells in tissue or an organ.

hypersensitivity (hy-pur-sen-sih-TIV-ih-tee)—excessive sensitivity to substances to which a normal individual does not react.

hyperthyroidism (hy-pur-THY-roy-diz-um)—excessive activity of the thyroid gland.

hypertrichosis (hy-pur-trih-KOH-sis)—also known as *hirsuties*; condition of abnormal growth of hair, characterized by the growth of terminal hair in areas of the body that normally grow only vellus hair.

hypertrophica, acne (hy-pur-TRAHF-ih-kuh, AK-nee)—acne scars that are raised and stay within the boundary of the original wound and can reduce in size with the passage of time.

hypertrophy (hy-PUR-troh-fee)—abnormal growth of the skin.

hypo (HY-poh)—a prefix denoting under; beneath; lowered state.

hypoallergenic (hy-poh-al-ur-JEN-ik)—having a lower than usual tendency to cause allergic reactions.

hypodermal (hy-poh-DUR-mul)—lying beneath the epidermis.

hypodermic (hy-poh-DUR-mik)—of or relating to parts beneath the skin; placed or introduced beneath the skin.

hypodermis (hy-poh-DUR-mis)—in human anatomy, the subcutaneous tissue.

hypoglossal nerve (hy-poh-GLAHS-ul NURV)—also known as *twelfth cranial nerve*; motor nerve located under the tongue.

hypoglycemia (hy-POH-gly-see-me-uh)—a condition in which blood glucose or blood sugar drops too low; caused by either too much insulin or low food intake.

hyponychium (hy-poh-NIK-eeum)—slightly thickened layer of skin that lies between the fingertip and free edge of the nail plate. It forms a protective barrier that prevents microorganisms from invading and infecting the nail bed.

hypopigmentation (hy-POH-pig-men-tay-shun)—absence of pigment, resulting in light or white splotches.

hypothalamus (hy-poh-THAL-uh-mus)—the part of the brain that regulates many metabolic body processes.

hypothenar (hy-poh-THEEN-ur)—the fleshy eminence on the palm of the hand over the metacarpal bone of the little finger; also the prominences of the palm at the base of the fingers.

hypothermia (hy-poh-THER-mee-uh)—a condition of abnormally low body temperature.

hypothesis (hy-PAHTH-uh-sis)—an assumption or theory proposed to account for facts.

I

ice pick scars (YS PIK SKARZ)—large, visible open pores that look as if the skin has been punctured with an ice pick or similar object; this scar is caused by a deep pimple or cyst that has destroyed the follicle.

ichthyosis (ik-thee-OH-sis)—also known as *fish skin disease*; a skin disease in which the skin is dry, thickened, scaly, or flaky.

imbalance (im-BAL-ens)—the state of being out of balance.

imbibition (im-buh-BISH-un)—the act of absorbing moisture.

imbricated (IM-brih-kayt-ud)—overlapped, as scales in skin disease.

imbrications (im-bruh-KAY-shunz)—cells arranged in layers overlapping one another; tiny overlapping scales found in the hair cuticle; overlapping of layers of tissue in the closure of wounds or repair of defects.

immersion (ih-MUR-shun)—plunging or dipping into a liquid especially so as to cover completely.

immiscible (im-IS-uh-bul)—liquids that are not capable of being mixed together to form stable solutions.

immobile (ih-MOH-bul)—incapable of being moved; motionless.

immune (ih-MYOON)—safe from attack; protected from disease by vaccination or natural defenses.

immunity (im-YOO-net-ee)—the ability of the body to destroy and resist infection. Immunity against disease can be either natural or acquired and is a sign of good health.

immunodermatology (im-yoo-noh-dur-muh-TAHL-uh-jee)—the study of the immune system as related to skin disorders and their treatment.

immunology (im-yoo-NAHL-uh-jee)—the branch of medical science that studies the immune systems in organisms.

impair (im-PAYR)—to make worse; to render less than perfect; to cause to lose quality.

impermeable (im-PUR-mee-uh-bul)—impenetrable; not capable of being penetrated; impervious to moisture.

impervious (im-PUR-vee-us)—impenetrable; incapable of being passed through.

impetigo (im-puh-TEE-goh)—contagious bacterial skin infection characterized by clusters of small blisters or crusty lesions.

implant (im-PLANT)—to imbed; to insert and fix firmly.

implements (IM-pluh-mentz)—tools used to perform services. Implements can be reusable or disposable.

impregnated (im-PREG-nayt-ud)—fertilized; saturated.

inactive electrode (in-AK-tiv ee-LEK-trohd)—the opposite pole from the active electrode.

inactive stage (IN-ac-tif STAYJE)—also known as *spore-forming stage*; the stage in which bacteria do not grow or reproduce.

incandescent (in-kan-DES-ent)—white, glowing, clear, or luminous with intense heat.

inch (INCH)—a measure of length equal to one twelfth of a foot; 2.54 centimeters.

incision (in-SIZH-un)—a cut; a division of soft body tissue made with a knife or similar instrument.

incombustible (in-kahm-BUS-tih-bul)—fireproof; not flammable.

increase layering (in-KREES LAY-ur-ing)—cutting to produce a layered effect with progressively longer lengths.

increasing graduation (in-KREES-ing graj-yoo-WAY-shun)—graduation within two nonparallel lines; it increases as it moves back from the face.

incretion (in-KREE-shun)—the secreting of a substance such as oil from the sebaceous glands.

incrust (in-KRUST)—also known as *encrust*; to form a crust or a coating.

incrustation (in-krus-TAY-shun)—the state of having crusts or scales; the formation of a crust or hard coating.

incubation (in-kyoo-BAY-shun)—the act or process of hatching or developing; the period of time between infection of an individual with an infectious disease and the appearance of symptoms.

incurable (in-KYOOR-uh-bul)—not capable of being cured.

indelible (in-DEL-ih-bul)—cannot be removed, erased, blotted out, or eliminated; permanent; lasting.

indentation (in-den-TAY-shun)—the curved depth, valley, or hollowness created by the formation of curls or waves in the hair.

indentation curl (in-den-TAY-shun KURL)—the point where curls of opposite directions meet, forming a recessed area.

indentation roller (in-den-TAY-shun ROHL-ur)—setting technique in which the stem is combed flat against the scalp and the roller is rolled upward, away from the head; used to create a hollow or valley in the finished style.

independent contractor (IN-dee-pen-dant CON-tract-uhr)—someone who sets his or her own fees, controls his or her own hours, has his or her own business card, and pays his or her own taxes.

indicator (IN-dih-kay-tur)—an apparatus or instrument used to show changes in conditions such as color or the degree of acidity or alkalinity.

indirect division (IN-dih-rekt dih-VIH-zshun)—also known as *mitosis*; the method by which a mature cell reproduces in the body.

I

indirect point (IN-dih-rekt POYNT)—partings of an oval shape using curved or straight lines; the first parting is out of the circumference, then intersections all form one point.

indirect transmission (IN-dih-rekt trans-MISH-un)—transmission of blood or body fluids through contact with an intermediate contaminated object such as a razor, extractor, nipper, or an environmental surface.

individual eyelashes (in-dih-VIJ-oo-ul EYE-lash-ez)—separate, artificial eyelashes that are applied to the eyelids one at a time.

individualize (in-dih-VIJ-oo-uh-lyz)—to distinguish from others; to give a client a particular hairstyle or haircut.

induction, electromagnetic (in-DUK-shun ee-LEK-troh-MAG-net-ik)—the process by which an electrified or magnetic state is produced through proximity to a charged body or presence in a magnetic field.

inductor (in-DUK-tur)—an electrical apparatus or part that acts inductively on another.

indurata, acne (in-dyoo-RAH-tuh AK-nee)—deeply seated acne with large papules and pustules that can cause severe scarring.

induration (in-dyuh-RAY-shun)—the process or act of hardening; a spot or area of hardened tissue.

inefficiency (in-ih-FISH-un-see)—quality, state, or fact of being wasteful of time or energy, or not producing the effect intended or desired within a given expenditure of time or energy.

inelasticity (in-ih-las-TIS-ih-tee)—in cosmetology, the ability to stretch but not return to its former shape as in porous or limp hair; aging skin or muscles.

inert (in-URT)—inactive; lacking the power to move.

inert tissues (in-URT TISH-yoos)—that which is not contractile such as bones, ligaments, and nerves.

infect (in-FEKT)—to cause infection; to contaminate.

infection (in-FEK-shun)—the invasion of body tissues by disease-causing or pathogenic bacteria.

infection control (in-FEK-shun CON-trol)—the methods used to eliminate or reduce the transmission of infectious organisms.

infection, general (in-FEK-shun, JEN-ur-ul)—the result of germs gaining entrance into the bloodstream and circulating throughout the entire body.

infection, local (in-FEK-shun, LOH-kul)—infection confined to only certain portions of the body such as an abscess.

infectious (in-FEK-shus)—caused by or capable of being transmitted by infection.

infectious allergy (in-FEK-shus AL-ur-jee)—delayed allergic reactivity that can accompany an infectious disease.

infectious dermatitis (in-FEK-shus dur-muh-TY-tis)—an inflamed irritation of the skin resulting from an allergic reaction to a specific substance.

infectious disease (in-FEK-shus DIZ-eez)—disease caused by pathogenic (harmful) microorganisms that enter the body. An infectious disease may or may not be spread from one person to another person.

infectious mononucleosis (in-FEK-shus mahn-uh-noo-klee-OH-sis)—also known as *glandular fever* or *kissing disease*; contagious disease characterized by a swelling of the lymph nodes, fever, and sore throat.

inferior (in-FEER-ee-or)—situated lower down or nearer the bottom or base; of lesser quality.

inferior alveolar nerve (in-FEER-ee-or al-VEE-oh-lar NURV)—a nerve servicing the teeth.

inferior labial artery (in-FEER-ee-ur LAY-bee-al ART-ur-ee)—artery that supplies blood to the lower lip.

inferior labial nerve (in-FEER-ee-ur LAY-bee-al NURV)—a nerve in the skin of the lower lip.

inferior labial vein (in-FEER-ee-ur LAY-bee-al VAYN)—a vein that drains the region of the lower lip into the facial vein.

inferior maxilla (in-FEER-ee-ur mak-SIL-uh)—the lower jawbone or mandible.

inferior ophthalmic vein (in-FEER-ee-ur ahf-THAL-mik VAYN)—a vein that supplies blood to the eye, orbit, and adjacent facial structures.

inferior palpebral nerve (in-FEER-ee-ur PAL-puh-brul NURV)—a nerve that receives stimuli for the lower eyelid.

inferior palpebral vein (in-FEER-ee-ur PAL-puh-brul VAYN)—a vein that drains blood from the lower eyelids to the facial veins.

inferior terbinate (in-FEER-ee-ur TUR-bih-nayt)—the nasal concha; an irregular scroll-shaped bone situated on the lateral wall of the nasal cavity.

inferior vena cava (in-FEER-ee-ur VEE-nuh KAYV-uh)—the large vein that carries blood to the heart from the abdomen, feet, and legs.

infiltration (in-fil-TRAY-shun)—the process or act of passing through or into another substance such as cells or fluid passing into tissues or other cells.

I

inflammable (in-FLAM-uh-bul)—tending to be easily ignited.

inflammation (in-fluh-MAY-shun)—a condition in which the body reacts to injury, irritation, or infection; characterized by redness, heat, pain, and swelling.

inflate (in-FLAYT)—to swell or distend by filling with air or gas.

influenza (in-floo-EN-zuh)—also known as *flu*; an acute, highly contagious viral disease characterized by sudden onset, fever, exhaustion, weakness, and severe aches and pains.

information interview (IN-for-may-shun IN-ter-vyuw)—a scheduled meeting or conversation whose sole purpose is to gather information.

infra (IN-fruh)—a prefix denoting below; lower.

inframandibular (in-fruh-man-DIB-yuh-lur)—below the lower jaw.

infraorbital (in-fruh-OR-bih-tul)—nerve located below the orbit; a sensory and motor nerve affecting the skin of the cheek muscles, side of the nose, upper lip, and mouth.

infraorbital artery (in-fruh-OR-bih-tul ARE-ter-ee)—supplies blood to the muscles of the eye.

infraorbital nerve (in-fruh-OR-bih-tul NURV)—affects the skin of the lower eyelid, side of the nose, upper lip, and mouth.

infrared (in-fruh-RED)—pertaining to that part of the spectrum lying outside the visible spectrum and below the red rays; deepest penetration, and produces the most heat.

infrared light (in-fruh-RED LYT)—also known as *infrared rays*; infrared light has longer wavelengths, penetrates more deeply, has less energy, and produces more heat than visible light; makes up 60 percent of natural sunlight.

infratrochlear nerve (in-frah-TRAHK-lee-ur NURV)—sensory nerve affecting the lacrimal sac, the skin of the nose, and the oblique muscle of the eye.

ingestion (in-JES-chun)—the act of taking substances, especially food, into the body.

ingredient (in-GREE-dee-unt)—any part of a compound; that which enters into the composition of a mixture.

ingrown (IN-grohn)—growing inward; an ingrown hair or nail.

ingrown hair (IN-grohn HAYR)—a hair that has grown so that the normally free end is embedded in or underneath the skin, sometimes causing an infection.

ingrown nail (IN-grohn NAYL)—a nail that has grown into the flesh instead of toward the tip of the finger or toe, sometimes causing an infection.

inhalation (in-huh-LAY-shun)—breathing in through the nose or mouth.

inhale (in-HAYL)—to draw in breath.

inhibit (in-HIB-it)—to check or restrain; prohibit.

inhibition layer (in-hih-BISH-un LAY-ur)—the tacky surface left on the nail after a UV gel has cured.

initiators (in-ISH-ee-ate-ors)—substance that starts the chain reaction that leads to the creation of very long polymer chains.

injectable fillers (in-JEK-tuh-bul FIL-urz)—substances used in nonsurgical procedures to fill in or plump up areas of the skin. Botox® and dermal fillers are injectables.

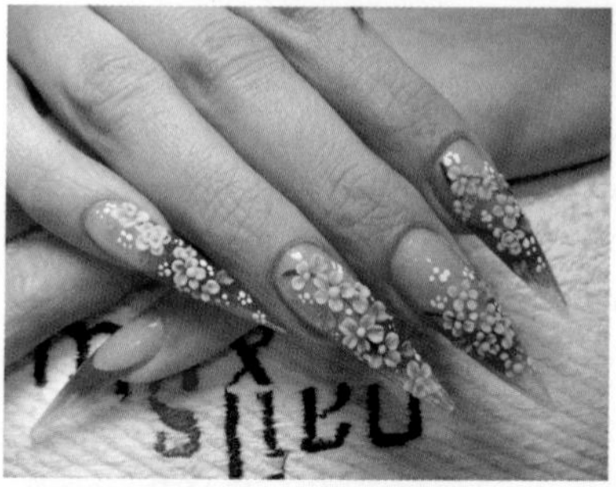

Nails by Massimiliano Braga

inlaid design

inlaid designs (IN-layd dis-EYNS)—designs inside a nail enhancement that are created when nail art is sandwiched between two layers of product while the nail enhancement is being formed.

inner perimeter (IN-ur puh-RIM-ih-tur)—in hairstyling, the hair length and density in the inner area excluding the hairline.

innermost (IN-ur-mohst)—the inmost part; the farthest inward from the outermost part.

innervation (in-ur-VAY-shun)—distribution of nerves to a part of the body.

innominate artery (in-AHM-uh-nut ART-uh-ree)—an artery that distributes blood to the right side of the head and to the right arm.

innominate bone (in-AHM-uh-nut BOHN)—one of two large irregular bones that form the pelvis; hipbone.

innominate veins (in-AHM-uh-nut VAYNZ)—veins of the neck; brachiocephalic veins.

inoculation (in-ahk-yuh-LAY-shun)—the injection of a vaccine to cause a mild form of the disease to build immunity to that disease.

inorganic (in-or-GAN-ik)—composed of matter not arising from natural growth or living organisms; without carbon.

inorganic chemistry (in-or-GAN-ik KEM-is-tree)—the study of substances that do not contain the element carbon, but may contain the element hydrogen.

inorganic hair dye (in-or-GAN-ik HAYR DYE)—a nonvegetable, non-animal hair-coloring material.

inorganic nutrients (in-or-GAN-ik NOO-tree-ents)—minerals needed in the daily diet.

inseparable (in-SEP-ar-uh-bul)—incapable of being separated.

insert (in-SURT)—to put or thrust in; to set, so as to be within.

insertion (in-SUR-shun)—act of inserting; that which is put in; point where the skeletal muscle is attached to a bone or other more movable body part.

inside curve (IN-syd KURV)—a concave (inward) curve cut in the hair.

inside movement (IN-syd MOOV-ment)—pertaining to an indentation, a curve, or movement keeping the hair close to the head.

insolation (in-suh-LAY-shun)—a measure of solar radiation.

insoluble (in-SAHL-yuh-bul)—incapable of being dissolved or very difficult to dissolve.

instant conditioners (IN-stant con-DISH-on-uhrs)—conditioners that typically remain on the hair from one to five minutes and are rinsed out.

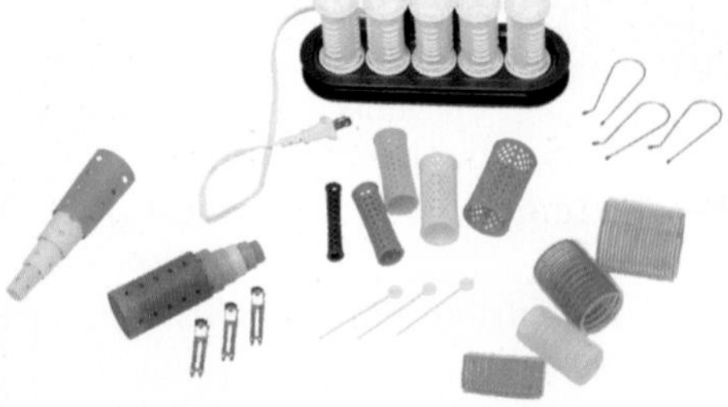
© Milady, a part of Cengage Learning. Photography by Paul Castle.

instant hair roller

instant hair roller (IN-stant HAYR ROHL-ur)—also known as *hot roller*; an electronically heated hair roller used to style the hair while it is dry.

instep (IN-step)—the dorsal part of the

human foot on the medial side; the arched upper part of the foot.

instrument **(IN-struh-ment)**—device or tool for performing cosmetology work.

insulate **(IN-suh-layt)**—to separate by nonconductors; to prevent transfer of electricity of heat.

insulation **(in-suh-LAY-shun)**—nonconducting substance; resisting the passage of an electric current.

insulator **(IN-suh-layt-ur)**—a nonconducting material or substance used to cover electric wires.

insulin **(IN-suh-lin)**—a hormone secreted by the pancreas that regulates carbohydrate and fat metabolism, and regulates the movement of glucose across cell membranes.

I

insurance **(in-SHUR-ens)**—guarantees protection against financial loss from malpractice, property liability, fire, burglary and theft, and business interruption.

integration hairpiece **(IN-tah-gray-shun HAYR-peace)**—hairpiece that has openings in the base through which the client's own hair is pulled to blend with the hair (natural or synthetic) of the hairpiece.

integument **(in-TEG-yuh-ment)**—a covering, especially the skin.

integumentary system **(in-TEG-yuh-ment-uh-ree SIS-tum)**—the skin and its accessory organs, such as the oil and sweat glands, sensory receptors, hair, and nails; serves as a protective covering and helps regulate the body's temperature.

intense pulse light (IPL) **(in-TENS PULSE LYHT)**—a medical device that uses multiple colors and wavelengths (broad spectrum) of focused light to treat spider veins, hyperpigmentation, rosacea and redness, wrinkles, enlarged hair follicles and pores, and excessive hair.

intensity **(in-TEN-sih-tee)**—the amount of force per unit area, as of heat, light, or current; the quality of being intense; used in haircoloring to describe the strength of the color's tonality.

intercellular **(in-tur-SEL-yuh-lur)**—between or among cells.

intercellular matrix **(in-tur-SEL-yuh-lur MAY-tricks)**—lipid substances between corneum cells that protect the cells from water loss and irritation.

intercostal **(in-tur-KAHS-tul)**—between the ribs.

intercostal muscles **(in-tur-KAHS-tul MUS-uhlz)**—muscles lying between adjacent ribs.

intercostal nerves (in-tur-KAHS-tul NURVZ)—the branches of the thoracic nerves in the intercostal spaces (spaces between the ribs).

interior (in-TEER-ee-ur)—inner or internal part of anything; situated within; occurring or functioning on the inside.

interior graduation (in-TEER-ee-ur grad-jyoo-AY-shun)—the hair underneath is shortened and covered by progressively increasing lengths.

interior guide (in-TEER-ee-ur GUYD)—guideline that is inside the haircut rather than on the perimeter.

interlace (in-tur-LAYS)—to weave strands of hair.

intermediate (in-tur-MEE-dee-ut)—between two extremes; being or occurring at the middle place or degree.

I

intermediate supraclavicular nerve (in-tur-MEE-dee-ut soo-pruh-kluh-VIK-yuh-lur NURV)—nerve that receives stimuli from the skin of the anterior part of the neck and chest wall.

intermittent heat (in-tur-MIT-ent HEET)—interrupted heating period; electric current turned on and off during a steaming procedure.

intermuscular (in-tur-MUS-kyuh-lur)—situated between the muscles.

internal absorption (in-TUR-nul ab-SORP-shun)—the normal digestive assimilation of foods and liquids.

internal carotid artery (in-TUR-nul kuh-RAHT-ud ART-uh-ree)—supplies blood to the brain, eyes, eyelids, forehead, nose, and internal ear.

internal carotid nerve (in-TUR-nul kuh-RAHT-ud NURV)—a sympathetic nerve (stimulated by activity) serving the internal carotid artery and its branches.

internal jugular vein (in-TUR-nul JUG-yuh-lur VAYN)—also known as *jugular*; vein located at the side of the neck, collects deoxygenated blood from the brain and parts of the face and neck and brings it back to the heart via the superior vena cava.

internal respiration (in-TUR-nul res-pih-RAY-shun)—an exchange of gases between the blood and the capillaries and tissues of the body.

interneuron (in-tur-NUHR-ahn)—carries impulses from one neuron to another.

interosseous (in-tur-AHS-ee-us)—lying between or connecting bones.

interosseous artery, anterior (in-tur-AHS-ee-us ART-uh-ree, an-TEER-eeur)—artery that supplies blood to the muscles of the deep anterior part of the forearm.

interosseous artery, posterior (in-tur-AHS-ee-us ART-uh-ree, poh-STEER-ee-ur)—artery that supplies blood to the posterior forearm.

interosseous membrane of the forearm (in-tur-AHS-ee-us MEM-brayn UV THE FOR-arm)—pertaining to the strong, fibrous membrane between the radius and the ulna; forearm.

interosseous membrane of the leg (in-tur-AHS-ee-us MEM-brayn UV THE LEG)—the strong, fibrous sheet between the margins of the tibia and the fibula.

interosseous nerve (in-tur-AHS-ee-us NURV)—a somatic, sensory nerve distributed in the ankle joint.

interparietal (in-tur-puh-RY-eh-tul)—between walls; between parietal bones.

interpenetrate (in-tur-PEN-uh-trayt)—to pervade; permeate; penetrate thoroughly.

interphase (IN-tur-fayz)—stage in cell division.

interstice (in-TUR-stus)—a narrow opening between adjoining parts.

interstitial fluid (INTER-stih-shall FLU-id)—blood plasma found in the spaces between tissues.

intervascular (in-tur-VAS-kyuh-lar)—between blood or lymph vessels.

interweave (in-tur-WEEV)—to blend a weft or faux hair with natural hair.

intestine (in-TES-tin)—body organ that, along with the stomach, digests food.

intraarterial (in-truh-ar-TEER-ee-ul)—within or directly into an artery.

intraarticular (in-truh-ar-TIK-yuh-lar)—within a joint.

intracardiac (in-truh-KAR-dee-ak)—occurring within or situated in the heart.

intracellular (in-truh-SEL-yuh-lur)—occurring or within a cell or cells.

intracorneal (in-truh-KOR-nee-ul)—within the horny layer of the skin; also, within the cornea of the eye.

intracranial (in-truh-KRAY-nee-ul)—occurring within the cranium.

intracuticular (in-truh-kyoo-TiK-yuh-lur)—within the dermis.

intradermal (in-truh-DUR-mul)—within the dermis.

I

intradermal nevus (in-truh-DUR-mul NEE-vus)—a skin lesion containing melanocytes located in the dermis.

intraepidermal (in-truh-ep-ih-DUR-mul)—within the epidermis.

intramuscular (in-truh-MUS-kyuh-lur)—within the muscle.

intraneural (in-truh-NUR-ul)—within a nerve.

intrinsic factors (IN-trin-sick FAK-turs)—belonging to the essential nature or constitution of a thing; in esthetics; skin-aging factors over which we have little control.

invasion (in-VAY-zhun)—occurs when bacteria or other microorganisms enter the body.

inventory (IN-ven-tor-ee)—a list of stock items; an accounting of products on hand; a record of supplies used and to be reordered.

I

inversion (in-VUR-zhun)—the act of turning inward.

inverted triangle (in-VUR-tud TRY-ang-gul)—a face shape having a narrow chin, broad cheeks, and broad forehead.

inverter (in-VUR-tur)—a device for converting direct current into alternating current.

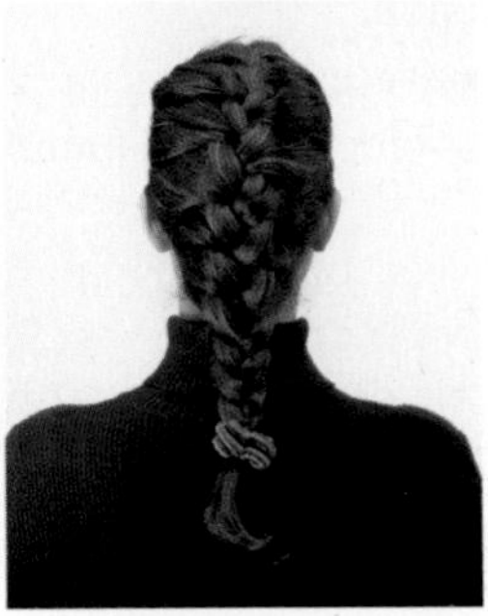
© Milady, a part of Cengage Learning. Photography by Paul Castle.
invisible braid

invisible braid (in-VIZ-ih-bul BRAYD)—also known as *inverted braid* or *French braid*; a three-strand braid that is produced with an overhand technique.

invisible light (in-VIZ-ih-bul LYT)—light at either end of the visible spectrum of light that is invisible to the naked eye.

involuntary (in-VAHL-un-tair-ee)—functioning or acting independently of the will or conscious control.

involuntary muscle (in-VAHL-un-tair-ee MUS-uhl)—a muscle that functions automatically without conscious will.

involute (IN-vuh-loot)—in hairdressing, having ends rolling upward; curving; spiraling.

inward (IN-ward)—toward the inside.

iododerma (eye-oh-duh-DUR-muh)—a skin eruption caused by the injection of iodine compounds.

iodoform (eye-OH-duh-form)—a yellow crystalline compound formed by the action of iodine on alcohol and potash; used as an antiseptic for wounds and sores.

ion (EYE-ahn)—an atom or molecule that carries an electrical charge.

ionic bond (eye-AHN-ik BAHND)—the chemical bond between charged atoms or ions.

ionization (eye-ahn-ih-ZAY-shun)—the separation of an atom or molecule into positive and negative ions.

ionto mask (eye-AHN-toh MASK)—a mask of spongy material that covers the face; used with a galvanic machine during the process of the ionization or desincrustation facial treatment.

ionto rollers (eye-AHN-toh ROHL-urz)—metal rollers attached to a galvanic machine used to aid the penetration of creams or lotions into the skin during a facial treatment.

iontophoresis (eye-ahn-toh-foh-REE-sus)—the process of introducing water-soluble products into the skin with the use of electric current such as the use of the positive and negative poles of a galvanic machine or microcurrent device.

iris (EYE-ris)—the colored muscular disk-like diaphragm of the eye that regulates the size of the pupil.

iron (EYE-urn)—a metallic element with the symbol Fe; required in the human diet with a recommended amount of approximately 10 milligrams daily.

irons (EYE-umz)—heated implements designed to wave or curl the hair while it is dry.

irrigate (IHR-ih-gayt)—to flush with water; to spray; to refresh with water.

irritant (IHR-ih-tent)—something that irritates, excites, or stimulates.

irritant contact dermatitis (ICD) (IHR-ih-tent CON-tact derma-TIH-tus)—occurs when irritating substances temporarily damage the epidermis.

irritation (ihr-ih-TAY-shun)—the reaction of tissues or nerves to overstimulation.

ischemia (is-KEE-mee-uh)—deficient supply of blood to a body part (as the heart or brain) that is due to obstruction of the inflow of arterial blood.

ischemic compression (is-KEE-mik kuhm-PRES-shun)—a therapeutic massage technique for trigger points; blood flow to an area is temporarily blocked so that when the area is released blood rushes to the area.

Islets of Langerhans (EYE-letz OF LAN-gur-hahns)—a region of the pancreas that has insulin-producing cells.

isometric contraction (eye-soh-MET-rik kun-TRAK-shun)—occurs when a muscle contracts and the ends of the muscle do not move.

isometric exercise (eye-soh-MET-rik EKS-ur-syz)—an exercise for the muscles in which contractions are counteracted by equal force exerted by the opposing muscles, and the body part affected does not move.

isopropyl alcohol (eye-soh-PROH-pul AL-kuh-hawl)—a volatile flammable alcohol used especially as a solvent and rubbing alcohol.

isopropylamine (eye-soh-PROH-pal-ah-mene)—a substance produced from acetone; an emulsifier used in many hair grooming creams and lotions.

isotonic contraction (eye-soh-TAHN-ik kahn-TRAK-shun)—contraction that occurs when a muscle contracts and the distance between the ends of the muscle changes.

ivy dermatitis (EYE-vee derma-TIH-tus)—a skin inflammation caused by exposure to the poison ivy, poison oak, or poison sumac.

J

Japanese thermal straighteners (JAP-an-eez THER-muhl STRATE-ners)—also known as *thermal reconditioning, TR,* or *thermal ionic reconstructors*; a method of permanently straightening curly hair which combines the use of a thioglycolate relaxer with flat ironing the hair.

jaundice (JAHN-dus)—yellowness of the skin, tissues, and body fluids; caused by deposits of bile pigments.

jaw clamp (JAW KLAMP)—also known as *butterfly clamp* or *butterfly clip*; a hair clip with teeth to secure large sections of hair.

Jessner's peel (JEZZ-nuhrz PEEL)—light to medium peel of lactic acid, salicylic acid, and resorcinol in an ethanol solvent.

job description (JOHB des-CRIP-shun)—specified list of duties and responsibilities that are required of an employee in the performance of his or her job.

joint (JOYNT)—a connection between two or more bones of the skeleton.

joint movement (JOYNT MOOV-ment)—articulations of the bones on either side of the joint.

jostling (JAH-sling)—massage movement used to release muscle tension and increase blood circulation, performed by grasping the entire muscle, lifting it slightly away from its position, and shaking it quickly across its axis.

Journeymen barber groups (JUHR-knee-men BAR-ber GROOPS)—barber employee unions.

jowl (JOWL)—the hanging part of a double chin; lower cheeks and jaw.

jugal (JOO-gul)—pertaining to the cheek.

jugular (JUG-yuh-lur)—pertaining to the neck or throat; the large veins in the neck.

jugular bulb (JUG-yuh-lur BULB)—bulb of the internal jugular vein.

jugular fossa (JUG-yuh-lur FAHS-uh)—the depression or cavity between the carotid canal and the stylomastoid (slender and pointed) opening containing the superior bulb of the internal jugular vein.

jugular nerves (JUG-yuh-lur NURVZ)—pertaining to nerves in the jugular area.

jugular trunk (JUG-yuh-lur TRUNK)—one of two connecting lymph trunks on the right and left sides of the head and neck; the right drains into the right lymphatic duct; the left drains into the thoracic duct.

jugular vein (JUG-yuh-lur VAYN)—one of the two large veins on each side of the neck that returns blood from the brain, neck, and parts of the face to the heart.

jugular vein, anterior (JUG-yuh-lur VAYN, an-TEER-ee-ur)—vein located in the middle of the neck that drains the anterior part of the neck.

jugular vein, external (JUG-yuh-lur VAYN, eks-TUR nul)—vein located parallel to arteries on the sides of the neck that returns blood to the heart from the face, head, and neck.

jugular vein, internal (JUG-yuh-lur VAYN, in-TUR nul)—vein that returns blood to the heart from the brain, face, and neck.

jugular vein, posterior (JUG-yuh-lur VAYN, poh-STEER-ee-ur)—vein situated in the occipital region that serves the skin and muscles in the upper back area of the neck.

junction nevus (JUNK-shun NEE-vus)—a benign skin lesion containing neuro cells; located at the junction of the epidermis and dermis.

K

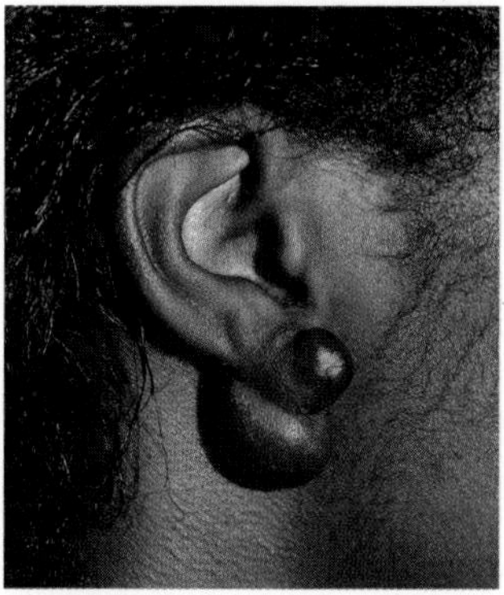
Courtesy of www.dermnet.com

keloids

keloid (KEE-loyd)—a thick scar resulting from excessive growth of fibrous tissue; a skin disorder caused by an overgrowth of collagen; marked by whitish hardened patches surrounded by a pinkish or purplish border.

keloid acne (KEE-loyd AK-nee)—a follicular infection with pustules that causes keloidal scarring; frequently affects black skin.

kanekalon (CANE-kuh-lon)—a manufactured, synthetic hair fiber used for adding length to the hair during braiding or hair extension services.

keratin (KAIR-uht-in)—fibrous protein of cells that is also the principal component of skin, hair, and nails; provides resiliency and protection.

keratin proteins (KAIR-uht-in PRO-teens)—long, coiled polypeptide chains.

keratin straightening treatments (KAIR-uht-in STRAYT-uhning TREAT-ments)—also known as *smoothing treatment, Brazilian keratin treatment,* or *Brazilian straightening treatment*; straightening treatment that contains silicone polymers and formalin or similar ingredients, which release formaldehyde gas when heated to high temperatures with a flat iron.

keratinization (kair-uh-tin-y-ZAY-shun)—process by which newly formed cells in the hair bulb mature, fill with keratin, move upward, lose their nucleus, and die.

keratinocytes (kair-uh-TIN-oh-syts)—epidermal cells composed of keratin, lipids, and other proteins.

keratitis (kair-uh-TY-tis)—inflammation of the cornea of the eye.

keratoacanthoma (kair-uh-toh-ak-an-THOH-muh)—a skin nodule or tumor that usually occurs in elderly white males; resembles squamous cell cancer of the skin.

keratoderma (kair-uh-tuh-DUR-muh)—a horny condition of the skin, especially of the palms of the hands and soles of the feet.

keratoid (KAIR-uh-toyd)—hornlike; horny tissue.

keratolytic therapy (kair-uh-tuh-LIT-ik THAYR-uh-pee)—treatment to remove warts and other lesions in which the epidermis produces excess skin. In this therapy, salicylic acid is put on the lesion. Keratolytic therapy thins the skin on and around the lesion. It causes the outer layer of the skin to loosen and shed.

keratoma (kair-uh-TOH-muh)—also known as *callus*; acquired, superficial, thickened patch of epidermis, caused by continued, repeated pressure or friction on any part of the skin, especially the hands and feet.

keratonosis (kair-uh-toh-NOH-sis)—an anomaly in the horny structure of the epidermis.

keratoprotein (kair-uh-toh-PROH-teen)—the protein of the horny tissues of the body that make up such structures as the hair, nails, and epidermis.

keratosa, acne (kair-uh-TOH-puh, AK-nee)—a rare form of acne consisting of horny plugs projecting from the hair follicles, accompanied by inflammation, usually at the angles of the mouth.

keratosis (kair-uh-TOH-sis)—abnormally thick buildup of cells.

keratosis pilaris (kair-uh-TOH-sis PILL-are-us)—a condition where keratin builds up and blocks the follicle; causes redness and bumpiness in the skin of the cheeks or upper arms.

ketone (KEE-tohn)—also known as *acetone, methyl,* or *ethyl*; substance obtained by the oxidation of secondary alcohols; used as a solvent in nail polish and polish remover.

kidney (KID-nee)—one of the body organs that supports the excretory system by eliminating water and waste products.

kilo (KEE-loh)—a prefix meaning thousand.

kilocalorie (KIL-uh-kal-uh-ree)—the quantity of heat required to raise the temperature of one kilogram of water one degree centigrade.

kilowatt (KIL-uh-wat)—Abbreviated as K; one thousand (1,000) watts.

kinesics (kih-NEE-siks)—also known as *body language*; the study of nonverbal body movements.

kinetics (kuh-NET-iks)—the branch of physics dealing with the effect of forces on the motion of physical objects, or with changes on physical or chemical systems.

kit (KIT)—in cosmetology, a case containing the implements the cosmetologist needs to perform services.

knead (NEED)—to work and press with the hands as in massage.

knit (NIT)—to cause to draw together, as in the healing of bone.

knot (NAHT)—also known as *chignon*; in hairdressing, a technique used for formal hairstyling that creates the look of a knot or bun; to intertwine and loop strands of hair, fabric, rope, and the like to form a flat or oval mass.

knotted hair (NAHT-id HAYR)—also known as *trichonodrosis*; hair that has tangled, snarled lumps.

knuckling (NUK-ling)—a massage movement made by using the knuckles of the four fingers of the hand to lightly tap the skin.

koilonychia (koy-loh-NIK-ee-ah)—also known as *spoon nails*; a malformation of the fingernails associated with nutritional deficiencies such as of iron and calcium; the nails become thin and concave in shape.

kojic acid (KOO-jick ASUD)—skin-brightening agent.

Kolinsky sable (KUH-lin-skee SAY-buhl)—a type of natural bristle that comes from mink found in the cold climates of China and Siberia; it is amongst the finest, softest, and most expensive material from which makeup brushes are made.

kosmetikos (kahz-MET-ih-kohs)—a Greek word meaning "skilled in the use of cosmetics" and from which the word *cosmetology* is derived.

kyphoscoliosis (ky-foh-skoh-lee-OH-sis)—backward and lateral curvature of the spinal column.

kyphosis (ky-FOH-sus)—also known as *humpback*; anterior concave curvature of the spine.

L

labia majora (LAY-bee-uh MAH-jor-uh)—the outer folds of the vulva on either side of the vagina.

labia minora (LAY-bee-uh MIN-ore-uh)—the inner folds of the vulva on the edge of the vaginal opening.

labial artery, inferior (LAY-bee-ul ART-uh-ree, in-FEER-ee-ur)—artery that supplies blood to the lower lip.

labial artery, superior (LAY-bee-ul ART-uh-ree, soo-PEER-ee-ur)—artery that supplies blood to the upper lip, septum, and wing of the nose.

labial nerve, inferior (LAY-bee-ul NURV, in-FEER-ee-ur)—nerve that distributes stimuli to the lower lip.

labial nerve, superior (LAY-bee-ul NURV, soo-PEER-ee-ur)—nerve that distributes stimuli to the skin of the upper lip.

labium (LAY-bee-um); pl., labia (LAY-be-uh)—lip; a fleshy border or edge; pertaining to the lips.

lace-front (LAYS-front)—in barbering; popular hair solution style used for off-the-face styles.

lacerate (LAS-uh-rayt)—to tear the skin or tissue.

laceration (las-uh-RAY-shun)—a tear of the skin or tissue.

lacing, French (LAYS-ing, FRENCH)—also known *as French braid*; a style of braiding.

lacquer (LAK-ur)—also known as *nail polish*, *polish*, or *colored lacquer*; a solution of nitrocellulose in a volatile solvent used on the nails.

lacrimal (LAK-ruh-mul)—pertaining to tears or weeping, and the glands that secrete tears.

lacrimal artery (LAK-ruh-mul ART-uh-ree)—artery supplying blood to the eye and eyelid area.

lacrimal bone (LAK-ruh-mul BOHN)—small, thin bones located at the front inner wall of the orbits (eye sockets).

lacrimal duct (LAK-ruh-mul DUKT)—either of the two tear ducts of the eyes.

lacrimal glands (LAK-ruh-mul GLANDZ)—glands situated in the orbit of the eye in the depression of the frontal bone that secrete tears.

lacrimal nerves (LAK-ruh-mul NURVZ)—nerves distributed in the area of the upper eye and eyelid, and affecting the tear glands.

lacteals (LAK-tee-ulz)—any one of the lymphatic capillaries located in the small intestine that helps absorb fats.

lactic acid (LAK-tik AS-ud)—a clear, syrupy organic acid; used in skin-freshening lotions; an alphahydroxy acid.

lamp dry (LAMP DRY)—to style the hair and dry it at the same time under an infrared heat lamp.

lamp, hot quartz (LAMP, HAHT KWORTZ)—a general all-purpose lamp used for skin tanning, and other cosmetics and germicidal purposes.

lamp, infrared (LAMP, IN-fruh-red)—a lamp producing infrared rays; used in skin-care treatments.

lamp, magnifying (LAMP, MAG-nih-fy-ing)—an apparatus with a magnifying glass and source of light; used to examine the skin or scalp.

lamp, ultraviolet (LAMP, ul-truh-VY-oh-let)—tone of the three types of lamps used in cosmetology (glass bulb, hot quartz, and cold quartz).

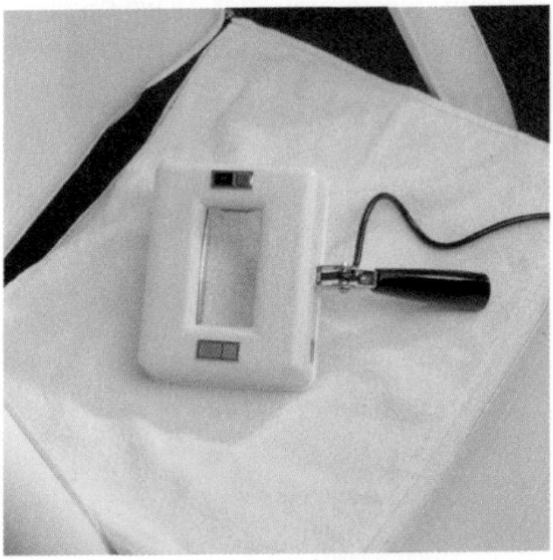

© Milady, a part of Cengage Learning. Photography by Paul Castle.

Wood's lamp

lamp, Wood's (LAMP, WOODZ)—a lamp developed by Robert W. Wood, an American physicist, used as a diagnostic tool dermatology by which ultraviolet light is shone onto the skin of the patient; a technician then observes any subsequent fluorescence. For example, bacterial infections show as coral pink; *Pseudomonas* is yellowish-green; Propionibacterium acnes, the bacteria responsible for acne, exhibits an orange glow under a Wood's lamp.

lancet (LAN-set)—a small, sharp-pointed surgical blade used by estheticians and physicians to pierce a pustule.

Langerhans immune cells (LAN-ger-han IM-yoon SELLS)—guard cells of the immune system that patrol and recognize invaders as foreign and initiate further immune system activity against the invader.

L

lanolin (LAN-ul-un)—emollient with moisturizing properties; also an emulsifier with high water-absorption capabilities.

lanthionine (lan-THEE-oh-nyn)—a nonessential form of amino acid.

lanthionine bonds (lan-THEE-oh-nyn BAHNDZ)—the bonds created when disulfide bonds are broken by hydroxide chemical hair relaxers after the relaxer is rinsed from the hair.

lanthionization (lan-THEE-ohn-iz-ay-shun)—process by which hydroxide relaxers permanently straighten hair; they remove a sulfur atom from a disulfide bond and convert it into a lanthionine bond.

lanugo hair (luh-NOO-goh HAYR)—the fine, soft, downy hair that covers most of the body, aiding in efficient evaporation of perspiration.

large intestine (LARJ in-TES-tin)—the distal portion of the intestine that extends from the ileum to the anus, and consists of the cecum, colon, and rectum.

larynx (LAIR-inks)—the organ of voice production above the trachea or windpipe.

laser (LAY-zur)—acronym for *light amplification stimulation emission of radiation*; a medical device that uses electromagnetic radiation for hair removal and skin treatments.

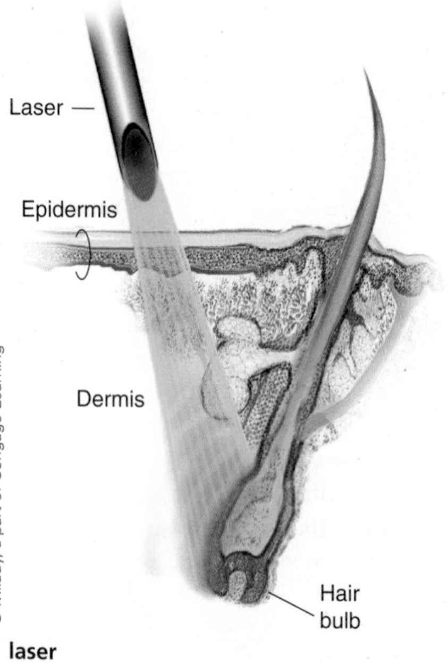

© Milady, a part of Cengage Learning

laser

L

laser hair removal (LAY-zur HAYR ree-MOOV-uhl)—photoepilation hair reduction treatment in which a laser beam is pulsed on the skin using one wavelength at a time, impairing hair growth; an intense pulse of electromagnetic radiation.

laser resurfacing (LAY-zur re-SUR-fas-ing)—procedure used to smooth wrinkles or lighten acne scars. Collagen remodeling stimulates the growth of new collagen in the dermis.

lateral cutaneous nerve (LAT-ur-ul kyoo-TAY-nee-us NURV)—nerve that receives stimuli from the skin of the lateral side of the forearm.

lateral nail fold (LAT-ur-uhl NAIL FOLD)—folds of normal skin that line the sides of the nail plate.

lateral nasal cartilage (LAT-ur-ul NAYZ-ul KART-ul-ij)—the upper lateral cartilage of the nose.

lateral palpebral artery (LAT-ur-ul PAL-puh-brul ART-uh-ree)—artery that supplies blood to the eyelids and surrounding area.

lateral pterygoid (LAT-ur-ul TARE-uh-goyd)—also known as *chewing muscles*; muscles that coordinate with the masseter, temporalis, and medial pterygoid muscles to open and close the mouth and bring the jaw forward.

lateral vibration (LAT-ur-ul vy-BRAY-shun)—a massage movement using the palms of the hands to press firmly on the muscles while moving them from side to side in a vibrating motion; primarily for shoulder and back massage.

latissimus dorsi (lah-TIS-ih-mus DOR-see)—a broad, flat superficial muscle covering the back of the neck and upper and middle region of the back, controlling the shoulder blade and the swinging movements of the arm.

law of color (LAW uv kulur)—system for understanding color relationships.

layer (LAY-ur)—a single thickness, fold, or stratum.

layers (LAY-urz)—create movement and volume in the hair by releasing weight.

layered haircut (LAY-urd HAYR-cut)—graduated effect achieved by cutting the hair with elevation or overdirection; the hair is cut at higher elevations, usually 90 degrees or above, which removes weight.

layering (LAY-ur-ing)—graduated effect achieved by cutting the hair with elevation or overdirection. Each subsequent subsection is slightly shorter than the guide when allowed to fall naturally.

leave-in conditioners (LEEV-in KAHN-dish-uhn uhr)—conditioners and thermal protectors that can be left in the hair without rinsing.

leiodermia (ly-oh-DUR-mee-uh)—a condition of abnormal smoothness and glossiness of the skin.

lentigenes (singular: lentigo) (len-tih-JEE-neez)—technical term for freckles; small yellow-brown colored spots. Lentigenes that result from sunlight exposure are actinic, or solar, lentigenes Patches are referred to as large macules.

lesion (LEE-zhun)—mark on the skin; may indicate an injury or damage that changes the structure of tissues or organs. There are three types of skin lesions: primary, secondary, and tertiary.

lesser multangular (LES-ur mul-TANG-gyuh-lur)—bone of the wrist.

lesser occipital (LES-ur ahk-SIP-ut-ul)—the nerve-supplying muscles at the back of the ear.

leucine (LOO-seen)—an essential amino acid that must be ingested and it is the only dietary amino acid that has the capacity to stimulate muscle protein synthesis.

leucocyte, leukocyte (LOO-koh-syt)—white blood cells that have enzymes to digest and kill bacteria and parasites. These white blood cells also respond to allergies.

leucoderma (loo-koh-DUR-muh)—skin disorder characterized by light abnormal patches (hypopigmentation); caused by a burn or congenital disease that destroys the pigment-producing cells. Vitiligo and albinism are leukodermas.

leuconychia (loo-koh-NIK-ee-ah)—also known as *white spots*; whitish discolorations of the nails, usually caused by injury to the matrix area; not related to the body's health or vitamin deficiencies.

leucotrichia (loo-koh-TRIK-ee-uh)—whiteness of the hair; canities.

levator (lih-VAYT-ur)—a muscle that elevates a part.

levator anguli oris muscle (lih-VAYT-ur ANG-yoo-ly OH-ris MUS-uhl)—also known as *caninus muscle*; muscle that raises the angle of the mouth and draws it inward.

levator labii superioris muscle (lih-VAYT-ur LAY-bee-eye soo-peer-ee-OR-is MUS-uhl)—also known as *quadratus labii superioris muscle*; muscle that elevates the lip and dilates the nostrils, as in expressing distaste.

levator palpebrae (lih-VAYT-ur PAL-puh-bree)—muscle that raises the upper eyelid.

level (LEV-ul)—the unit of measurement used to identify the lightness or darkness of a color.

level system (LEV-ul SIS-tum)—a system colorists use to analyze the lightness or darkness of a hair color.

liability insurance (ly-uh-BIL-ih-tee in-SHUR-ans)—the act or system of insuring against personal damage.

lice (LYS)—plural of *louse*; also known as *pediculosis capitis*; any of various small wingless, usually flattened, insects that are parasitic on warm-blooded animals, once infected with lice, can be found living on the hair of human beings.

license (LYS-uns)—an official document granting permission to engage in a specified activity or to perform certain services.

lichen (LY-kun)—a type of skin lesion with solid papules.

lichenification (ly-kun-ih-fih-KAY-shun)—the process by which the skin becomes hard and leathery.

lichenoid eczema (LIK-uh-noyd EG-zuh-muh)—eczema characterized by papules on a reddened base, accompanied by a tingling and itching sensation.

life skills (LIYF SKILZ)—tools and guidelines that prepare you for living as an adult in a challenging world.

lift (LIFT)—a term used in haircoloring to indicate the lightening action of a color or lightening product on the hair's pigment; to raise or cause to raise to a higher plane or position.

lift, face (LIFT, FAYS)—also known as *rhytidectomy*; a technique used by a surgeon to lift the skin of the face to create a more youthful appearance.

ligament (LIG-uh-munt)—a strong fibrous connective tissue that connects bone to bone.

lighten (LYT-un)—in haircoloring, to make the hair color lighter.

lightener (LYT-un-ur)—chemical compounds that lighten hair by dispersing, dissolving, and decolorizing the natural hair pigment.

lightening (LYT-un-ing)—process using chemical compounds to lighten hair by dispersing, dissolving, and decolorizing the natural hair pigment.

lightening retouch (LYT-un-ing REE-tuch)—the application of a lightening agent to the hair that has grown out since the first lightening application.

light-emitting diode (LYT EE-mitt-ing DYE-ode) (LED)—a medical device used to reduce acne, increase skin circulation, and improve the collagen content in the skin.

light therapy (LYT THAIR-uh-pee)—also known as *phototherapy*; the application of light rays for treatment of disorders. May be applied to the skin for the treatment of acne, wrinkles, capillaries, pigmentation, or hair removal.

limp (LIMP)—weak; lacking firmness or strength.

line (LYN)—thin continuous mark used as a guide; can be straight or curved, horizontal, vertical, or diagonal.

line of demarcation (LYN UV dee-mar-KAY-shun)—a visible line separating colored hair from new growth; an obvious line on the face where foundation starts or stops.

lineal albicantes (LYN-ee-ul al-bih-KAN-teez)—also known as *stretch marks*; shiny white lines in the skin due to rupture of elastic fibers; often due to rapid weight loss.

linear (LIN-ee-ur)—pertaining to or resembling a line or lines; straight.

linen (LIN-un)—closely woven, heavy material used for nail wraps.

linen wraps (LIN-un RAPS)—a strengthening procedure used over nail extensions to complete a nail enhancement service.

liner brush (LYN-uhr BRUSH)—in nail art, a detail brush preferred for creating straight lines, outlining, and lettering.

liniment (LIN-uh-mint)—a medicated liquid applied to the skin to relieve sore or inflamed conditions.

linoleic acid (lin-uh-LEE-ik AS-ud)—also known as *Omega 6*, an essential fatty acid used to make important hormones; also part of the skin's lipid barrier.

lip color (LIP KUL-ur)—also known as *lipstick* or *lip gloss*; a paste-like cosmetic used to change or enhance the color of lips.

lip color sealer (LIP KUL-ur SEEL-ur)—a product used to keep lip color from seeping into fine lines around the lips.

liparotrichia (LIP-uh-roh-trik-ee-uh)—abnormal oiliness of the hair.

lip gloss (LIP GLAWS)—a product formulated to add lubricating oil to the lips. Contains many of the same ingredients as lipsticks and is packaged in a small jar or tube.

lip liner (LIP LYN-ur)—colored pencil used to outline the lips and to help keep lip color from bleeding into the small lines around the mouth.

lipectomy (lih-PEK-tuh-mee)—a surgical procedure to eliminate excessive fatty tissue.

lipid (LIP-id)—any of a large class of organic substances insoluble in water, including fats, sterols, and waxes.

lipophilic (ly-puh-FIL-ik)—having an affinity or attraction to fat and oils; oil-loving.

liposuction (ly-POH-suk-shun)—a surgical procedure used to remove stubborn areas of fat.

liquefying cream (LIK-wuh-fy-ing KREEM)—a cream that becomes liquid-like on contact with the warmth of the skin.

liquid dry cleaner (LIK-wud DRY KLEEN-ur)—a product used to clean wigs and hairpieces.

liquid-dry shampoo (LIK-wud DRY sham-POO)—liquid shampoos that evaporate quickly and do not require rinsing.

liquid gels (LIK-wud JELZ)—also known as *texturizers*; styling products that are lighter and less viscous than firm hold gels, used for easy styling, defining, and molding.

liquid tissue (LIK-wud TISH-oo)—body tissue that carries food, waste products, and hormones by means of blood and lymph.

litmus paper (LIT-mus PAYP-ur)—also known as *nitrozine paper*; strips of chemically treated paper containing coloring matter used in testing acidity or alkalinity of a product; red turns blue to indicate alkalinity, and blue turns red to indicate acidity.

liver (LIV-ur)—one of the organs which supports the excretory system by removing toxic waste products of digestion.

liver spots (LIV-ur SPAHTS)—also known as *chloasma*; flat, macular lesions presenting as increased deposits of pigment in the skin.

lobe (LOHB)—a curved or rounded projection of a body organ or part; ear lobe.

local infection (LOHK-al in-FECK-shun)—an infection, such as a pimple or abscess, that is confined to a particular part of the body and appears as a lesion containing pus.

locks (LOKZ)—also known as *dreadlocks*; separate networks of curly, textured hair that have been intertwined and meshed together.

logarithm (LAWG-uh-rith-um)—the power to which a fixed number, the base, is raised in order to produce a given number; used in calculating pH, indicating each change by one full digit equals a ten-fold change of acidity.

LOHAS (LOW-hahs)—acronym for *lifestyle of health and sustainability*; forward-thinking consumers who consider the impact on the environment and society when making purchasing decisions.

long face (LAWNG FAYS)—a face that is longer in proportion than an oval shape; a long, oval- or rectangular-shaped face.

long-layered haircut (LAWNG lay-UHRD HAYR-cut)—haircut in which the hair is cut at a 180-degree angle; the resulting shape has shorter layers at the top and increasingly longer layers toward the perimeter.

loofah (LOO-fah)—a fibrous fruit of the gourd family; used as a sponge when bathing to stimulate circulation and to remove dead surface cells from the skin.

loop rod (LUYP rahd)—also known as *circle rod;* tool that is usually about 12 inches long with a uniform diameter along the entire length of the rod, used in permanent waving.

lordosis (lor-DOH-sis)—a forward curvature of the lumbar spine.

lotion wrap (LOH-shun RAP)—application of permanent wave solution to a working panel or section of hair just prior to wrapping with rods for the purpose of presoftening resistant hair.

low elevation (LOH el-uh-VAY-shun)—haircutting technique using slight layering.

low frequency (LOH FREE-kwen-see)—in electricity, pertaining to current characterized by a low rate of oscillation.

low lighting (LOH LYT-ing)—the technique of coloring strands of hair darker than the natural color.

L

low molecular weight (LOH muh-LEK-yuh-lur WAYT)—term used in cosmetology to indicate the ability of a substance to penetrate hair or skin tissue.

low-pH waves (LOH-P-H wayves)—perms that use sulfates, sulfites, and bisulfites as an alternative to ammonium thioglycolate; they have a low pH.

lower-grit abrasives (LOH-uhr GRIT UH-bras-ifs)—boards and buffers less than 180 grit that quickly reduce the thickness of any surface.

Lucas sprayer (LOO-kus SPRAY-uhr)—atomizer designed to apply plant extracts and other ingredients to the skin.

lucid layer (LOO-sid LAY-ur)—also known as the *stratum lucidum*; the clear layer of the skin; located below the stratum corneum and above the stratum granulosum.

lucidum (LOO-sih-dum)—the clear layer of the epidermis.

lumbar plexus (LUM-bar PLEX-us)—formed from the first four lumbar nerves.

lumbar region (LUM-bar REE-jun)—the area of the back lying lateral to the vertebral column.

lumbar vertebrae (LUM-bar VUR-tuh-bree)—the bones that make up the vertebral column located in the lower part of the back; the five vertebrae associated with the lower part of the back.

lunate bone (LOO-nayt BOHN)—semilunar; a bone of the wrist.

lung (LUNG)—spongy organ composed of microscopic cells in which inhaled air is exchanged for carbon dioxide during one breathing cycle; organs of respiration.

lunula (LOO-nuh-luh)—whitish, half-moon shape at the base of the nail plate, caused by the reflection of light off the surface of the matrix.

lupus erythematosus (LOO-pus uh-rith-muh-TOH-sis)—a chronic, inflammatory autoimmune disease of the connective tissue.

lupus vulgaris (LOO-pus vul-GAIR-is)—tuberculosis of the skin.

lye (LYE)—a solution of sodium or potassium hydroxide; a strong alkali substance used in making soap and other cleansing products.

lymph (LIMF)—colorless fluid that circulates in the lymph spaces (lymphatic) of the body; carries waste and impurities away from the cells.

lymph capillaries (LIMF cap-ill-air-eez)—blind-end tubes that are the origin of lymphatic vessels.

lymph channels (LIMF CHAN-ulz)—the lymph sinuses around lymphatic glands and vessels; a lymph channel that surrounds a nerve trunk.

lymph drainage massage (LIMF DRAYN-ij muh-SAHZH)—a method of massage that works on lymph vessels and glands to eliminate watery stagnation of tissues (edema) and to stimulate the flow of body fluids.

lymph node (LIMF NOHD)—any of the gland-like bodies found in the lymphatic vessels.

lymph vessels (LIMF ves-uhl)—located in the dermis, these supply nourishment within the skin and remove waste.

lymphatic (lim-FAT-ik)—pertaining to, containing, or conveying lymph.

lymphatic blockage (lim-FAT-ik BLAHK-ij)—obstruction of lymphatic drainage.

lymphatic glands (lim-FAT-ik GLANDZ)—the glands that produce white corpuscles and filter the lymph as it passes through them.

lymphatic/immune system, (lim-FAT-ik/IH-muyn SIS-tum)—body system made up of lymph, lymph nodes, the thymus gland, the spleen, and lymph vessels. It carries waste and impurities away from the cells and protects the body from disease by developing immunities and destroying disease-causing microorganisms.

lymphocytes (LIM-foh-syts)—lymph cells that neutralize and filter away harmful bacteria and toxic substances collected in lymph.

lymphoderma (lim-fuh-DUR-muh)—a disease of the lymphatics of the skin.

lymphoid tissue (LIM-foyd TISH-oo)—tissue found in nodes, tonsils, and adenoids.

lysine (LY-seen)—an amino acid essential in nutrition to ensure growth; used to improve protein content.

M

macrofollicular (mak-roh-fah-LIK-yuh-lur)—pertaining to or having large follicles.

macronutrients (MAK-row NEW-tree-entz)—nutrients that make up the largest part of the nutrition we take in; the three basic food groups: protein, carbohydrates, and fats.

macronychia (mak-roh-NIK-ee-uh)—excessively large nails.

macule (MAK-yuhl) (plural: maculae)—flat spot or discoloration on the skin, such as a freckle or a red spot left after a pimple has healed.

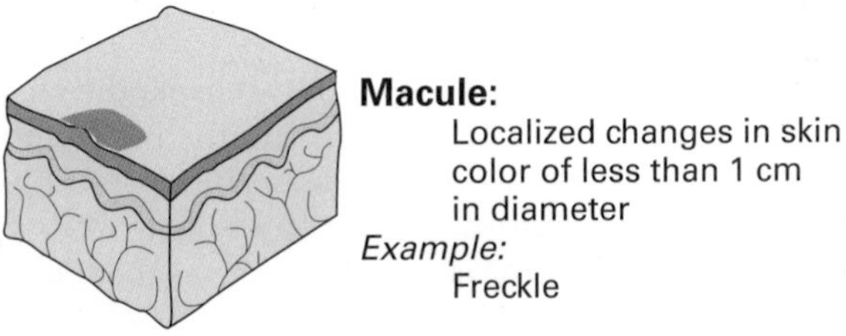

Macule:
Localized changes in skin color of less than 1 cm in diameter
Example:
Freckle

© Milady, a part of Cengage Learning

macule

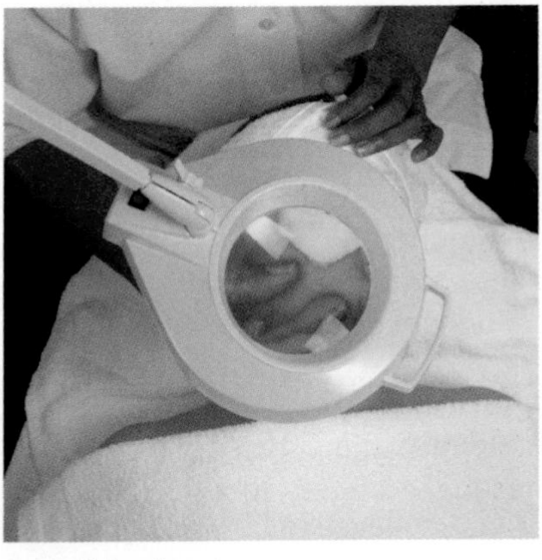

© Milady, a part of Cengage Learning. Photography by Paul Castle.

magnifying lamp

madarosis (mad-uh-ROH-sus)—loss of the eyelashes or eyebrows.

magnify (MAG-nuh-fy)—increase in fact or in appearance by placement under a microscope; increase in size by use of a mirror or lens.

magnifying lamp (MAG-nuh-fy-ing LAMP)—an apparatus with a magnifying glass and source of light; used to examine the skin or scalp.

magnum (MAG-num)—the largest bone in the distal row of the carpus located at the center of the wrist; capitate bone.

M

maintenance (MAY-ten-ance)—also known as *fill, backfill, refill,* or *rebalance*; in nail technology, term for when a nail enhancement needs to be serviced after two or more weeks from the initial application of the nail enhancement product. The maintenance service allows the professional to apply the enhancement product onto the new growth of nail, and it allows the professional to structurally correct the nail to ensure its strength, shape, and durability.

makeup (MAYK-up)—cosmetic products used to groom, color, or beautify the face.

makeup base (MAYK-up BAYS)—also known as *foundation* and *base*; a clear or colored cosmetic in liquid or cream form, applied to the face as a foundation before the application of powder and cheek color.

makeup cape (MAYK-up KAYP)—a garment made of cloth or plastic designed to be draped across the chest and shoulders of a client to protect clothing during a makeup application or other salon service.

malar (MAY-lur)—of or pertaining to the cheek; the cheekbone.

malassezia (mal-uh-SEEZ-ee-uh)—naturally occurring fungus that is present on all human skin, but is responsible for dandruff when it grows out of control.

malformation (mal-for-MAY-shun)—an abnormal or badly formed shape or structure.

malignant (muh-LIG-nent)—a growth or condition endangering health; not benign.

malignant melanoma (muh-LIG-nent mel-ahn-OH-ma)—most serious form of skin cancer; often characterized by black or dark brown patches on the skin that may appear uneven in texture, jagged, or raised.

malnutrition (mal-noo-TRISH-un)—poor nutrition resulting from inadequate consumption of nutrients.

malpighian layer (mal-PIG-ee-un LAY-ur)—also known as *stratum mucosum, stratum germinativum* or *basal layer*; the deepest layer of the epidermis.

M

malpractice (mal-PRAK-tis)—in cosmetology, the negligent or improper treatment of a client while performing a service.

mammoplasty (MAYM-oh-plas-tee)—surgery to alter the shape or contours of the breast.

mandible (MAN-duh-bul)—the lower jaw bone; largest and strongest bone of the face.

mandibular nerve (man-DIB-yuh-lur NURV)—branch of the fifth cranial nerve that affects the muscles of the chin, lower lip, and external ear.

manicure (MAN-ih-kyoor)—the artful treatment and care of the hands and nails.

manicure bowl (MAN-ih-kyoor BOHL)—a vessel shaped to fit the hand and fingers; warm, sudsy, water is placed in the bowl and the fingers are allowed to soak so that the cuticles are softened before treatment.

manicure chair (MAN-ih-kyoor CHAYR)—a chair designed to allow the manicurist to sit comfortably during the manicure treatment.

manicure implements (MAN-ih-kyoor IM-pluh-ments)—the tools or equipment used for the manicuring procedure such as nail file, cuticle pusher, cuticle scissor, cuticle nipper, emery board, and buffer.

manicure kit (MAN-ih-kyoor KIT)—a case or kit designed to carry the implements, equipment, and supplies used for the manicure procedure.

manicure lamp (MAN-ih-kyoor LAMP)—a flexible light fixture attached to the manicure table to provide adequate light during the manicure.

manicure oil heater (MAN-ih-kyoor OYL HEET-ur)—a thermostatically controlled electric heating cup used to heat the oil or cream used on the hands and nails during the manicure treatment.

manicure table (MAN-ih-kyoor TAY-bul)—a small table especially designed for the manicure treatment.

manicurist (MAN-ih-kyoor-ist)—also known as *nail technician*; one who professionally attends to the care of the hands and nails.

mannequin (MAN-ih-kun)—also known as *manikin*; in cosmetology, a model of the human head manufactured with hair to be used for practice work; in fashion, a model of a human figure used for display purposes.

mannequin case (MAN-ih-kun KAYS)—a box-like carrying case designed to hold the mannequin head and holder.

mannequin holder (MAN-ih-kun HOHL-dur)—a clamp-like implement designed to be used to secure a mannequin head to a tabletop while it is in use.

mannequin, slip-on (MAN-ih-kun, SLIP-awn)—a glove-like mannequin form that can be slipped over another mannequin head to allow more varied practice routines.

mantle (MAN-tul)—also known as *nail mantle*; the deep fold of the skin into which the nail root is lodged.

manual lymph drainage (MLD) (MAN-yoo-ul LIMF drayn-IHJE)—gentle, rhythmic pressure on the lymphatic system to detoxify and remove waste materials from the body more quickly; reduces swelling and is used before and after surgery for pre- and post-op care.

manus (MAN-us); pl., mani (MAN-ee)—the hand.

marbleizer (MAR-bul-yz-uhr)—also known as *stylus*; in nail technology, a tool with wooden handles and a rounded ball tip that can range in size and is excellent for dotting small circles of color on a nail.

marbleizing (MAR-bul-yz-ing)—in haircoloring, intertwining sections of light and dark shades of hair on one head; in nail technology, a swirled effect when you combine two or more colors together when wet and mix them on the nail with a marbleizing tool known as a stylus.

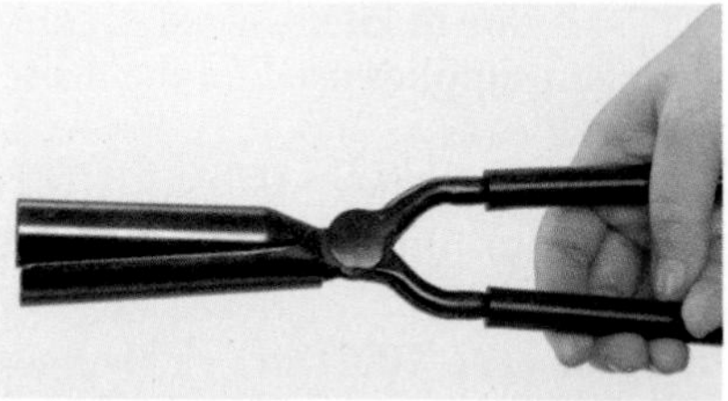

© Milady, a part of Cengage Learning. Photography by Paul Castle.

Marcel iron

Marcel irons (mar-SEL EYE-urnz)—a curling (thermal) iron with a rod and groove attached to a handle that opens and closes; the iron is heated and strands of hair are placed between the rod and groove to create curls or waves.

Marcel wave (mar-SEL WAYV)—a wave resembling a natural hair wave produced by a thermal iron either electrically heated or stove heated using special manipulative techniques; originated by Francois Marcel, a French hairdresser.

marginal blepharitis (MAR-jin-ul blef-uh-RY-tus)—inflammation of the sebaceous glands and hair follicles that line the margins of the eyelids.

marginal mandibular nerve (MAR-jin-ul MAN-dib-yoo-lar NURV)—branch of the seventh cranial nerve that affects the muscles of the chin and lower lip.

marketing (MAR-KET-ing)—a strategy for how goods and services are bought, sold, or exchanged.

M

marrow (MAYR-oh)—connective tissue filling in the cavities of bones which forms red and white blood cells.

mascara (mas-KAIR-uh)—cosmetic preparation used to darken, define, and thicken the eyelashes.

masks (MASKS)—also known as *masques* or *packs*; concentrated treatment products often composed of mineral clays, moisturizing agents, skin softeners, aromatherapy oils, beneficial extracts, and other beneficial ingredients to cleanse, exfoliate, tighten, tone, hydrate, and nourish the skin.

masotherapy (mas-oh-THAIR-uh-pee)—the treatment of the body by massage.

mass (MAS)—a quantity of matter in any given body, relatively large in size with no particular shape.

massage (muh-SAHZH)—manual or mechanical manipulation of the body by rubbing, gently pinching, kneading, tapping, and other movements to increase metabolism and circulation, promote absorption, and relieve pain.

massage compression (muh-SAHZH kahm-PRESH-un)—pressure used in massage movements.

massage creams (muh-SAHZH KREEMZ)—also known as *tissue cream* or *nourishing cream*; lubricants used to make the skin slippery during massage.

massage movement direction (muh-SAHZH MOOV-ment dih-REK-shun)—in massage, the direction of movement toward the origin of a muscle in order to avoid damage to muscular tissue.

massage movements (muh-SAHZH MOOV-ments)—specific movements used in facial and body massage; basic movements include friction, joint, percussion, petrissage, stroking, and vibration.

massage therapist (muh-SAHZH THAIR-uh-pist)—a professionally trained massage practitioner.

masseter (muh-SEET-ur)—also known as *chewing muscles*; muscles that coordinate with the temporalis, medial pterygoid, and lateral pterygoid muscles to open and close the mouth and bring the jaw forward.

masseteric artery (mas-uh-TAIR-ik ART-uh-ree)—the artery supplying blood to the muscles of the jaw (masseter).

masseteric nerve (mas-uh-TAIR-ik NURV)—a nerve in the face supplying the masseter muscle.

masseur (muh-SUR); fem., masseuse (muh-SOOZ)—one who practices or gives massage.

masticate (MAS-tih-kayt)—to chew or grind food with the teeth.

mastoid process (MAS-toyd PRAH-ses)—a conical projection of the temporal bone.

material safety data sheet (MSDS) (muh-TEE-ree-uhl SAYF-tee DAY-tuh SHEETS)—information compiled by the manufacturer about product safety, including the names of hazardous ingredients, safe handling and use procedures, precautions to reduce the risk of accidental harm or overexposure, and flammability warnings.

matrix (MAY-triks)—area where the nail plate cells are formed; this area is composed of matrix cells that produce the nail plate.

matte (MAT)—nonshiny; dull.

matter (MAT-ur)—any substance that occupies space and has mass (weight).

matting (MAT-ing)—also known as *teasing*, *ratting*, or *backcombing*; tangling the hair into a thick mass; another term for back-combing.

maturation (match-urAY-shun)—in skin care, the ripening or coming to a head of a pimple or other blemish.

maturity (muh-CHOOR-ih-tee)—the quality of being responsible, self-disciplined, and well-adjusted; fully developed.

maxillae pl. (mak-SIL-uh)—bones of the jaw.

maxillary artery (MAK-suh-lair-ee ART-uh-ree)—artery that supplies blood to the lower regions of the face.

maxillary nerves (MAK-suh-lair-ee NURVZ)—branch of the fifth cranial nerve that supplies impulses to the upper part of the face.

mechanical (muh-KAN-ih-kul)—relating to a machine; performed by means of some apparatus; not manual.

mechanical exfoliation (muh-KAN-ih-kul EX-foly-ay-shun)—physical method of rubbing dead cells off of the skin.

medial; median (MEE-dee-ul; MEE-dee-un)—pertaining to the middle.

medial pterygoid (MEE-dee-ul THER-ih-goyd)—also known as *chewing muscles*; muscles that coordinate with the masseter, temporalis, and lateral pterygoid muscles to open and close the mouth and bring the jaw forward.

median nerve (MEE-dee-un NURV)—sensory-motor nerve, smaller than the ulnar and radial nerves that, with its branches, supplies the arm and hand.

medical aesthetics (MED-ih-kul ESS-thet-icks)—also known as *medical esthetics*; the integration of surgical procedures and esthetic treatments.

M

medical nail technician (MNT) (MED-ih-kul NAYL teck-NISH-un)—a salon-based nail technician who has completed advanced training in how to work safely with at-risk clients or patients of podiatrists.

medicamentosus (med-ih-kuh-men-TOH-sus)—a skin eruption caused by a drug.

medicated ingredient (MED-ih-kayt-ud in-GREE-dee-ent)—a substance added to cosmetics to promote healing.

medicated scalp lotion (MED-ih-kayt-ed SKALP LOW-shun)—conditioner that promotes healing of the scalp.

medicated shampoo (MED-ih-kayt-ed sham-POO)—shampoo containing special chemicals or drugs that are very effective in reducing dandruff or relieving other scalp conditions.

medium elevation (MEE-dee-um el-uh-VAY-shun)—a term used in hair dressing to indicate hair held at approximately a 45° angle to the head while it is being cut.

medium-grit abrasives (MEE-dee-um GRIT uh-bray-siffs)—180 to 240 grit abrasives that are used to smooth and refine surfaces and shorten natural nails.

medium hair (MEE-dee-um HAYR)—a hair fiber neither especially large nor small in circumference, but of a thickness about halfway between fine and coarse.

medium press (MEE-dee-um PRES)—technique that removes 60 to 75 percent of the curl by applying a thermal pressing comb once on each side of the hair, using slightly more pressure than in the soft press.

medius (MEE-dee-us)—the middle finger.

medulla (muh-DUL-uh)—also known as *pith* or *core*; innermost layer of the hair.

medulla oblongata (muh-DUL-uh ob-lawng-GAY-tuh)—the lowest or posterior part of the brain continuous with the spinal cord.

medullary space (MED-yoo-lair-ee SPAYS)—the cavity through the shaft of the long bones.

megalonychosis (meg-uh-lon-ih-KOH-sus)—non-inflammatory hypertrophy (thickening) of the nails.

melanin (MEL-uh-nin)—tiny grains of pigment (coloring matter) that are produced by melanocytes and deposited into cells in the stratum germinativum layer of the epidermis and in the papillary layers of the dermis. There are two types of melanin: pheomelanin, which is red to yellow in color, and eumelanin, which is dark brown to black.

melanism (MEL-uh-niz-um)—excessive pigmentation of the hair, skin, eyes, tissues, or organs.

melanochroi (mel-uh-NAHK-ruh-wy)—a term used to describe the very fair skin and very dark hair of Caucasians.

melanocyte (muh-LAN-uh-syt)—cells that produce skin pigment granules in the basal layer.

melanocytic nevi (mel-uh-noh-SIT-ik NEE-vye)—also known as *mole*; brown spots sometimes having hair growing from them.

melanocytoma (mel-uh-noh-sy-TOH-muh)—a benign, heavily pigmented tumor.

melanoderma (mel-uh-noh-DUR-muh)—also known as *dark spots* or *skin spots*; abnormal darkening of the skin, usually in patches caused by accumulation or deposits of melanin.

melanodermatitis (mel-uh-noh-DUR-muh-TY-tis)—an inflamed skin condition characterized by increased skin pigmentation.

melanogenesis (mel-uh-noh-JEN-uh-sis)—the formation of melanin.

melanoid (MEL-uh-noyd)—having dark pigment.

melanoma (mel-uh-NOH-muh)—a black or dark brown pigmented tumor.

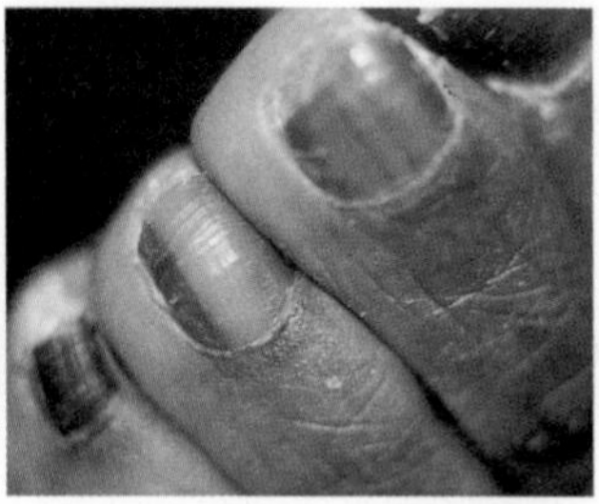

Courtesy of Godfrey F. Mix, DPM, Sacramento, CA.

melanonychia

melanonychia (mel-uh-nuh-NIK-ee-uh)—significant darkening of the fingernails or toenails; may be seen as a black band within the nail plate, extending from the base to the free edge.

melanoprotein (mel-uh-noh-PROH-teen)—a protein complex containing melanin.

melanosis (mel-uh-NOH-sis)—a condition in that pigment is deposited in the skin or other tissues.

melanosome (MEL-uh-noh-sohm)—pigment granules that produce the complex protein melanin.

melanotic sarcoma (mel-uh-NAHT-ik sar-KOH-muh)—a fatal skin cancer that starts with a mole.

melasma (mel-AZ-muh)—also known as *pregnancy mask* or *chloasma gravidarum*; skin condition that is triggered by hormones that causes darker pigmentation in areas such as on the upper lip and around the eyes and cheeks.

membrane (MEM-brayn)—a thin sheet or layer of pliable tissue surrounding a part, separating adjacent cavities, lining a cavity, or connecting adjacent structures.

meningitis (men-in-JEYE-tus)—a serious and often deadly disease in which an outside layer of the brain or spinal cord becomes infected and swollen.

Mehndhi makeup (men-dee MAYK-up)—the art of decorating the body with henna.

mental artery (MEN-tul ART-uh-ree)—artery that supplies blood to the lower lip and the chin.

mentalis muscle (men-TAY-lis MUS-uhl)—muscle that elevates the lower lip and raises and wrinkles the skin of the chin.

mental nerve (MEN-tul NURV)—affects the skin of the lower lip and chin.

menthyl salicylate (MEN-thil suh-LIS-ih-layt)—an organic compound that is used as a filtering agent in sunburn preventives; produces an even tan by removing the majority of the ultraviolet rays.

mentoplasty (MEN-toh-plas-tee)—chin surgery involving a small incision made inside the mouth or just underneath and behind the most prominent part of the chin to change a person's profile by building up a small chin.

merchandising (MER-chen-dyz-ing)—how retail products are arranged and displayed in your salon.

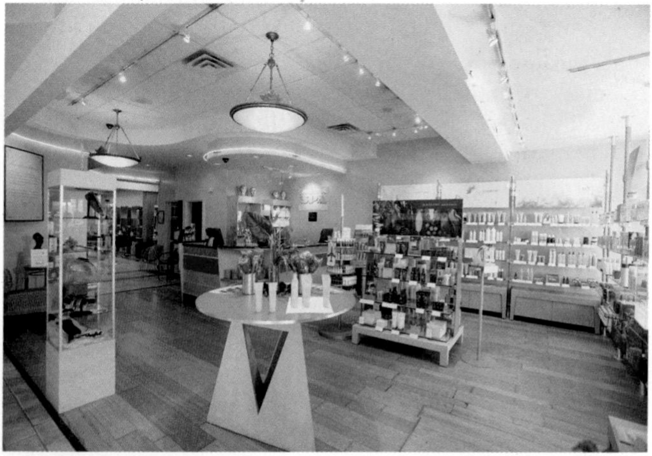

© Milady, a part of Cengage Learning. Photography by Dino Petrocelli.

merchandising

mercurochrome (mur-KYUR-uh-krohm)—a germicide, 3 to 5 percent solution of iodine, used for cuts.

mesh (MESH)—an open-weave foundation used to attach hair in a hairpiece; a wig foundation or base made of a net material.

mesoderm (MES-oh-durm)—middle layer of cells of the skin.

mesomorph (MES-uh-morf)—a body type characterized by a sturdy body structure and great strength.

mesorrhine (MES-uh-ryn)—pertaining to a broad, high-bridged nose.

M

mesothelium (mes-uh-THEE-lee-um)—smooth tissue that allows the movement of organs to take place with little or no friction.

metabolism (muh-TAB-uh-liz-um)—chemical process that takes place in living organisms through which the cells are nourished and carry out their activities.

metacarpal (met-uh-KAR-pul)—pertaining to the long, slender bones of the palm of the hand.

metacarpal, dorsal (met-uh-KAR-pul, DOR-sul)—the vein that draws blood from the back of the hand.

metacarpal, palmar (met-uh-KAR-pul, PAHL-mur)—the main vein that draws blood from the palm of the hand.

metacarpus (met-uh-KAR-pus)—the bones of the palm of the hand; the part of the hand containing five bones between the carpus and phalanges.

metal hydroxide relaxers (muh-TAL HY-drox-ide re-LAX-ors)—ionic compounds formed by a metal (sodium, potassium, or lithium), which is combined with oxygen and hydrogen.

metal pusher (muh-TAL PUSH-uhr)—a reusable implement, made of stainless steel; used to push back the eponychium but can also be used to gently scrape cuticle tissue from the natural nail plate.

metallic haircolors (muh-TAL-ik HAYR KULL-ehrz)—also known as *gradual haircolors*; haircolors containing metal salts that change hair color gradually by progressive buildup and exposure to air creating a dull, metallic appearance.

metallic salts (muh-TAL-ik SAHLTS)—a compound of a base and an acid.

metastasis (muh-TAS-tuh-sus)—the migration or transference of a disease from one site in the body to another by the conveyance of cells in blood vessels or lymph channels.

metatarsal (met-uh-TAR-sull)—one of three subdivisions of the foot; long and slender bones, like the metacarpal bones of the hand.

M

metatarsus (met-uh-TAR-sus)—the bones that make up the instep of the foot; the part of the foot between the phalanges and the tarsus containing five bones.

meter (MEE-tur)—an instrument for measuring the strength of an electric current in amperes; the basic metric unit of length equal to 39.37 inches.

methacrylate (METH-ACK-ruh-late)—a type of acrylic monomer (cross-linking) that has very good adhesion to the natural nail plate and polymerizes in minutes; used to make all liquid/powder systems and at least one type of UV gel.

methicillin-resistant staphylococcus aureus (MRSA) (METH-eh-sill-en-ree-ZIST-ent staf-uh-loh-KOK-us-OR-ee-us)—a type of infectious bacteria that is highly resistant to conventional treatments such as antibiotics.

methyl methacrylate monomer (MMA) (METH-ul METH-ACK-ruh-late MON-uh-mer)—a substance in wide use around the world for many applications, such as bone repair cement for implantation into the body.

methylparaben (METH-ul-para-bin)—one of the most frequently used preservatives because of its very low sensitizing potential; combats bacteria and molds; noncomedogenic.

metric system (MET-rik SIS-tum)—a decimal system of weights and measures based on the gram from which measures of weights and mass are derived, and the meter from which measures of area, length, and volume are derived.

mica (MY-kuh)—a mineral occurring in the form of thin, shining, transparent plates.

micro (MY-kroh)—a prefix denoting very small; slight; millionth part of.

microbicide (my-KROH-bih-syd)—an agent that destroys microbes.

microbraids (mi-kroh-braydz)—also known as *minibraids*; thin strands of hair woven to form small braids.

microcirculation (my-kroh-sur-kyoo-LAY-shun)—pertaining to the microvasculature; circulation of blood in the body's system of five vessels, 100 microns or less in diameter.

microcurrent (mi-kroh-CUR-ent)—an extremely low level of electricity that mirrors the body's natural electrical impulses.

microcurrent device (mi-kroh-CUR-ent dee-VICE)—a device that mimics the body's natural electrical energy to reeducate and tone facial muscles; improves circulation and increases collagen and elastin production.

microdermabrasion (MI-kroh-DERMA-bray-shun)—mechanical exfoliation that involves pressurized delivery of aluminum oxide or other crystals to the skin with a handheld device that also uses vacuum and suction to exfoliate the skin.

microdermabrasion scrubs (MI-kroh-DERMA-bray-shun SK-RUBZ)—scrubs used in microdermabrasion treatments, may or may not contain aluminum oxide crystals.

microfollicular (my-kroh-fah-LIK-yoo-lur)—characterized by very small follicles.

micronutrients (MY-kroh-new-tree-ents)—nutrients required by humans and other living things throughout life in small quantities to orchestrate a whole range of physiological functions, but which the organism itself cannot produce.

micronychia (my-kroh-NIK-ee-uh)—the presence of abnormally small fingernails or toenails.

microorganism (mi-kroh-ORGAN-iz-um)—also known as *microbe*; any organism of microscopic or submicroscopic size.

microscope (MY-kruh-skohp)—an instrument for enlarging views of minute objects.

microscopic (mi-kroh-SKAHP-ik)—extremely small; visible only with the aid of a microscope; not visible to the naked eye.

microshattering (MY-kroh-shat-ter-ing)—tiny cracks in nail enhancements as they age with wear and become brittle; can also be caused by aggressive filing with or without an electric file.

microtrauma (MI-kroh-tro-mah)—the act of causing tiny unseen openings in the skin that can allow entry by pathogenic microbes.

middle temporal artery (MID-ul TEM-puh-rul ART-uh-ree)—the artery that supplies blood to the temporal muscles.

midfrontal (mid-FRUN-tul)—pertaining to the middle of the forehead.

mildew (MIL-doo)—a type of fungus that affects plants or grows on inanimate objects, but does not cause human infections in the salon.

milia (MIL-ee-ah)—epidermal cysts; small, firm papules with no visible opening; whitish, pearl-like masses of sebum and dead cells under the skin. Milia are more common in dry skin types and may form after skin trauma, such as a laser resurfacing.

miliaria (mil-ee-AIR-ee-ah)—an eruption of minute vesicles due to retention of fluid at the mouths of the sweat follicles.

miliaria profunda (mil-ee-AIR-ee-ah proh-FUN-dah)—a skin reaction in the sweat retention syndrome, characterized by papules located at the sweat pores.

miliaria rubra (mil-ee-AIR-ee-ah ROOB-rah)—also known as *prickly heat*; an acute inflammatory disorder of the sweat glands, characterized by the eruption of small red vesicles and accompanied by burning, itching skin.

miliary fever (MIL-ee-air-ee FEE-vur)—sweating sickness; an infectious disease characterized by fever, profuse sweating, and the production of papular vesicular and other eruptions.

milium (MIL-ee-um); pl., milia (MIL-ee-uh)—a small, whitish pear-like mass in the epidermis due to retention of sebum; a whitehead.

milliameter (mil-ee-AM-uh-tur)—an instrument that registers electric current in milliamperes; used to measure the amount of current required for a given treatment.

mind-mapping (MYND MAP-ing)—a graphic representation of an idea or problem that helps to organize one's thoughts.

mineral (MIN-ur-ul)—any inorganic material found in the earth's crust.

mineral makeup (MIN-ur-ul MAYK-up)—contains nonbacterial, finely ground particles from the earth; contains fewer chemicals and dyes than most traditional makeup; most are talc-free and less likely to cause allergic reactions.

mineral oil (MIN-ur-ul OYL)—white oil; oil found in the rock strata of the earth; a colorless, tasteless oil derived from petroleum; used in creams, lotions, moisturizing products, powders, lip and eye makeup, hairdressings, and many other cosmetics; it is a widely used cosmetic lubricant and binder.

minibraid (MIH-nee-brayd)—also known as *microbraid*; thin strands of hair woven to form small braids; type of hair extensions.

minifall (MIH-nee-fawl)—a loose-hanging hairpiece (shorter than a regular fall) attached at the crown.

mini-shears (MIH-nee-sheerz)—small scissors used to cut and layer hair in small graduations.

Minoxidil (MIN-ox-ih-dil)—topical medication used to promote hair growth or reduce hair loss.

minute (my-NOOT)—very small; tiny.

miscible (MIS-uh-bul)—liquids that are mutually soluble, meaning that they can be mixed together to form stable solutions.

mission statement (MISH-uhn STATE-ment)—a statement that establishes the values that an individual or institution lives by, as well as future goals.

mitosis (my-TOH-sis)—usual process of cell reproduction of human tissues that occurs when the cell divides into two identical cells called *daughter cells*.

mitral valve (MY-trill VALV)—also known as *bicuspid valve*; the valve between the left atrium and the left ventricle of the heart.

mixed media (MICKST MEE-dee-ah)—description used for nail art when more than one nail art medium is used to create the design.

mixed melanin (MIKST MEL-uh-nin)—combination of natural hair color that contains both pheomelanin and eumelanin.

mixed nerves (MIKST NURVZ)—nerves that contain both sensory and motor fibers, and have the ability to send and receive messages.

mixture (MIKS-chur)—a preparation made by incorporating an insoluble ingredient in a liquid vehicle; sometimes used to identify an aqueous solution containing two or more solutes; a combination of two or more substances that are not chemically united.

mnemonics (NEW-mon-icks)—any memorization technique that helps a person to recall information.

mobility (moh-BIL-ih-tee)—the quality of being movable.

modalities (MOH-dal-ih-tees)—the specific measures of electricity used in electrical facial and scalp treatments.

modelage masks (MAHD-ul-ahj MASKZ)—also known as *thermal masks*; thermal heat masks.

moderate porosity (MAHD-ur-ut por-AHS-ih-tee)—category of normal hair in which the cuticle is close to the hair shaft.

modifier (MAHD-ih-fy-ur)—anything that will change the form or characteristics of an object or substance; a chemical found as an ingredient in permanent haircolors whose function is to alter the dye intermediates.

moist (MOYST)—slightly wet; damp.

moist heat packs (MOYST HEET PAKS)—chemical gel packs that are heated in a water bath, wrapped in a terry cover, and placed on the body.

moisture (MOYST-yur)—water or other liquid spread in very small drops in the air or on a surface.

moisture gradient (MOYST-yur GRAY-dee-unt)—the amount of moisture in the skin or hair.

moisturizer (MOYST-yur-yz-ur)—a product formulated to add moisture to dry skin or hair; to promote the retention of moisture.

mold (MOHLD)—a superficial growth produced especially on damp or decaying organic matter or on living organisms by a fungus.

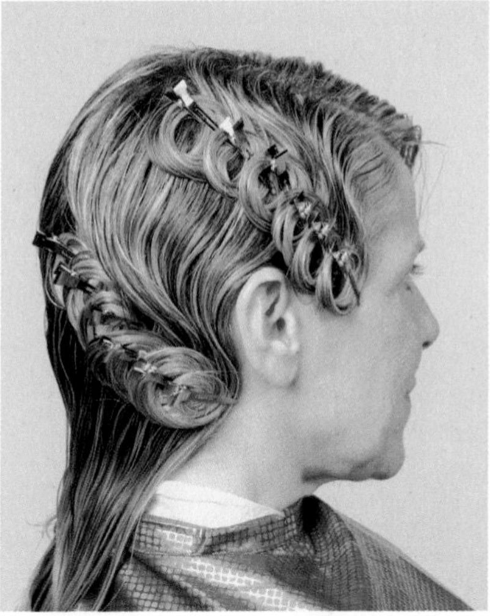

© Milady, a part of Cengage Learning. Photography by Yanik Chauvin.

molded curl

molded curl (MOHLD-ud KURL)—also known as *sculptured curls* or *carved curls*; pin curls sliced from a shaping and formed without lifting the hair from the head.

molding (MOHLD-ing)—the act of forming or directing hair into a desired pattern.

mole (MOHL)—small, brownish, spot or blemish on the skin, ranging in color from pale tan to brown or bluish black.

molecular attraction (muh-LEK-yuh-lur uh-TRAK-shun)—the force exerted between two unlike molecules tending to draw them together and to resist separation.

molecular breakdown (muh-LEK-yuh-lur BRAYK-down)—the disrupting or disuniting of a molecular unit.

molecular weight (muh-LEK-yuh-lur WAYT)—the sum of the weights of the atoms of a molecule.

molecule (MAHL-uh-kyool)—a chemical combination of two or more atoms in definite (fixed) proportions.

molluscum (mah-LUS-kum)—a skin disease having soft, dome-shaped nodules.

molluscum fibrosum (mah-LUS-kum fy-BROH-sum)—a cutaneous tumor of the dermis, characterized by fibrous papules.

monilethrix (mah-NIL-ee-thriks)—technical term for beaded hair.

monochromatic (mahn-uh-kroh-MAT-ik)—consisting of one color or color family; displaying shades and tints of the same color.

monochromatism (mahn-uh-KROH-muh-tiz-um)—total color blindness.

monosaccharides (mahn-uh-SACK-uhr-ides)—carbohydrates made up of one basic sugar unit.

monomer liquid (MAHN-oh-mur LICK-wid)—chemical liquid mixed with polymer powder to form the sculptured nail enhancement.

monomer liquid and polymer powder nail enhancements (MAHN-oh-mur LICK-wid AND PAHL-imer POW-der NAYL EN-HANZ-mentz)—also known as *acrylic nails*, or *sculptured nails*; nail enhancements created by combining monomer liquid and polymer powder.

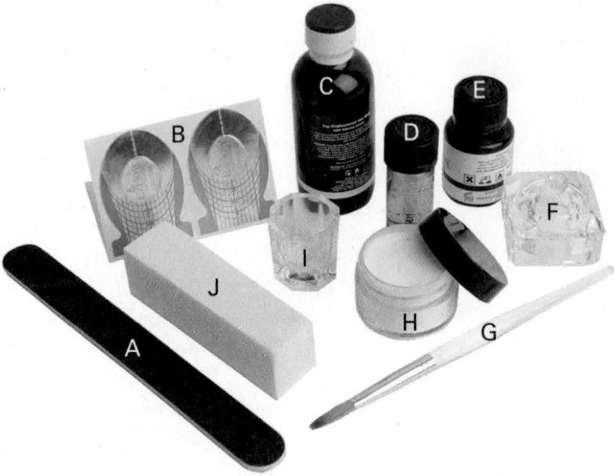

© Milady, a part of Cengage Learning. Photography by Dino Petrocelli.

Products used in monomer liquid and polymer powder nail enhancements: (a) medium-grit nail abrasive; (b) nail forms; (c) monomer liquid; (d) nail primer; (e) nail dehydrator; (f) dappen dish for polymer powder; (g) application brush; (h) polymer powder; (i) dappen dish for monomer liquid; and (j) buffer.

monomers (MAHN-oh-murs)—unit called a *molecule*.

moons (MOONZ)—crescent-shaped areas at the base of the fingernails.

morphology (mor-FAHL-uh-jee)—the branch of biology that deals with structure and form; it includes anatomy, histology, and cytology of the organism at any stage of its life history.

M

motile (MOH-tul)—having the power of movement, as do certain bacteria.

motility (MOH-till-it-ee)—self-movement.

motivation (MOW-tih-vay-shun)—a desire for change.

motor (MOH-tur)—of or relating to muscular movement.

motor nerve fibers (MOH-tur NURVZ FY-burz)—fibers of the motor nerves that are distributed to the arrector pili muscles attached to hair follicles. Motor nerves carry impulses from the brain to the muscles.

motor nerves (MOH-tur NURVZ)—also known as *efferent nerves*; carry impulses from the brain to the muscles or glands. These transmitted impulses produce movement.

motor neuron (MOH-tur NUHR-ahn)—carries nerve impulses from the brain to the effectors.

motor oculi (MOH-tur AHK-yoo-ly)—also known as *third cranial nerve*; the nerve controlling most of the eye muscles.

motor point (MOH-tur POYNT)—point on the skin over the muscle where pressure or stimulation will cause contraction of that muscle.

motor units (MOH-tur YOO-nits)—muscle neurons and all the muscle fibers they control.

mousse (MOOS)—a light, airy, whipped hair styling and sculpturing product resembling shaving foam.

movement (MOOV-ment)—the change of place or position of hair; the rhythmic quality or motion of hair.

mucopolysaccharides (MYOO-koh-poly-sack-uhr-ides)—carbohydrate–lipid complexes that are also good water binders.

mucosa (myoo-KOH-suh)—mucous membrane.

mucosum, stratum (myoo-KOH-sum, STRAY-tum)—mucous or malpighian layer of the skin.

mucus (MYOO-kus)—a thick, slippery secretion produced by the mucous membranes to lubricate and cleanse.

mudpack (MUD-pak)—a thick, spreadable product, usually containing clay; used for facial and body treatments.

multicellular (mul-tih-SEL-yoo-lur)—having many cells.

multicolor (mul-tih-KUL-ur)—having many colors.

multidimensional (mul-tih-dih-MEN-shun-ul)—having several dimensions.

multidirectional (mul-tih-dih-REK-shun-ul)—extending in many directions.

multilayered (mul-tih-LAY-urd)—having several layers.

multiuse (mul-tih-YUS)—also known as *reusable*; items that can be cleaned, disinfected, and used on more than one person, even if the item is accidentally exposed to blood or body fluid.

muscle-bound (MUS-uhl-bownd)—having tight, inflexible muscles.

muscle energy technique (MUS-uhl EN-ur-jee tek-NEEK)—technique utilizing neurophysiological muscle reflexes to improve functional mobility of joints.

muscle fatigue (MUS-uhl fuh-TEEG)—cessation of muscle response due to oxygen deprivation from rapid or prolonged muscle contractions.

muscle insertion (MUS-uhl in-SUR-shun)—the distal point of muscle attachment.

muscle origin (MUS-uhl OR-ih-jin)—the proximal point of muscle attachment.

muscle spasm (MUS-uhl SPAZ-um)—a sudden, involuntary contraction of muscles.

muscle strains (MUS-uhl STRAYNZ)—torn or pulled muscles; most common injury to muscles.

muscle strapping (MUS-uhl STRAP-ing)—a heavy massage treatment used to reduce fatty deposits.

muscle tone (MUS-uhl TOHN)—the normal degree of tension in a healthy muscle, even at rest.

muscle tissue (MUS-uhl TISH-yoo)—tissue that contracts and moves various parts of the body.

muscles (MUS-uhlz)—fibrous tissues that have the ability to stretch, contract, and produce all body movements.

muscular (MUS-kyuh-lur)—relating to a muscle or the muscles.

muscular system (MUS-kyuh-lur SIS-tum)—body system that covers, shapes, and holds the skeleton system in place; muscular system contracts and moves various parts of the body.

muscular tissue (MUS-kyuh-lur TISH-oo)—contracts and moves various parts of the body.

musculi colli (MUS-kyoo-ly KOH-lih)—the anterior muscles of the neck.

musculi dorsi (MUS-kyoo-ly DOR-see)—the muscles of the back.

muslin (MUZ-lin)—used in waxing; any of several plain-weave cotton fabrics of varying fineness, used to remove unwanted hair.

mustache (MUS-tash)—the growth of hair on the upper lip.

mustache brush (MUS-tash BRUSH)—a small brush designed to groom the mustache.

mustache comb (MUS-tash KOHM)—a small comb with fine teeth designed to groom the mustache.

mutation (myoo-TAY-shun)—a change as in quality, form, or nature.

myalgia (my-AL-jee-uh)—pain in the muscles.

myasthenia (my-us-THEE-nee-uh)—muscular weakness.

mycetoma (my-suh-TOH-mah)—any disease or infection caused by actinomycetes or fungus.

mycobacterium fortuitum (MY-CO-bac-tear-ee-um for-TWO-it-uhm)—a microscopic germ that normally exists in tap water in small numbers.

myocardial infarction (my-oh-KAR-dee-uhl in-FARK-shun)—also known as *heart attack*; result of a reduced blood flow in the coronary arteries supplying the heart muscle with adequate oxygen.

myocardium (my-oh-KAR-dee-um)—cardiac muscle.

myodystrophy (my-uh-DIS-truh-fee)—degeneration of muscles.

myoedema (my-oh-eh-DEE-muh)—edema (swelling) of a muscle.

myofibrils (my-oh-FYB-rulz)—muscle fibers containing filaments; give muscles their contractible ability.

myofibrosis (my-oh-FYB-roh-sis)—condition characterized by the replacement of muscle tissue by fibrous tissue with a consequent reduction in muscle function.

myology (my-AHL-uh-jee)—study of the nature, structure, function, and diseases of the muscles.

myomalacia (my-oh-muh-LAY-shee-ah)—degeneration with softening of muscle tissue.

myoneural (my-oh-NOO-ral)—relating to nerve endings in muscle tissue.

myopalmus (my-oh-PAL-mus)—twitching and quivering of muscles.

myopathic (my-oh-PATH-ik)—pertaining to disease of the muscles.

myoplasty (MY-oh-plas-tee)—plastic surgery on a muscle or group of muscles.

myosin (MY-oh-sin)—muscular filament; gives contractile ability.

myositis (my-oh-SY-tis)—inflammation of muscle tissue.

myotasis (MY-ot-uh-sis)—stretching and extending of muscle.

myotrophy (MY-ot-ruh-fee)—nutrition of the muscles.

N

naevus; nevus (NEE-vus); pl., naevi, nevi (NEE-vy)—a birthmark; a congenital skin blemish caused by abnormal pigmentation or dilated capillaries.

nail (NAYL)—an appendage of the skin; horny protective plate at the end of the finger or toe.

nail art competitions (NAYL ART COM-puh-tish-uhns)—opportunities for licensed professionals or nail students to compete in a specified category where the art and theme of the nails are part of the judging criteria.

nail bed (NAYL BED)—portion of the living skin that supports the nail plate as it grows toward the free edge.

nail biting (NAYL BYT-ing)—also known as *onychophagia*; the habit of biting off the tips of the nails to the nail bed.

nail bleach (NAYL BLEECH)—a product used in manicuring to remove stains and to whiten the nails.

nail body (NAYL BAHD-ee)—the horny nail plate resting on and attached to the nail bed.

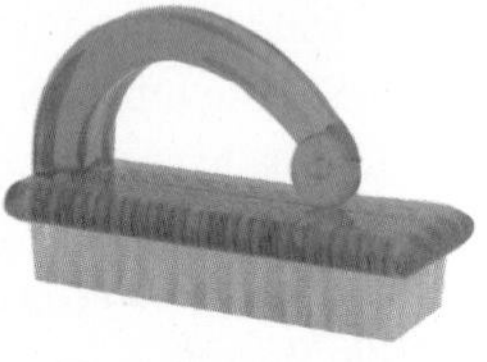

© Milady, a part of Cengage Learning. Photography by Dino Petrocelli.

nail brush

nail brush (NAYL BRUSH)—a small brush used to clean under and around the nails.

nail buffer (NAYL BUF-ur)—an instrument made of leather or chamois; used with a polishing powder to polish the nails to a high luster.

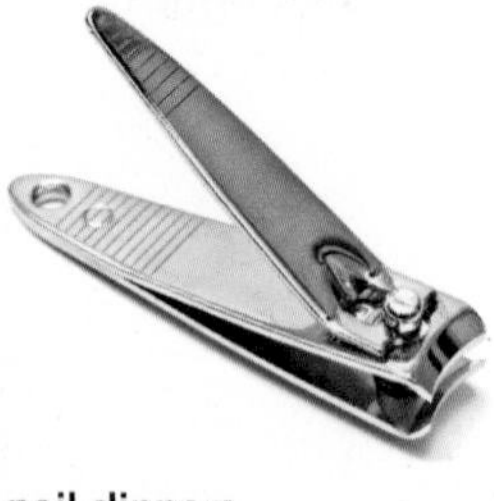

© Ingvar Bjork/www.Shutterstock.com

nail clippers

nail clippers (NAYL klip-urz)—a reusable implement used to shorten the nail plate quickly and efficiently.

nail corrugations (NAYL kohr-ruh-GAY-shuns)—wavy ridges caused by uneven growth of the nails, usually the result of illness or injury.

nail creams (NAYL KREEMZ)—barrier products that contain ingredients designed to seal the surface and hold subdermal moisture in the skin.

nail cuticle (NAYL CYOO-tik-uhl)—dead, colorless tissue attached to the natural nail plate.

nail dehydrator (NAYL dee-HY-drat-uhr)—a substance used to remove surface moisture and tiny amounts of oil left on the natural nail plate.

nail disorder (NAYL dis-ORDER)—condition caused by an injury or disease of the nail unit.

nail enamel (NAYL ee-NAM-ul)—also known as *nail polish*; a liquid coating applied to protect and beautify the nails.

nail extension (NAYL EX-ten-shun)—also known as *nail tip*; plastic, pre-molded nails shaped from a tough polymer made from ABS plastic, affixed to the natural nail to add length.

nail extension underside (NAYL EX-ten-shun UNDER-side)—the actual underside of the nail extension.

nail file (NAYL FYL)—a metal instrument with a specially prepared surface used to file and shape the nails.

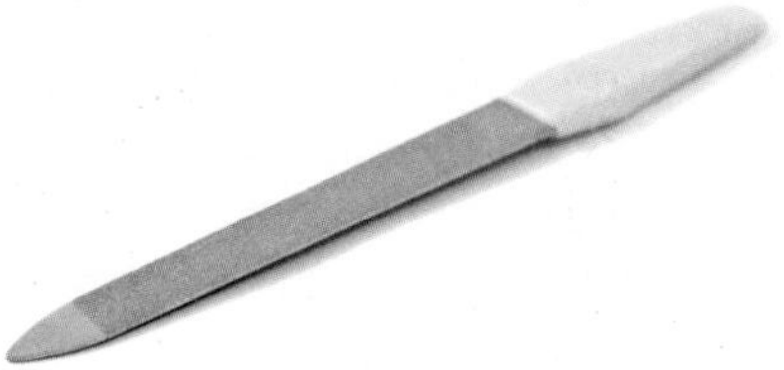

© oksana2010/www.Shutterstock.com

nail file

nail fold (NAYL FOHLD)—folds of normal skin that surround the natural nail plate.

nail mold (NAYL MOHLD)—also known as *nail form*; a metal or paper substance used to create a nail extension from nail enhancement product.

nail grooves (NAYL GROOVZ)—slits or furrows on the sides of the sidewall.

nail lacquer (NAYL LAK-ur)— also known as *nail polish*; a liquid coating applied to protect and beautify the nails.

nail mantal (NAYL MAN-tul)— also known as *mantle*; the deep fold of the skin into which the nail root is lodged.

nail matrix (NAYL MAY-triks)—also known as *matrix*; area where the nail plate cells are formed; this area is composed of matrix cells that produce the nail plate.

nail oils (NAYL OY-ills)—designed to absorb into the nail plate to increase flexibility and into the surrounding skin to soften.

nail plate (NAYL PLAYT)—hardened keratin plate that sits on and covers the natural nail bed. It is the most visible and functional part of the natural nail unit.

nail polish remover (NAYL PAHL-ish ree-MOOV-ur)—a solution used to remove polish from the nails.

nail psoriasis (NAYL sore-EYE-uh-sis)—a non-infectious condition that affects the surface of the natural nail plate, causing it to appear rough and pitted, as well as causing reddish color spots on the nail bed and onycholysis.

nail pterygium (NAYL TAH-jeer-ee-um)—abnormal condition that occurs when the skin is stretched by the nail plate; usually caused by serious injury, such as burns, or an adverse skin reaction to chemical nail enhancement products.

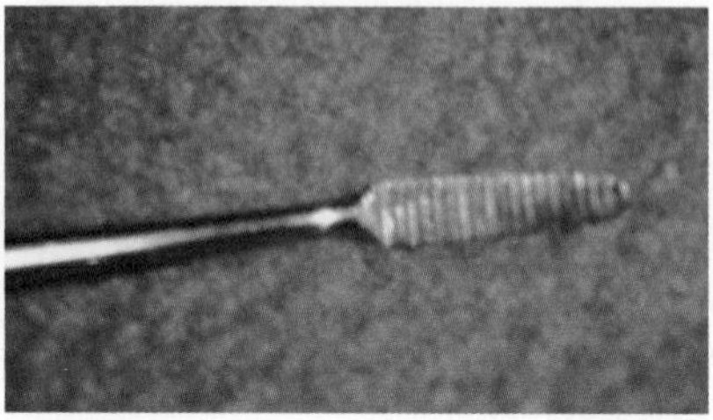
© Milady, a part of Cengage Learning. Photography by Michael Dzaman.
nail rasp

nail rasp (NAYL RASP)—metal file with an edge that can file the nail plate in only one direction.

nail technology (NAYL TECK-nol-o-jee)—the art and science of beautifying and improving the nails and skin of the hands and feet.

nail tip adhesive (NAYL TIP add-HEES-if)—the bonding agent used to secure the nail tip to the natural nail.

nail tips (NAYL TIPS)—also known as *nail extensions*; plastic, pre-molded nails shaped from a tough polymer made from ABS plastic.

nail unit (NAYL YOO-nit)—all the anatomical parts of the fingernail necessary to produce the natural nail plate.

nail wall (NAYL WAWL)—also known as *side walls*; the fold of skin overlapping the sides of the nail.

nail white (NAYL WHYT)—a nail cosmetic used to whiten the free edge of the nails.

nail wrap (NAYL RAP)—a method of securing a layer of fabric or paper on and around the nail tip to ensure its strength and durability.

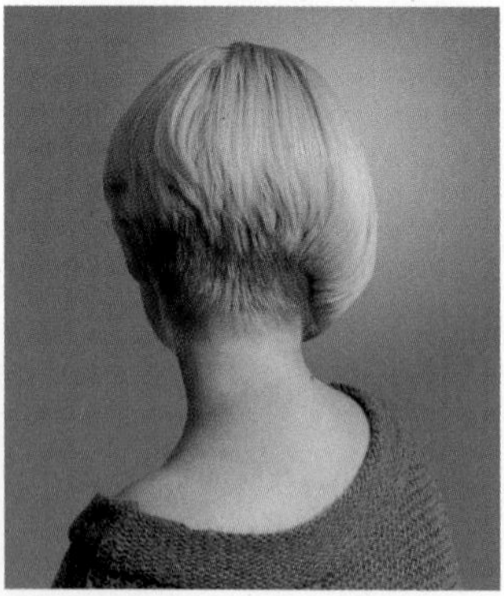
© chsherbakova yuliya/www.Shutterstock.com
nape

nail wrap resin (NAYL RAP REZ-in)—used to coat and secure fabric wraps to the natural nail and nail tip.

nanotechnology (nan-o-tek-nol-o-je)—the art of manipulating materials on an atomic or molecular scale.

nape (NAYP)—back part of the neck; the hair below the occipital bone.

N

nape line **(NAYP LYN)**—the hairline at the nape of the neck; nape section.

nasal **(NAY-zul)**—pertaining to the nose.

nasal bones **(NAY-zul BOHNZ)**—bones that form the bridge of the nose.

nasal nerve **(NAY-zul NURV)**—affects the point and lower side of the nose.

nasal turbinates **(NAY-zul TUR-buh-nitz)**—areas of bone and mucosa projecting from the lateral walls of the nasal cavity that warm and humidify inhaled air; sometimes can cause nasal airway obstruction.

nasalis **(nay-ZAY-lis)**—a muscle of the nose.

nasalis muscle **(NAY-sal-iz MUS-uhl)**—two-part muscle which covers the nose.

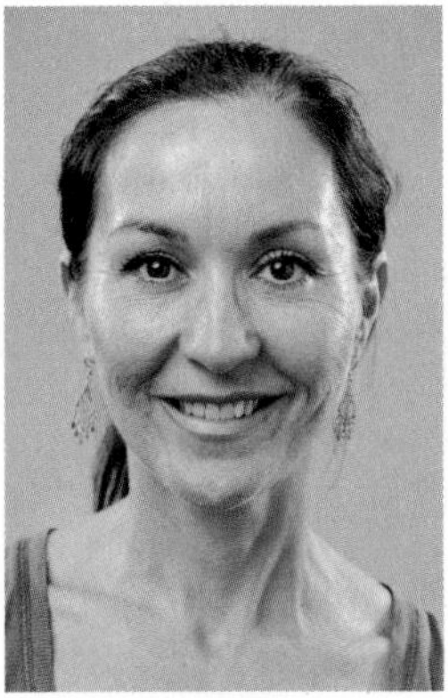
© Warren Goldswain/www.Shutterstock.com

nasolabial folds

nasolabial folds **(NAY-so-lay-bee-ole FOLDZ)**—the lines extending from the nostrils to the corners of the mouth.

nasolabial groove **(NAY-so-lay-bee-ole GROOV)**—laugh lines.

nasolabial lines **(NAY-so-lay-bee-ole LYNS)**—dynamic wrinkles that connect the nose to the mouth.

natural bristle brush **(NATCH-uh-rul BRIS-ul BRUSH)**—a brush with bristles made from the hairs of an animal, not from synthetic hair or fibers.

natural distribution **(NATCH-uh-rul dis-truh-BYOO-shun)**—the direction hair assumes as it grows out from the scalp.

natural growth pattern **(NATCH-uh-rul GROHTH PAT-urn)**—the direction in which hair grows naturally; usually in a large circle from the crown.

natural haircolors **(NATCH-uh-rul HARE-colorz)**—also known as *vegetable haircolors*; colors, such as henna, obtained from the leaves or bark of plants.

natural hairstyling **(NATCH-uh-rul HARE-styl-ing)**—also known as *braiding*; hairstyling that uses no chemicals or dyes and does not alter the natural curl or coil pattern of the hair.

natural immunity **(NATCH-uh-rul im-YOO-net-ee)**—immunity that is partly inherited and partly developed through healthy living.

natural ingredients **(NATCH-uh-rul in-GREED-ee-antz)**—ingredients found in nature, such as plants, minerals, and water.

natural nail **(NATCH-uh-rul NAYL)**—also known as *onyx*; the hard protective plate is composed mainly of keratin, the same fibrous protein found in skin and hair. The keratin in natural nails is harder than the keratin in skin or hair.

natural nail unit (NATCH-uh-rul NAYL YOO-nit)—composed of several major parts of the fingernail including the nail plate, nail bed, matrix, cuticle, eponychium, hyponychium, specialized ligaments, and nail fold. Together, all of these parts form the nail unit.

natural neckline (NACH-uh-rul NEK-lyn)—in haircutting, allowing the hair to follow its natural growth tendency at the neckline, rather than forcing an unnatural pattern into the hair.

navicular (nuh-VIK-yuh-lur)—boat-shaped; a bone of the wrist.

neck duster (NEK DUS-tur)—a brush used to remove hair from the neck after a haircut.

neck shave (NEK SHAYV)—shaving the areas behind the ears, down the sides of the neck, and at the back neckline.

neck strips (NEK STRIPS)—soft, flexible strips of paper placed around the client's neck to keep the cape from touching the skin while a service is being given.

neckline (NEK-lyn)—also known as *hairline*; in haircutting, the line where the hair growth of the head ends and the neck begins.

negative pole (NEG-uh-tiv POHL)—the pole from which negative galvanic current flows.

negative skin test (NEG-uh-tiv SKIN TEST)—having no reaction to a skin test for allergy, indicating safety in performing the service.

negative terminal (NEG-uh-tiv TUR-mih-nul)—the end of the conducting circuit of the electric current manifesting alkaline reaction; the zinc plate in a battery.

neoplasm (NEE-oh-plaz-um)—an abnormal growth or tumor.

nephron (NEF-rahn)—the functional unit of the kidney.

nerve (NURV)—whitish cords made up of bundles of nerve fibers held together by connective tissue, through which impulses are transmitted.

nerve cell (NURV SEL)—also known as *neuron*; the fundamental cellular unit of the nervous system.

nerve center (NURV SEN-tur)—also known as *command center*; an aggregation of neurons with a specific function for a part of the body.

nerve fiber (NURV FY-bur)—threadlike processes (axons and dendrites) arising from a neuron that make up a nerve.

nerve impulse (NURV IM-puls)—an electrical wave transmitted along a nerve that has been stimulated.

nerve reflex (NURV REE-flex)—the path traveled by a nerve impulse through the spinal cord and brain in response to a stimulus.

nerve tissue (NURV TISH-oo)—tissue that carries messages to and from the brain and controls and coordinates all body functions.

nervous cutaneous (NUR-vus kyoo-TAY-nee-us)—any nerve supplying an area of the skin.

nervous system (NUR-vus SIS-tum)—body system composed of the brain, spinal cord, and nerves; controls and coordinates all other systems of the body and makes them work harmoniously and efficiently.

net (NET)—a fabric of thread or cord woven in an open pattern or meshwork; a fabric of this type is used to cover the hair and hold a wet set in place while drying under a hood dryer.

net profit (NET PROF-it)—the real income of a business after all of the expenses associated with operation are subtracted.

networking (NET-work-ing)—establishing contacts that may eventually lead to a job and that help you gain valuable information about the workings of various establishments.

neural tube (noo-RAL TOOB)—a layer of the ectoderm germ layer; it provides most of the central nervous system.

neuralgia (noo-RAL-juh)—acute pain along the course of a nerve.

neurasthenia (nur-us-THEE-nee-uh)—a condition of weakness and depression due to exhaustion that affects the nervous system.

neurofilament (NOO-row-FILL-ah-ment)—an intermediate filament found in nerve cells.

neurohormones (NOO-row-HORE-moanes)—hormones secreted by the hypothalamus that control many pituitary hormone secretions.

neurology (nuh-RAHL-uh-jee)—scientific study of the structure, function, and pathology of the nervous system.

neuromuscular junction (nuh-roh-MUS-kyuh-lur JUNK-shun)—the point where the motor neuron and muscle join.

neuron (NOO-rahn)—also known as a *nerve cell*; primary structural unit of the nervous system, consisting of cell body, nucleus, dendrites, and axon.

neurotransmitter (NOO-row-trans-mit-uhr)—a chemical that modifies or causes the transmission of nerve impulses across synapses to act on or inhibit a target cell.

neutral (NOO-trul)—neither positive nor negative, indifferent; in chemistry, neither acid nor alkaline with a pH of 7; a color balanced between warm and cool that does not reflect a highlight of any primary or secondary color.

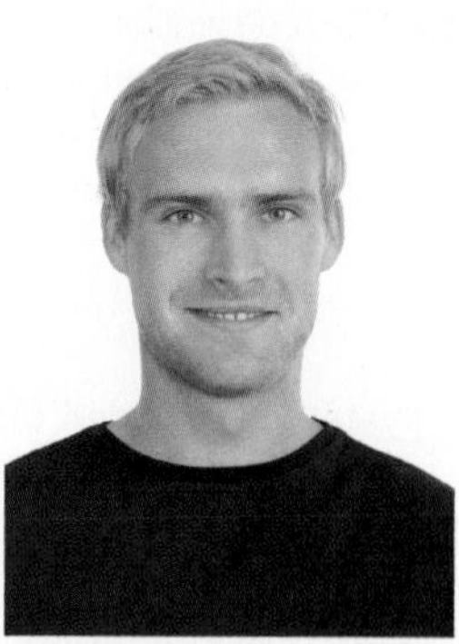
© courtyardpix/www.Shutterstock.com
neutral blonde

neutral blonde (NOO-trul BLAHND)—a beige-blond that is neither gold nor ash.

neutralization (noo-truh-ly-ZAY-shun)—the process that counterbalances or cancels an action of an agent or color; in chemistry, reaction forming a substance that is neither alkaline nor acid; a chemical reaction between an acid and a base; rehardening the hair in permanent waving or in chemical hair relaxing.

neutralize (NOO-truh-lyz)—to render ineffective; to effect neutralization; counterbalance of an action or influence.

neutralizer (NOO-trul-yz-ur)—an agent capable of neutralizing another substance.

neutralizing (NOO-truh-lyz-ing)—the process of stopping the action of a permanent wave solution and hardening the hair in its new form by the application of a chemical solution.

neutrons (NEW-trahns)—subatomic particles found in the nucleus of the atom that carry no charge.

nevus (NEE-vus) (plural: nevi)—also known as a *birthmark*; small or large malformation of the skin due to abnormal pigmentation or dilated capillaries.

nevus pilosus (NEE-vus py-LOH-sus)—hairy mole; a birthmark characterized by hair growing from the dark area.

new growth (NOO GROHTH)—part of the hair shaft between the scalp and the hair that has been previously colored.

Nikolsky sign (ne-KOHL-skee SIGN)—an indication of a skin reaction; the clinical manifestations observed are perifollicular edema, erythema or blistering, or an epidermal separation caused by lateral pressure on the skin.

ninth cranial nerve (NYNTH KRAY-nee-ul NURV)—pertains to the pharynx and tongue, controls the sense of taste.

nipper (NIP-ur)—a stainless-steel implement used to carefully trim away dead skin around the nails.

nit (NIT)—the egg of a louse, usually attached to a hair.

nitrate (NEYE-trayt)—an oxidizing agent.

nitric acid (NEYE-trik AS-ud)—concentrated acid employed as a caustic.

nitrite (NEYE-tryt)—a reducing agent; sodium nitrite is used as a sanitizing agent and acts as an anti-rusting agent.

nitrogen **(NY-truh-jun)**—a colorless gaseous element that makes up about four-fifths of the air in our atmosphere and is found chiefly in ammonia and nitrates.

nitrous **(NY-trus)**—designating a compound of nitrogen.

no-base relaxer **(NOH-BAYS ree-LAKS-ur)**—relaxers that do not require application of a protective base cream.

no stem curl **(NOH STEM CURL)**—curl placed directly on its base; produces a tight, firm, long-lasting curl and allows minimum mobility.

node **(NOHD)**—a knot or knob; a circumscribed swelling; a knuckle or finger joint.

nodule **(NAHD-yul)**—a solid bump larger than 0.4 inches (1 centimeter) that can be easily felt. These are often referred to as tumors, but these are smaller bumps caused by conditions such as scar tissue, fatty deposits, or infections.

nominal hazard zone (NHZ) **(NOM-in-all HAZARD ZON)**—the zone in which direct, reflected, or scattered radiation, such as lasers, are used during normal operation or treatment. Exceeding the maximum permissible exposure (MPE) can cause injury to the skin or eyes.

noncertified colors **(NAHN-sir-tif-eyed COLORZ)**—colors that are organic, meaning they come from animal or plant extracts; they can also be natural mineral pigments.

noncomedogenic **(NAHN-com-ee-deo-GEN-ick)**—product that has been designed and proven not to clog the follicle.

nonconductor **(nahn-kun-DUK-tur)**—also known as *insulator*; a material that does not transmit electricity.

nonessential amino acids **(NAHN-ee-SENT-shul AMINO ASUDS)**—amino acids that can be synthesized by the body and do not have to be obtained from the diet.

noninfectious **(nahn-in-FEK-shus)**—not spread by contact; unable to spread disease.

nonpathogenic **(nahn-path-uh-JEN-ik)**—harmless microorganisms that may perform useful functions and are safe to come in contact with since they do not cause disease or harm.

nonporous **(nahn-pur-us)**—an item that is made or constructed of a material that has no pores or openings and cannot absorb liquids.

nonresistant **(nahn-ree-ZIS-tent)**—porous hair; the condition of the hair that absorbs moisture readily.

nonstriated muscles (nahn-STRY-ayt-ud MUS-uhlz)—also known as *smooth muscles*; these muscles are involuntary and function automatically, without conscious will.

nonstripping shampoo (nahn-STRIP-ing sham-POO)—a shampoo that cleanses the hair without removing artificial color from the hair.

nonvolatile (NAHN-vol-ih-til)—does not evaporate easily.

normal (NOR-mul)—regular; natural; conforming to some ideal norm or standard.

normal hair condition (NOR-mul HAYR kahn-DIH-shun)—an average condition in which hair is neither porous nor resistant, neither dry nor oily.

normal hair shampoo (NOR-mul HAYR sham-POO)—a shampoo formulated for hair that is neither too dry nor too oily.

normal skin (NOR-mul SKIN)—skin that is neither too dry nor too oily, and is free of conditions such as blackheads, whiteheads, acne, or disease.

normalize (NOR-mul-yz)—to make something conform to a norm or standard; return the pH of the skin or hair to normal.

normalizer (NOR-mul-yz-ur)—a solution used to return the hair to its normal pH of 4.5 to 5.5 or the skin to approximately 4.5 to 6.0.

normalizing conditioners (NOR-mul-yz-ing con-DISH-on-uhr)—conditioners with an acidic pH that restore the hair's natural pH after a hydroxide relaxer and for shampooing.

nostril (NAHS-trul)—one of the two external openings of the nose.

notching (NAH-ching)—version of point cutting in which the tips of the scissors are moved toward the hair ends rather than into them; creates a chunkier effect.

nourishing cream (NUR-ish-ing KREEM)—a cream formulated to nourish the skin; used in massage and facial treatments.

nourishment (NUR-ish-ment)—anything that nourishes; nutriment; food.

noxious (NAHK-shus)—harmful; poisonous.

nuclear membrane (NOO-cle-ear MEM-brayn)—the membrane surrounding the nucleus of eukaryotic cells.

nucleic acid (noo-KLEE-ik AS-ud)—one of a group of compounds found in cell nuclei and cytoplasm involved in building the proteins necessary to the formation of living matter.

nucleolus (NOO-klee-oh-lus)—a non-membrane-bound structure composed of proteins and nucleic acids found within the nucleus.

nucleoplasm (NEW-clee-oh-plasm)—fluid within the nucleus of the cell that contains proteins and DNA; determines our genetic makeup.

nucleus (NOO-klee-us); pl., nuclei (NOO-klee-eye)—the central part, core. (1) In histology the dense, active protoplasm found in the center of a eukaryotic cell that acts as the genetic control center; it plays an important role in cell reproduction and metabolism. (2) In chemistry, the center of the atom, where protons and neutrons are located.

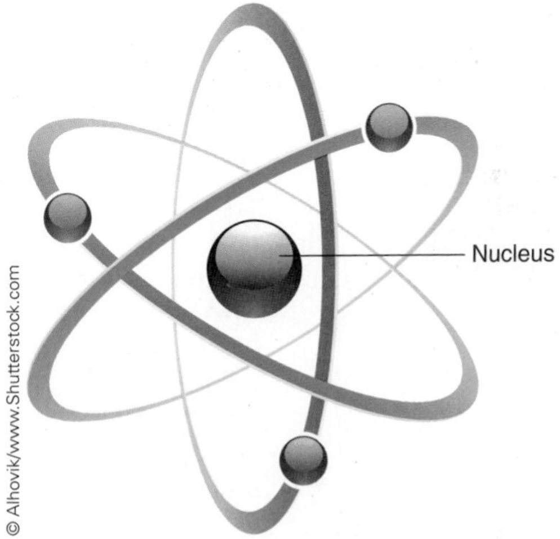

nucleus

nutrient (NOO-tree-ent)—a nourishing substance; nutritious.

nutrition (noo-TRISH-un)—the processes involved in taking in nutriments and assimilating and utilizing them.

nylon (NY-lahn)—a synthetic thermoplastic polyamide from which fibers and bristles are made.

nylon fiber (NY-lahn FY-bur)—a combination of clear polish with nylon fibers. It is first applied vertically and then horizontally on the nail plate.

O

O

O (OH)—in chemistry, the symbol for oxygen.

obese (oh-BEES)—also known as *stout, corpulent,* or *fat*; extremely overweight.

obesity (oh-BEE-sut-ee)—the condition of having excessive body weight over what is considered to be normal for one's height and bone structure.

objective symptoms (ub-JEK-tiv SIMP-tums)—symptoms that can be seen by anyone.

oblong (AHB-lawng)—longer than broad; rectangle whose horizontal sides are longer than its vertical sides.

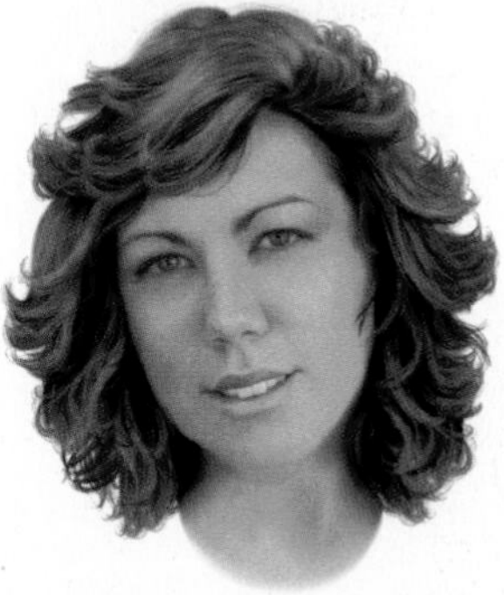

© Milady, a part of Cengage Learning

oblong-shaped face

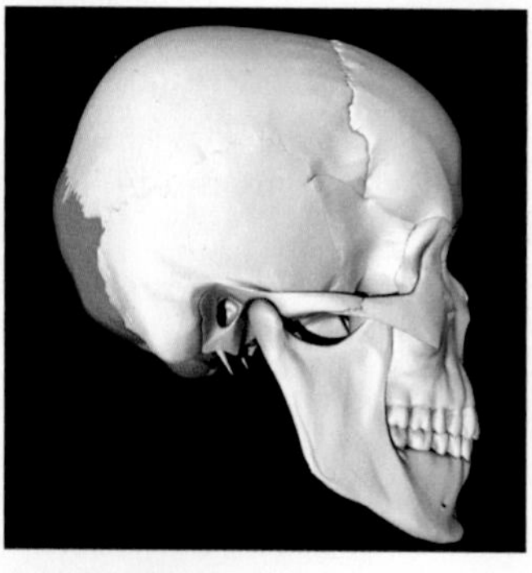

© JCElv /www.Shutterstock.com

occipital bone

oblong-shaped face (AHB-lawng SHAYPT FAYS)—a face characterized by a long, thin structure.

oblong shapings (AHB-lawng SHAYP-ings)—waves that remain the same width throughout the shaping.

obsolete (ahb-suh-LEET)—out of date; no longer in use; not current.

occipita (ahk-SIP-it-uh)—the back of the head or skull.

occipital (ahk-SIP-it-ul)—pertaining to the back part of the head; the bone that forms the back and lower part of the cranium.

occipital artery (ahk-SIP-it-ul AR-tuh-ree)—supplies blood to the skin and muscles of the scalp and back of the head up to the crown.

occipital bone (ahk-SIP-ih-tul BOHN)—hindmost bone of the skull, below the parietal bones; forms the back of the skull above the nape.

occipital frontalis (ahk-SIP-it-ul frun-TAY-lus)—epicranius; the scalp muscle.

occipital lobe (ahk-SIP-ih-tal LOHB)—one of the lobes of the cerebrum.

occipital nerve (ahk-SIP-ih-tul NURV)—also known as *major occipital nerve*; nerve that receives stimuli for the skin of the posterior portion of the scalp.

occipitalis (ahk-SIP-ih-tahl-is)—back of the epicranius; a muscle that draws the scalp backward.

occlusive (AHH-cluez-if)—products that are thick and lay on top of the skin to reduce transepidermal water loss (TEWL); helps hold in moisture, and protect the skin's top barrier layer.

occupational disease (ahk-yuh-PAY-shun-ul DIZ-eez)—illness resulting from conditions associated with employment, such as prolonged and repeated overexposure to certain products or ingredients.

Occupational Safety and Health Administration (OSHA) (ahk-yuh-PAY-shun-ul SAFE-tee and hellth ADD-min-is-tray-shun)—created as a part of the U.S. Department of Labor to regulate and enforce safety and health standards to protect employees in the workplace.

ocular (AHK-yuh-lur)—pertaining to the eye; the eyepiece of a microscope; the lens at the upper end of the microscope.

ocular rosacea (AHK-yuh-lur row-ZAY-shah)—a subtype of rosacea that affects the eyes, resulting in eye redness, swollen eyelids, and other eye lesions.

oculofacial (ahk-yuh-loh-FAY-shul)—pertaining to the eyes and face.

oculomotor nerve (ahk-yuh-loh-MOHT-ur NURV)—third cranial nerve that controls the motion of the eye.

oculus (AHK-yoo-lus); pl., oculi (AHK-yoo-lye)—the eye.

odontic (oh-DAHN-tik)—pertaining to the teeth.

odor (OH-dur)—also known as *scent*; the property of a substance that causes it to be perceptible to the sense of smell.

odorless (OH-dur-les)—having no odor.

odorless monomer liquid and polymer powder products (OH-dur-les MONO-mer LICK-wid and POL-ih-mer POW-der PRAH-dux)—nail enhancement products that have little odor.

off-base (AWF BAYS)—in hairstyling, the position of a curl or a roller completely off its base for maximum mobility and minimum volume.

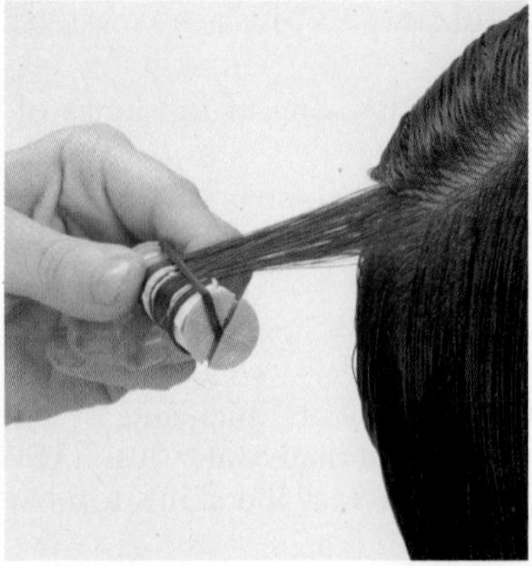
© Milady, a part of Cengage Learning. Photography by Paul Castle.
off-base placement

off-base placement (AWF BAYS PLAYS-ment)—base control in which the hair is wrapped at 45 degrees below the center of the base section, so the rod is positioned completely off its base.

off-color (AWF-KUL-ur)—lacking the correct or acceptable standard of color.

off-the-scalp lighteners (AWF-THE-SKALP LYT-un-urz)—also known as *quick lighteners*; powdered lighteners that cannot be used directly on the scalp.

ohm (OHM)—abbreviated *O*; a unit for measuring the resistance of an electric current.

Ohm's law (OHMZ LAW)—the simple statement that the strength of a current in an electric circuit is equal to the electromotive force divided by the resistance.

oil (OYL)—a greasy liquid of vegetable, animal, or mineral origin; soluble in alcohol and ether, but not in water; used in foods, cosmetics, and many other products.

oil bleach (OYL BLEECH)—a combination of sulfonated oil, ammonia water, and hydrogen peroxide.

oil gland (OYL GLAND)—also known as *sebaceous gland*; an oil-secreting gland; little sacs whose ducts open into hair follicles, lubricating skin and hair by the secretion of sebum.

oil heater (OYL HEET-ur)—machine used to heat oil and keep it warm when giving an oil manicure.

oil-in-water emulsions (OYL-IN-WAHT-ur ih-MUL-shuns)—oil droplets suspended in a water base.

oil soluble (OYL sol-yoo-bull)—compatible with oil.

oily hair (OYL-ee HAYR)—hair that has an excessive amount of oil due to overactivity of the sebaceous glands.

oily hair shampoo (OYL-ee HAYR sham-POO)—a preparation formulated for cleansing excessive oil from the hair and scalp.

oily skin (OYL-ee SKIN)—skin that is excessively oily due primarily to the overactivity of the sebaceous glands.

ointment (OYNT-ment)—a semisolid mixture of organic substances and a medicinal agent.

oleic acid (oh-LEE-ik AS-ud)—an oily, fatty acid used in soaps, shampoos, and some ointments.

olfaction (ohl-FAK-shun)—the sense of smell; the act or process of smelling.

olfactory glands (ohl-FAK-tuh-ree GLANDZ)—serous glands found in the mucous membranes of the nose.

olfactory nerve (ohl-FAK-tuh-ree NURV)—the first cranial nerve; sensory nerve fibers of the mucous membrane of the nose.

olfactory organ (ohl-FAK-tuh-ree OR-gan)—the sense organ located in the nasal cavity responsible for the ability to detect pleasant or unpleasant odors.

oligomer (UH-lig-uh-mer)—short chain of monomer liquids that is often thick, sticky, and gel-like and that is not long enough to be considered a polymer.

oligotrichia (ohl-ih-goh-TRIK-ee-uh)—scantiness or thinness of hair.

–ology (AHL-O-jee)—word ending meaning study of.

omega-3 fatty acids (OH-may-gah THREE FAHT-ee ASUDS)—also known as *alpha-linolenic acid*; a type of "good" polyunsaturated fat that may decrease cardiovascular diseases. It is also an anti-inflammatory and beneficial for skin.

on-base (AWN BAYS)—also known as *full base*; position of a curl or roller directly on its base for maximum volume.

on-base placement (AWN BAYS PLAYS-ment)—base control in which the hair is wrapped at a 45-degree angle beyond perpendicular to its base section, and the rod is positioned on its base.

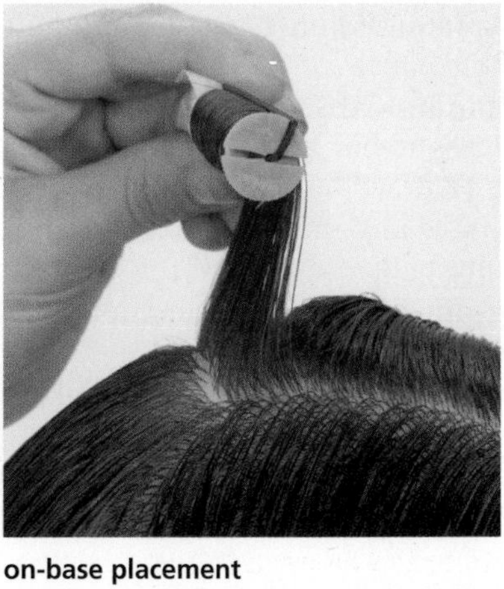

© Milady, a part of Cengage Learning. Photography by Paul Castle.

on-base placement

O

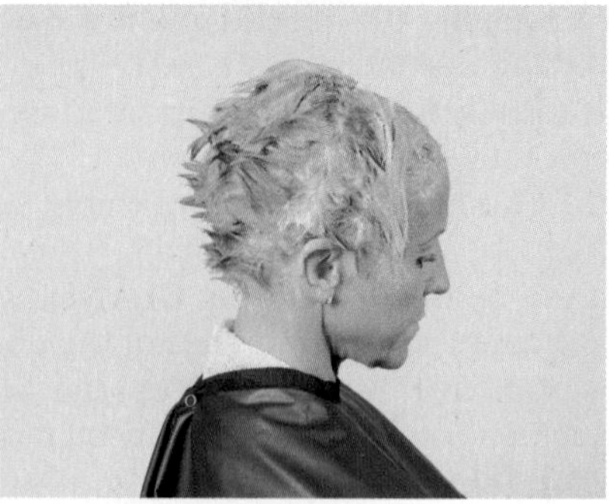
© Milady, a part of Cengage Learning. Photography by Yanik Chauvin.

on-the-scalp lightener

O

on-the-scalp lightener (AWN-THE-SKALP LYT-un-ur)—lighteners that can be used directly on the scalp by mixing the lightener with activators.

once-over shave (WONCE-ov-er-SHAYV)—single-lather shave in which the shaving strokes are made across the grain of the hair.

oncogenic (ahng-koh-JEN-ik)—tending to cause tumors; relating to tumor formation.

one-application process (WUN ap-lih-KAY-shun PRAH-ses)—a haircoloring process that decolorizes and colors in a single application.

one-color method (WUN-KULUR METH-id)—in nail technology; when one color of gel, usually clear, is applied over the entire surface of the nail.

onychatrophia (ahn-ih-kuh-TROH-fee-uh)—atrophy or wasting away of the nails.

onychauxis (ahn-ih-KAHK-sis)—overgrowth of the nail, usually in thickness rather than length; caused by a local infection; can be hereditary.

onychia (uh-NIK-ee-uh)—inflammation of the nail matrix, followed by shedding of the natural nail.

onychitis (uh-nih-KY-tis)—inflammation of the area around the nails.

onycho (UH-nih-kuh)—a prefix meaning relating to the nails.

onychoclasis (ahn-ih-KAHK-lah-sis)—breaking of a nail.

onychocryptosis (ahn-ih-koh-krip-TOH-sis)—also known as *ingrown nails*; nail grows into the sides of the tissue around the nail.

onychogryposis (ahn-ih-koh-gry-POH-sis)—thickening and increased curvature of the nail.

onychohelcosis (ahn-ih-koh-hel-KOH-sis)—ulceration of a nail.

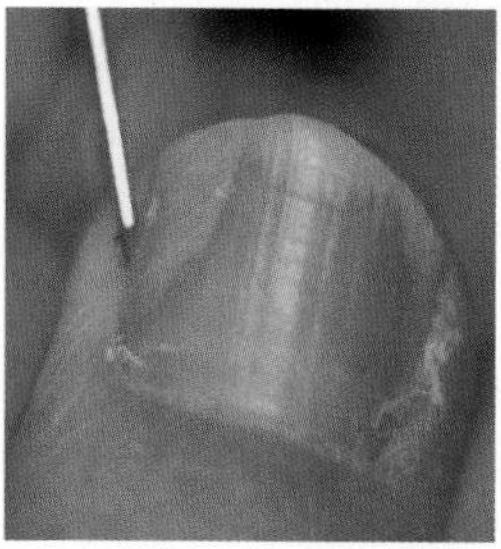
Robert Baran, MD (France)

onycholysis

onycholysis(ahn-ih-KAHL-ih-sis)—lifting of the nail plate from the nail bed without shedding, usually beginning at the free edge and continuing toward the lunula area.

onychomadesis (ahn-ih-koh-muh-DEE-sis)—the separation and falling off of a nail plate from the nail bed; affects fingernails and toenails.

onychomycosis (ahn-ih-koh-my-KOH-sis)—also known as *tinia unguium*; fungal infection of the natural nail plate.

onychophagia (ahn-ih-koh-FAY-jee-uh)—also known as *bitten nails*; result of a habit of chewing the nail or chewing the hardened skin surrounding the nail plate.

onychophagy (ahn-ih-koh-FAY-jee)—result of an acquired nervous habit that prompts an individual to chew the nail or the hardened cuticle.

onychophosis (ahn-ih-kahf-OH-sis)—growth of horny epithelium in the nail bed.

onychophyma (ahn-ih-koh-FY-muh)—swelling of the nails.

onychoptosis (ahn-ih-kahp-TOH-sis)—periodic shedding of one or more nails; in whole or in part.

onychorrhexis (ahn-ih-koh-REK-sis)—split or brittle nails that have a series of lengthwise ridges giving a rough appearance to the surface of the nail plate.

onychorrhiza (ahn-ih-koy-RY-zuh)—the root of the nail.

onychosis, onychonosus (ahn-ih-KOH-sis, ahn-ih-koh-NOH-sus)—any deformity or disease of the nails.

onychostroma (ahn-ih-koh-STROH-muh)—the matrix of the nail.

onychotrophy (ahn-ih-KAHT-ruh-fee)—nourishment of the nails.

onyx (AHN-iks)—technical term for nail of the fingers or toes.

onyxis (AHN-ik-sis)—ingrown toenail.

onyxitis (ahn-ik-SY-tis)—inflammation of the nail matrix.

opacity (oh-PAY-sit-ee)—in nail technology; the amount of colored pigment concentration in a gel, making it more or less difficult to see through.

O

opaque (oh-PAYK)—neither transparent nor translucent; allowing no light to shine through.

open center curls (OH-pen CEN-tur CURLZ)—pincurls that produce even, smooth waves and uniform curls.

open comedones (OH-pen COM-AH-donz)—also known as *blackheads*; follicles impacted with solidified sebum and dead cell buildup.

open end (OH-pen END)—the concave, indented end of a wave or shaping.

ophthalmic (ahf-THAL-mik)—pertaining to the eye.

ophthalmic artery (ahf-THAL-mik ART-uh-ree)—the main branch of the carotid artery supplying the eye and nearby structures.

ophthalmic nerve (ahf-THAL-mik NURV)—branch of the fifth cranial nerve that supplies impulses to the skin of the forehead, upper eyelids, and interior portion of the scalp, orbit, eyeball, and nasal passage.

ophthalmology (ahf-thal-MAHL-uh-jee)—the science dealing with the structure, functions, and diseases of the eye.

opponent muscles (uh-POH-nent MUS-uhlz)—muscles in the palm that act to bring the thumb toward the fingers.

opportunistic infection (ah-puhr-toon-IS-tic in-FEK-shun)—diseased caused by organisms commonly found in the environment and on the body which become deadly when the body's immune system is weakened.

opportunistic mycosis (ah-puhr-toon-IS-tic my-COH-sis)—a fungal infection caused by fungi that use breaks in the skin or abnormal immunity to infect the body.

optic (AHP-tik)—pertaining to the eye or to vision.

optic nerve (AHP-tik NURV)—the second cranial nerve; the nerve of sight that conducts impulses from the retina of the eye to the brain.

optician (ahp-TISH-un)—one who makes eyeglasses.

optometrist (ahp-TAHM-uh-trist)—a person who examines eyes and fits or prescribes glasses to correct visual defects.

orbicular (or-BIK-yuh-lur)—circular; a term applied to a muscle whose fibers are circularly arranged.

orbicularis oculi muscle (or-bik-yuh-LAIR-is AHK-yuh-lye MUS-uhl)—ring muscle of the eye socket; enables you to close your eyes.

orbicularis oris muscle (or-bik-yuh-LAIR-is OH-ris MUS-uhl)—orbicular muscle; flat band around the upper and lower lips that compresses, contracts, puckers, and wrinkles the lips.

orbicularis palpebrarum (or-bik-yuh-LAIR-is pal-puh-BRAIR-um)—a muscle of the face that closes the eyes.

orbit (OR-bit)—the bony cavity protecting the eyeball; the eye socket.

organ (OR-gun)—structures composed of specialized tissues designed to perform specific functions in plants and animals.

organelle (OR-gun-elle)—small structures or miniature organs within a cell that have their own function.

organic (or-GAN-ik)—relating to an organ; pertaining to substances having carbon-to-carbon bonds.

organic chemistry (or-GAN-ik KEM-is-tree)—the study of substances that contain the element carbon.

organic compound (or-GAN-ik KAHM-pownd)—a compound containing carbon exclusive of salts and carbonic acid.

organic cosmetics (or-GAN-ik kahz-MET-iks)—cosmetics made from animal or vegetable products.

organic ingredients (or-GAN-ik in-GREED-ee-antz)—ingredients derived from an agricultural product that has been produced, handled, and processed under the guidelines of the U.S. Department of Agriculture's National Organic Program.

organic shampoos (or-GAN-ih SHAM-poos)—shampoo formulated from natural organic ingredients.

organism (OR-gah-niz-um)—any living thing, plant, or animal. May be unicellular (bacteria, yeasts, protozoa) or multicellular (all complex organisms, including humans).

orifice (OR-uh-fus)—an opening; a mouth.

origin (OR-ih-jin)—part of the muscle that does not move; attached to the skeleton and usually part of a skeletal muscle.

originate (uh-RIJ-ih-nayt)—to produce as new; to create.

ornament (ORN-uh-ment)—in hairdressing, a ribbon, comb, pin, or other accessory added to the finished hairstyle.

O

orthopedics (or-thoh-PEED-iks)—the branch of surgery that deals with prevention and correction of problems of the skeletal system.

os (AHS)—means *bone* and is used as a prefix in many medical terms, such as osteoarthritis, a joint disease.

os magnum (AHS MAG-num)—bone in the lower row of the carpus.

oscillate (AHS-ul-ayt)—to swing back and forth like a pendulum; to vibrate.

oscillator (AHS-uh-layt-ur)—an apparatus that produces vibrating movements used in massage.

osmidrosis (ahz-mih-DROH-sis)—also known as *bromidrosis*; foul-smelling perspiration.

osmosis (ahz-MOH-sis)—the diffusion of a fluid or solution through a semipermeable membrane; especially the passage of a solvent through a membrane from a dilute solution into a more concentrated one.

osteoarthritis (ahs-tee-oh-arth-RY-tis)—a joint condition characterized by inflammation of weight-bearing joints.

osteodermia (ahs-tee-oh-DUR-mee-ah)—a condition characterized by bony formations in the skin.

osteology (ahs-tee-AHL-oh-jee)—the study of anatomy, structure, and function of the bones.

osteoporosis (ahs-tee-oh-puh-ROH-sis)—a thinning of bones, leaving them fragile and prone to fractures; caused by the reabsorption of calcium into the blood.

ostium (AHS-tee-um)—the opening of a follicle on the skin surface.

ounce (OWNS)—a unit of measure of weight; one-sixteenth of a pound; 30 milliliters.

outcrop (OWT-krahp)—in cosmetology, a new growth of hair.

outer ear (OW-tur EER)—the flared outer portion of the ear.

outer perimeter (OW-tur puh-RIM-ih-tur)—in cosmetology, the outer area of the hair length.

outline (OWT-lyn)—the line that defines a shape; the boundary of a figure or a body; the defining of the eyes or lips by use of a cosmetic pencil.

outlining (OWT-lyn-ing)—finish work of a haircut with shears, trimmers, or razor.

outside curve (OWT-syd KURV)—the convex; the outward curve in which hair may be cut.

oval design (OH-vul DE-zyn)—a hair design shaped like an ellipse; a hair design having an oval shape.

oval nail (OH-vul NAYL)—a conservative nail shape that is thought to be attractive on most women's hands. It is similar to a squoval nail with even more rounded corners.

O

oval-shaped face (OH-vul SHAYPT FAYS)—egg-shaped; resembling an ellipse; something having an oval shape; oval facial type.

ovaries (OH-var-ees)—female sexual glands that function in reproduction, as well as determining female sexual characteristics.

overdirection (oh-var-dih-REK-shun)—combing a section away from its natural falling position, rather than straight out from the head, toward a guideline; used to create increasing lengths in the interior or perimeter of a haircut.

overexposure (OH-var-ex-POH-zur)—prolonged, repeated, or long-term exposure that can cause sensitivity.

overfilling (OH-var-FYL-ing)—excessively roughing up the nail plate.

overhand technique (OH-vur HAND tek-NEEK)—a braiding technique in which the first side section goes over the middle one, then the other side section goes over the middle strand.

overhydration (oh-vur-hy-DRAY-shun)—the presence of excess fluids in the tissues of the body.

overlapping (oh-vur-LAP-ing)—in cosmetology, applying a chemical solution, such as a relaxer, tint or lightener, beyond the limits of the new growth of hair.

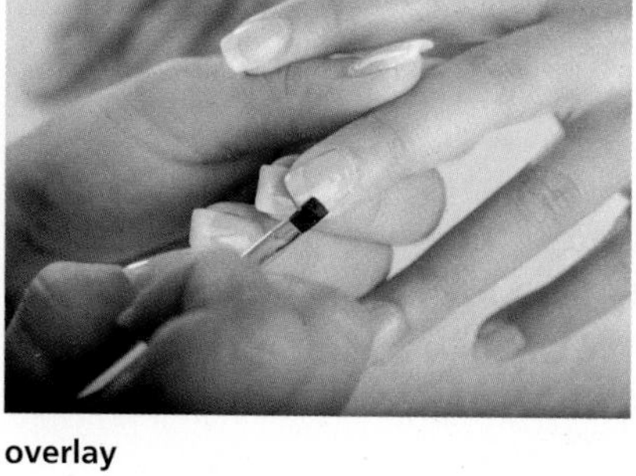

© Milady, a part of Cengage Learning. Photography by Dino Petrocelli.

overlay

overlapping curl (oh-vur-LAP-ing KURL)—a pincurl that partially covers its adjacent curl.

overlay (OH-vur lay)—a layer of any kind of nail enhancement product that is applied over the natural nail or nail and tip application for added strength.

overporosity (oh-vur-puh-RAHS-ih-tee)—excessive ability of the hair to absorb moisture; undesirable stage of porosity requiring correction.

overprocessing (oh-vur-PRAH-ses-ing)—overexposure of the hair to the chemical action of a chemical solution, usually resulting in weakened or damaged hair.

ovular (AHV-yuh-lur)—egg-like in shape; pertaining to the ovum or egg.

o/w—abbreviation for oil in water.

owner's equity (OWN-erz eck-WIT-ee)—the owner's interest in the assets of the company after all of the business's liabilities have been deducted.

oxidation (ahk-sih-DAY-shun)—a chemical reaction that combines a substance with oxygen to produce an oxide.

oxidation dye (ahk-sih-DAY-shun DYE)—aniline derivative dye; hair tint.

oxidation–reduction (ahk-sih-DAY-shun–ree-DUK-shun)—also known as *redox* and *oxidation–reduction reaction*; a chemical reaction in which the oxidizing agent is reduced (by losing oxygen) and the reducing agent is oxidized (by gaining oxygen).

oxidative haircolor (ahk-sih-DAY-tiv HAYR KUL-ur)—a product containing oxidation dyes that require hydrogen peroxide to develop the permanent color.

oxide (AHK-syd)—a compound of oxygen with another element or radical.

oxidize (AHK-sih-dyz)—to combine or to cause an element or radical to combine with oxygen.

oxidizing agent (AHK-sih-dyz-ing AY-jent)—a substance that releases oxygen, causing a chemical reaction; an example is hydrogen peroxide.

oxygen (AHK-sih-jin)—a gaseous element essential to animal and plant life; most abundant element.

oxygenated (ahk-sih-juh-NAY-ted)—rich in oxygen.

oxygenation (ahk-sih-juh-NAY-shun)—saturation with oxygen; to combine a substance with oxygen; the aeration of the blood with oxygen.

oxyhemoglobin (ahk-sih-HEE-muh-gloh-bin)—hemoglobin in red blood cells that has been oxygenated; a protein in red blood cells.

oxytalan (ok-SIT-ăh-lan)—an elastin-type fiber found in the dermis that contains only microfibrils and is 10 to 12 nm (0.10-0.12 cm) in diameter.

oxytocin (ahk-sih-TOH-cin)—hormone that causes the uterus to contract and triggers the letdown of breast milk.

ozone (OH-zohn)—a pale blue gas that is another form of oxygen; used as a deodorizing and bleaching agent; a form of oxygen used as a disinfectant.

P

P

pacinian corpuscle (PUH-sin-ee-an COR-pus-uhl)—also known as *lamellated corpuscle*; a sensory receptor in skin, muscles, body joints, body organs, and tendons that is involved with the vibratory sense and firm pressure on the skin.

pack (PAK)—also known as *mask* or *masque*; a special cosmetic formula used to benefit the skin.

packing (PAK-ing)—heavy back-combing, matted at the scalp, and extended along the hair strand, giving the strand of hair almost a rigid quality.

pad (PAD)—a small, soft cushion-like item, usually of cotton or sponge; used to apply makeup, remove nail polish, and so forth.

pain receptors (PAYN ree-SEP-turz)—sensory nerve fibers that respond to pain-causing stimuli.

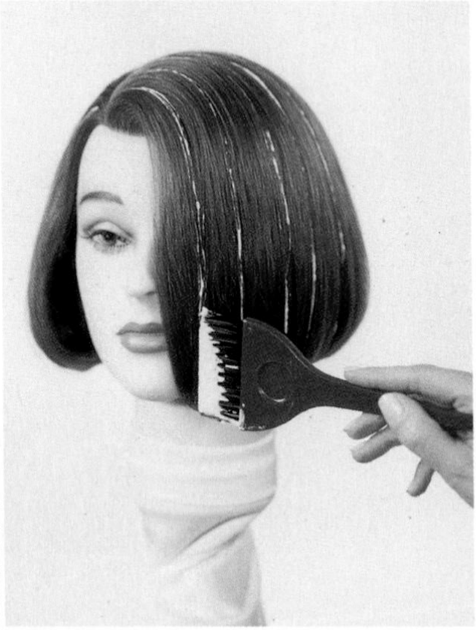

© Milady, a part of Cengage Learning. Photography by Paul Castle.

painting or baliage

painting (PAYNT-ing)—also known as *baliage*; a technique in haircoloring in which the hair is darkened or lightened in thin strands with a brush.

palate (PAL-ut)—the roof of the mouth and the floor of the nose.

palatine bones (PALL-uh-tyn BOHNZ)—bones form the floor and outer wall of the nose, roof of the mouth, and floor of the orbits.

palette (PAL-it)—a thin board usually with a hole for the thumb on which the artist places an assortment of paint colors; the selection of colors for an individual. Some artists use disposable waterproof parchment paper or artist paper as a palette.

pallor (PAL-ur)—paleness; deficiency of color, especially of the face.

palm (PAHM)—the inner surface of the hand between the wrist and base of the fingers.

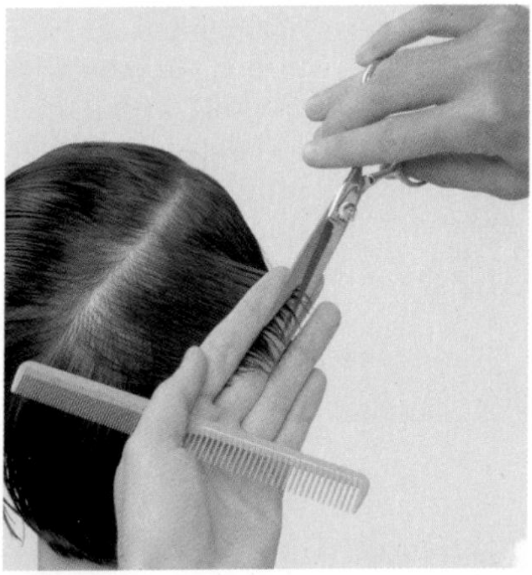

© Milady, a part of Cengage Learning. Photography by Paul Castle.

palm-to-palm cutting

palm-to-palm (PAHM-to-PAHM)—cutting position in which the palms of both hands are facing each other.

palmar (PAHL-mur)—of or pertaining to the palm or hollow of the hand.

palmar arch (PAHL-mur ARCH)—the branches of arteries in the palm that supply blood to the bones, joints, muscles, and skin of the palm of the hand and fingers.

palmar compression (PAHL-mur kum-PRES-shun)—massage movement using the whole hand or heel of the hand over a large area of the body.

palmar friction (PAHL-mur FRIK-shun)—a massage movement using the palm of the hand to apply pressure and a rubbing movement over underlying structures.

palmar kneading (PAHL-mur NEED-ing)—a massage movement in which the flesh is grasped with palms and fingers, squeezed, and released.

palmar manus (PAHL-mur MAN-us)—the palm of the hand.

palmar rotation (PAHL-mur roh-TAY-shun)—a massage movement in which the palms are moved in a circle over underlying tissues.

palmar stroking (PAHL-mur STROHK-ing)—also known as *effleurage*; a massage movement in which the palms are used to stroke large areas of the skin.

palming the comb (PAHM-ing THE KOM)—the technique used to hold the comb in the hand opposite of the hand that is cutting with the shears; should allow for holding and controlling the hair to be cut between the first and second fingers of the same hand.

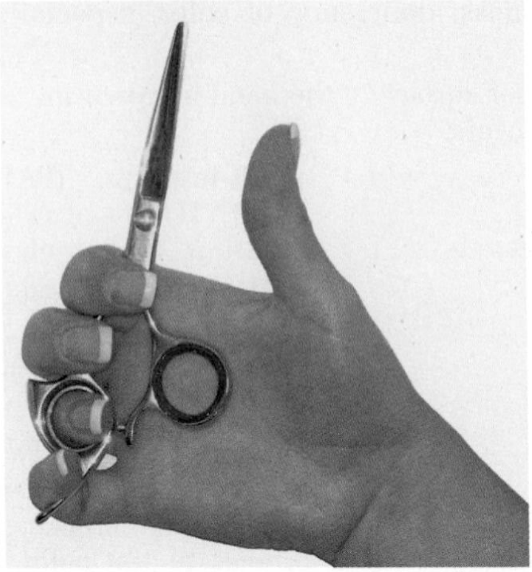
Copyright © 2010 Shark Fin Shear Company and www.sharkfinshears.com.

palming the shears

P

palming the shears (PAHM-ing THE SHEERZ)—the technique used to hold shears in a safe manner while combing through or otherwise working with hair.

palpebra (pal-PEE-bruh); pl., palpebrae (pal-PEE-breye)—the eyelid; eyelids.

palpebral artery (PAL-puh-brul ART-uh-ree)—the lateral artery that supplies blood to the upper and lower eyelids.

palpebral nerve, inferior (PAL-puh-brul NURV, in-FEER-ee-or)—nerve that receives stimuli from the lower eyelid.

palpebral nerve, superior (PAL-puh-brul NURV, soo-PEER-ee-or)—nerve that receives stimuli from the upper eyelid.

palpebrarum (pal-puh-BRAY-rum)—of or pertaining to the eyelids.

pancreas (PANG-kree-us)—a gland located in the abdomen that secretes enzyme-producing cells that are responsible for digesting carbohydrates, proteins, and fats. The islet of Langerhans cells within the pancreas control insulin and glucagon production.

panel (PAN-ul)—in hairdressing, the area between two parallel partings.

paper wraps (PAY-pur RAPS)—temporary nail wraps made of very thin paper; not nearly as strong as fabric wraps.

papilla (puh-PIL-uh); pl., papillae (puh-PIL-eye)—a small cone-shaped projecting body part.

papilla, hair (puh-PIL-uh, HAYR)—a small, cone-shaped elevation at the bottom of the hair follicle in the dermis.

papillary (PAP-uh-lair-ee)—relating to, resembling, or provided with papillae.

papillary layer (PAP-uh-lair-ee LAY-ur)—the outer layer of the dermis, directly beneath the epidermis.

papilloma (pap-uh-LOH-muh); pl., papillomata (pap-uh-LOH-mah-tah)—an epithelial tumor formed by hypertrophy of the papillae of the skin.

papular (PAP-yuh-lur)—characterized by papules.

papule (PAP-yool)—also known as *pimple*; small elevation on the skin that contains no fluid but may develop pus.

papulosis (pap-yuh-LOH-sis)—a condition involving multiple papules.

papulous (PAP-yuh-lus)—area of skin covered with papulae or pimples.

para tint (PAYR-uh TINT)—a tint made from an aniline derivative; oxidation dyes.

para-toluene-diamine (PAYR-uh-TAHL-yoo-ene-dye-AM-in)—a variety of aniline derivative dyes commonly used in preparations compounded to provide red and blond tones.

P

parabens (PAYR-uh-beenz)—one of the most commonly used groups of preservatives in the cosmetic, pharmaceutical, and food industries; provide bacteriostatic and fungistatic activity against a diverse number of organisms.

paradye (PAYR-uh-dye)—an aniline derivative hair tint.

paraffin (PAYR-uh-fin)—a petroleum by-product that has excellent sealing properties (barrier qualities) to hold moisture in the skin.

paraffin wax mask (PAYR-uh-fin WAKS MASK)—a specially prepared facial mask containing paraffin and other beneficial ingredients; typically used with treatment cream.

parallel (PAYR-uh-lel)—extending, as two lines, in the same direction and maintaining a constant distance apart.

parallel lines (PAYR-uh-lel LYNS)—repeating lines in a hairstyle; may be straight or curved.

paralysis (puh-RAL-ih-sis)—loss of muscle function or of sensation through injury to or disease of the nerves or neurons.

paraphenylenediamine (payr-uh-FEEN-ih-leen-dye-AM-in)—an aniline derivative used in oxidation dye; most permanent haircolors, often abbreviated as P.P.D.

paraplegia (payr-uh-PLEE-jee-uh)—paralysis of the legs caused by a stroke or injury to the spinal column.

parasites (PAYR-uh-sytz)—organisms that grow, feed, and shelter on or in another organism (referred to as the host) while contributing nothing to the survival of that organism. Parasites must have a host to survive.

parasitic (payr-uh-SIT-ik)—pertaining to parasites.

parasitic disease (payr-uh-SIT-ik DIZ-eez)—disease caused by parasites, such as lice and mites.

parasitical (payr-uh-SIT-ih-kul)—pertaining to living organisms that live on or within some other living being.

parasympathetic nervous system (payr-uh-sim-puh-THET-ik NUR-vus SIS-tum)—the part of the autonomic nervous system that is concerned with controlling the body during normal routine situations.

parathormone (payr-uh-THOHR-mohn)—hormone regulating metabolism of calcium and phosphorus.

parathyroid (payr-uh-THY-royd)—an endocrine gland located near the thyroid.

parathyroid gland (payr-uh THY-royd GLAND)—gland that regulates blood calcium and phosphorus levels so that the nervous and muscular systems can function properly.

parietal (puh-RY-ate-ul)—pertaining to the wall of a cavity; a bone at the side of the head.

parietal artery (puh-RY-ate-ul ART-uh-ree)—the artery that supplies blood to the side and crown of the head.

parietal bones (puh-RY-ate-ul BONZ)—bones that form the sides and top of the cranium.

parietal ridge (puh-RY-ate-ul RIJ)—also known as *crest*, *hatband*, *horseshoe*, or *temporal region*; widest area of the head, usually starting at the temples and ending at the bottom of the crown.

paronychia (payr-uh-NIK-ee-uh)—bacterial inflammation of the tissues surrounding the nail causing pus, swelling, and redness, usually in the skin fold adjacent to the nail plate.

part (PART)—a line dividing the hair at the scalp, separating one section of hair from another, creating subsections.

part base (PART BAYS)—the part or line in the hair toward which the hair is rolled or curled.

parting (PART-ing)—a line dividing the hair of the scalp that separates one section of hair from another or creates subsections from a larger section of hair.

partnership (PART-nur-ship)—form of business ownership in which two or more people share ownership, although this does not necessarily mean an equal arrangement. In a partnership, each partner assumes the other's unlimited liability for debt. Profits are shared among partners.

passive massage (PAS-iv muh-SAHZH)—a massage movement in which the part (hand, foot, finger, toe) is bent up, down, or forward to flex the joint though its range of motion.

paste-on (PAYST-AWN)—any item such as a jewel, flower, artificial eyelash, or nail that can be glued or pasted on the skin, hair, or nails as a decoration.

pat (PAT)—to tap lightly; to apply makeup by pressing lightly to the skin.

patch (PACH)—a blotch; an irregular spot or area.

patch test (PACH TEST)—also known as a *predisposition test, skin test*; or *allergy test*; test required by the Federal Food, Drug, and Cosmetic Act for identifying a possible allergy in a client.

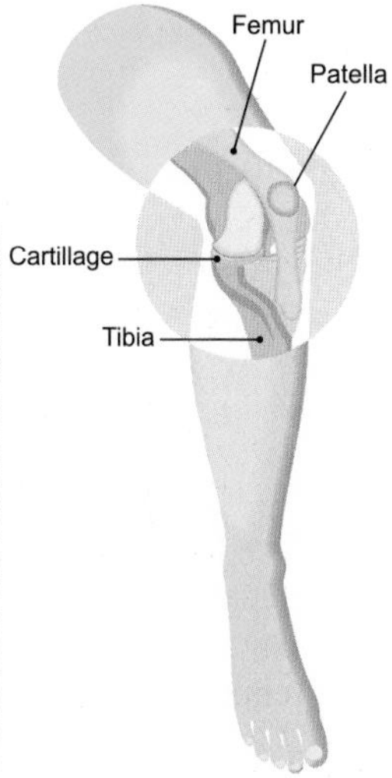

© Jose Elias da Silva Neto /www.Shutterstock.com

patella

patella (puh-TEL-uh)—also known as *accessory bone* or *kneecap*; forms the kneecap joint.

pathogenesis (path-uh-JEN-uh-sis)—the origin and course of the development of a disease.

pathogenic (path-uh-JEN-ik)—harmful microorganisms that can cause disease or infection in humans when they invade the body.

pathogenic disease (path-uh-JEN-ik DIZ-eez)—disease produced by organisms, including bacteria, viruses, fungi, and parasites.

pathological (path-uh-LAHJ-ih-kul)—relating to pathology; morbid; diseased; due to disease.

pathology (puh-THAHL-uh-jee)—the science that investigates modifications of the functions and changes in structure caused by disease.

pattern (PAT-urn)—in hairstyling, a diagram showing where and in which direction hair rollers or pin curls are placed in order to achieve the finished style; a form from which to model a replica; shape and location of an area with hair loss.

peak (PEEK)—also known as *widow's peak*; a point formed by the hair growth at the center of the forehead; named after a bonnet styled with a center point at the forehead worn by widows in the nineteenth century.

pear-shaped face (PAYR-SHAYPT FAYS)—a facial structure characterized by a wide jaw and a narrow forehead.

pectoral nerve (PEK-tuh-rul NURV)—lateral pectoral nerve; the nerve that stimulates the pectoralis major and minor.

pectoralis (pek-tor-AL-is)—a muscle of the chest assisting the swinging movements of the arm.

pectoralis major (pek-tor-AL-is MAY-jor)—muscles of the chest that assist the swinging movements of the arm.

pectoralis minor (pek-tor-AL-is MY-nur)—muscles of the chest that assist the swinging movements of the arm.

pediculosis (puh-dik-yuh-LOH-sis)—a skin disease caused by infestation of the head louse.

pediculosis capitis (puh-dik-ytth-LOH-sis KAP-ih-tus)—infestation of the hair and scalp with head lice.

pedicure (PED-ih-kyoor)—a cosmetic service performed on the feet by a licensed cosmetologist or nail technician; can include exfoliating the skin, callus reduction, as well as trimming, shaping, and polishing toenails. Often includes foot massage.

peel (PEEL)—a technique in facial treatments in which a product is applied to the face to remove dead cells from the surface of the skin.

peeling treatment (PEEL-ing TREET-ment)—a facial treatment using a chemical agent to remove the surface layer of skin, the epidermis, to eliminate lines and acne scars.

pelada (puh-LAH-duh)—also known as *alopecia areata*; a disease of the hair causing circumscribed patches of baldness.

pelage (PEL-aj)—the hair covering of the body of humans and animals.

pellagra (puh-LAG-ruh)—a syndrome due to niacin deficiency; characterized by scaling or peeling of the skin, and in later stages, by nervous and mental disorders.

pencils, makeup (PEN-silz, MAYK-up)—pencils manufactured with a wide assortment of colored leads; used for making up the eyes, lips, and for facial contouring.

penetrate (PEN-uh-trayt)—to pass into or through; to enter by overcoming resistance.

penetrating tint (PEN-uh-trayt-ing TINT)—a haircolor that enters or penetrates into the cortex and deposits color.

pepsin (PEP-sin)—an enzyme that digests protein.

peptide bond (PEP-tyd BAHND)—also known as *end bond*; chemical bond that joins amino acids to each other, end to end, to form a polypeptide chain.

peptides **(PEP-tydz)**—chains of amino acids that stimulate fibroblasts, cell metabolism, collagen and improve skin's firmness; Larger chains are called *polypeptides*.

percussion **(pur-KUSH-un)**—a form of massage consisting of repeated light taps, slaps, or hacks of varying force.

perfectionism **(PUR-fek-shun-izm)**—an unhealthy compulsion to do things perfectly.

perforate **(PUR-fuh-rayt)**—to pierce with holes.

performance ingredients **(per-FOR-manz in-GREED-ee-antz)**—ingredients in cosmetic products that cause the actual changes in the appearance of the skin.

pericardial cavity **(payr-ih-KAR-dee-al KAV-ih-tee)**—a space within the pericardium that contains a serous fluid (resembling serum) that cushions the heart.

P

pericardium **(payr-ih-KAR-dee-um)**—the double-layered membranous sac enclosing the heart; made of epithelial tissue.

perichondrium **(payr-ih-KAHN-dree-um)**—the membrane covering cartilage.

perifollicular inflammation **(PARE-ee-foe-LICK-u-lar in-FLAM-aye-shun)**—inflammation of the follicle walls inside of the follicle.

perimeter **(puh-RIM-ih-tur)**—the outer line of a hairstyle; the silhouette line.

perimysium **(payr-ih-MIS-ee-um)**—the sheath that encases bundles of muscle fibers.

perineum **(PAIR-uh-NEE-um)**—the area between the vulva and anus or scrotum and anus.

periodic table of the elements **(PEER-ee-ODD-ick TABLE UF THEE ELLA-mints)**—a chart of all the known chemical elements, including naturally occurring elements and synthetic elements.

perionychium **(payr-ee-uh-NIK-ee-um)**—the epidermis surrounding a nail.

perioral dermatitis **(PAIR-ee-or-tul DERM-uh-ty-tis)**—acne-like condition around the mouth. These are mainly small clusters of papules that could be caused by toothpaste or products used on the face.

periorbital fat **(PAIR-ee-or-bit-uhl FAT)**—the fat supporting the upper and lower eyelids.

periosteum **(PAIR-ee-AHS-tee-um)**—the fibrous membrane covering the surface of the bones; serves as an attachment of tendons and ligaments.

peripheral nervous system (PNS) (puh-RIF-uh-rul NUR-vus SIS-tum)—system of nerves and ganglia that connects the peripheral parts of the body to the central nervous system; has both sensory and motor nerves.

periphery (puh-RIF-ur-ee)—the part of the body away from the center; the outer part or surface.

peristalsis (payr-ih-STAWL-sis)—moving food through the digestive tract.

perm (PURM)—a permanent wave or a straightening treatment.

perm cap (PURM KAP)—a plastic head covering used during the processing time of a permanent wave to help speed up the action of the product being used.

P

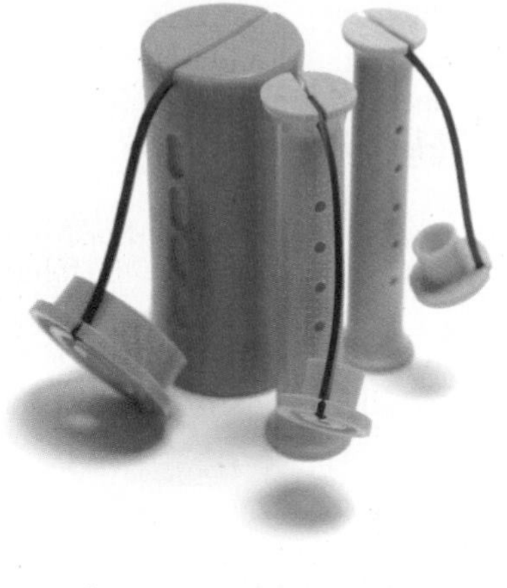

© Milady, a part of Cengage Learning. Photography by Yanik Chauvin.

perm rod

perm rod (PURM RAHD)—a cylindrical or concave rod used for winding the hair for permanent waves.

permanent (PUR-muh-nent)—lasting; enduring; not changing; term used to describe the two-step process of breaking down the internal structure (disulfide bonds) of the hair and rehardening the hair into a curl pattern defined by the size and shape of rod.

permanent, cold wave (PUR-muh-nent, KOHLD WAYV)—a system of permanent waving employing chemicals rather than heat.

permanent haircolors (PUR-muh-nent HAYR-KUL-urz)—lighten and deposit color at the same time and in a single process because they are more alkaline than no-lift deposit-only colors and are usually mixed with a higher-volume developer.

permanent makeup (PUR-muh-nent MAYK-up)—commonly called *permanent cosmetics* and also known as dermapigmentation, micropigmentation, and cosmetic tattooing; the introduction of lasting pigments, or dyes, into the dermal layer of skin for the enhancement of colors; similar to tattooing.

permanent, partial (PUR-muh-nent, PARSH-ul)—technique used to perm controlled sections of the hair for special effects.

permanent waving **(PUR-muh-nent WAYV-ing)**—a two-step process whereby the hair undergoes a physical change caused by wrapping the hair on perm rods, and then the hair undergoes a chemical change caused by the application of permanent waving solution and neutralizer.

peroneal brevis **(payr-uh-NEE-ul BREH-vis)**—muscle that originates on the lower surface of the fibula and bends the foot down and out.

peroneal longus **(payr-uh-NEE-ul LAWNG-gus)**—muscle that covers the outer side of the calf and inverts the foot and turns it outward.

peroneal muscle **(payr-uh-NEE-ul MUS-uhl)**—muscle located on the outer portion of the lower leg that assists in turning the foot downward and outward.

peroneal nerve **(payr-uh-NEE-ul NURV)**—nerve that receives stimuli from the skin of the lateral aspect of the leg.

peroxide **(pur-AHK-syd)**—common term for hydrogen peroxide.

peroxide residue **(pur-AHK-syd RES-ih-doo)**—traces of peroxide left in the hair after treatment with lightener or tint.

perpendicular **(pur-pen-DIK-yuh-lur)**—two lines that intersect at a 90-degree angle.

personal hygiene **(pur-sun-AL HY-jene)**—daily maintenance of cleanliness by practicing good healthful habits.

personal protective equipment (PPE) **(PUR-sun-uhl PRO-tect-if ee-QWIP-ment)**—protective clothing and devices designed to protect an individual from contact with bloodborne pathogens; examples include gloves; fluid-resistant lab coat, apron, or gown; goggles or eye shield; and face masks that cover the nose and mouth.

P

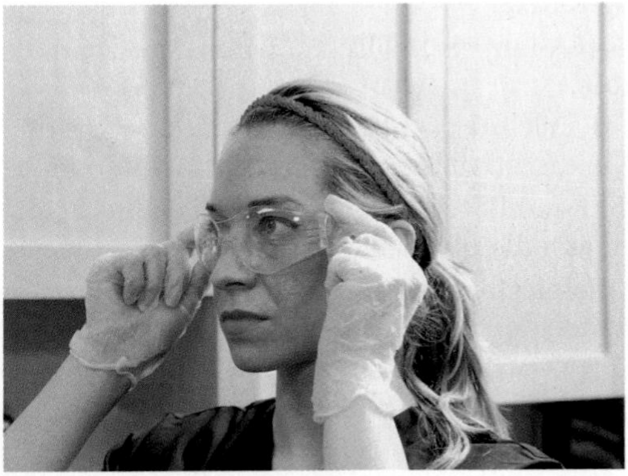

© Milady, a part of Cengage Learning. Photography by Dino Petrocelli.

personal protective equipment

personal selling (pur-SUN-UHL SELL-ing)—a marketing strategy that involves a one-to-one exchange or dialogue with the consumer.

personnel (PER-son-elle)—your staff or employees.

perspiration (pur-spih-RAY-shun)—also known as *sweat*; the fluid excreted from the sudoriferous (sweat) glands of the skin.

perspire (pur-SPYR)—to emit perspiration from the pores of the skin; to sweat.

persulfate (pur-SUL-fayt)—in haircoloring, a chemical ingredient commonly used in activators; it increases the speed of the decolorizing process.

P

pétrissage (PEH-treh-sahzh)—kneading movement performed by lifting, squeezing, and pressing the tissue with a light, firm pressure.

petroleum jelly (peh-TROH-lee-um JELL-ee)—occlusive agent that restores the barrier layer by holding in water; used after laser surgery to protect the skin while healing.

pH (P-H)—the abbreviation used for potential hydrogen. pH represents the quantity of hydrogen ions.

pH adjusters (P-H ah-JUST-uhrz)—acids or alkalis (bases) used to adjust the pH of products.

pH scale (P-H SKAYL)—a measure of the acidity and alkalinity of a substance; the pH scale has a range of 0 to 14, with 7 being neutral. A pH below 7 is an acidic solution; a pH above 7 is an alkaline solution.

pH-balanced shampoo (P-H BAL-unzt sham-POO)—shampoo that is balanced to the pH of skin and hair (4.5 to 5.5).

phagocyte (FAG-oh-site)—any cell that engulfs and devours microorganisms or other particles (a process known as phagocytosis).

phalanges (FA-lanj-eez)—also known as *digits*; bones of the fingers or toes.

pharynx (FAYR-inks)—also known as *throat*; the upper portion of the digestive tube behind the nose and mouth.

phenol (FEE-nohl)—a corrosive and poisonous acidic compound used as a disinfectant.

phenolic disinfectants (FEE-nohl dis-in-FECT-antz)—powerful tuberculocidal disinfectants. They are a form of formaldehyde, have a very high pH, and can damage the skin and eyes.

pheomelanin (fee-oh-MEL-uh-nin)—a type of melanin that is red to yellow in color. People with light-colored skin mostly produce pheomelanin. There are two types of melanin; the other type is eumelanin.

phlebitis (fluh-BYT-us)—inflammation of a vein accompanied by pain and swelling.

phoresis (fuh-REE-sis)—the process of forcing chemical solutions into unbroken skin by way of a galvanic current.

phospholipids (FAHS-foe-lip-id)—compounds that contain fatty acid and phosphoric acid groups.

phosphorus (FAHS-fohr-us)—an element found in bones, muscles, and nerves.

photodamage (FOE-toe-dam-aje)—skin damage caused by exposure to the sun's rays; it can be as simple as fine lines or as serious as hyperpigmentation, actinic keratosis, deep rhytids, facial laxity, and invasive skin cancers.

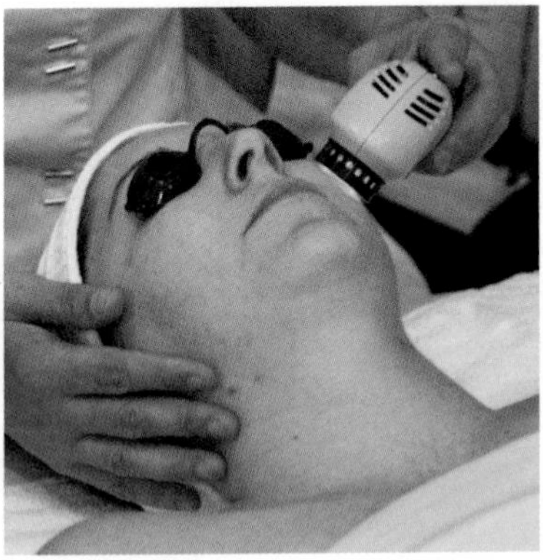

© Milady, a part of Cengage Learning. Photography by Rob Werfel.

photoepilation

photoepilation (FOTO-epp-ihl-aye-shun)—also known as *Intense Pulsed Light*; permanent hair removal treatment that uses intense light to destroy the growth cells of the hair follicles.

photoinitiator (FOTO-in-ish-ee-ate-uhr)—a chemical which, in combination with resins and the proper curing lamp, causes UV gels to cure.

photomodulation (FOTO-mod-yoo-lay-shun)—LED technology that uses energy-producing packets of light to enhance fibroblast collagen synthesis.

photons (FOE-TONS)—in quantum theory, the elemental unit of light; a particle of energy that has motion and travels in waves.

photorejuvenation (FOTO-re-jewv-en-aye-shun)—a series of laser or IPL facial treatments conducted to improve vascular and pigmented lesions and induce collagen stimulation.

photosensitivity (FOTO-sensa-tiv-it-ee)—responsiveness to sunlight.

photothermolysis (FOTO-ther-moll-ih-sis)—process that turns the light from the laser into heat.

phototoxic (FOTO-tock-sick)—describes a toxic effect triggered by exposure of light to the skin, sometimes as a result of topical or oral medications.

phyma (FEYE-ma) pl., phymata (feye-MAY-ta)—circumscribed swelling on the skin larger than a tubercle.

phymatous rosacea (FEYE-may-tuss roe-ZAY-shah)—a subtype of rosacea in which the nose has a thickened appearance and the individual sometimes has rhinophyma, which is a substantial enlargement of the nose.

physical change (FIZ-ih-kuhl CHAYNJ)—a change in the form or physical properties of a substance, without a chemical reaction or the creation of a new substance.

physical mixture (FIZ-ih-kuhl mix-CHUR)—a physical combination of matter in any proportions.

physical presentation (FIZ-ih-kuhl pres-ent-TAY-shun)—a person's physical posture, walk, and movements.

physical properties (FIZ-ih-kuhl PRAH-per-tees)—characteristics that can be determined without a chemical reaction and that do not cause a chemical change in the substance.

P

physiology (fiz-ih-OL-oh-gee)—the study of the functions or activities performed by the body's structures.

phytotherapy (FY-TO-thair-uh-pee)—use of plant extracts for therapeutic benefits.

pia mater (PEE-ah MAY-tur)—the innermost layer of the brain.

picealis (pih-see-AH-lis)—type of acne caused by an allergy to tar products.

piggyback (PIG-gee-BAK)—the double-rod wrapping method used in perming long hair to produce a more uniform wave pattern; two rods are used for one strand of hair.

pigment (PIG-ment)—any organic coloring matter such as that of the red blood cells, the hair, skin, and iris; any substance or matter used as coloring for natural or artificial hair.

pigmentary (PIG-men-tair-ee)—pertaining to producing or containing pigment.

pigmentation (pig-men-TAY-shun)—the deposition of pigment in the skin or tissues.

pigmented UV gels (PIG-ment-ed YOO-VEE JELZ)—in nail technology; any building or self-leveling gel that includes color pigment.

pileous (PY-lee-us)—pertaining to hair; hairy.

pili; pilar (PY-leh; PIH-lur)—hair; related to hair.

pili incarnati (PY-leh in-kar-NAY-tye)—ingrown hairs.

pili multigemini (PY-leh mul-tih-JEM-ih-nye)—several hairs growing from a single follicle opening.

pili tactiles (PY-leh TAK-tih-leez)—tactile hairs; associated with the sense of touch.

pili torti (PY-leh TOR-tye)—a congenital deformity of the hair characterized by short, broken hairs that resemble stubble.

piliation (pih-lee-AY-shun)—the formation and production of hair.

piloerection (py-luh-ih-REK-shun)—also known as *goosebumps* or *gooseflesh*; characterized by erection of hair and a bump around the follicle.

pilomotor (py-luh-MOH-tur)—causing movement of the hair.

pilomotor muscle (py-luh-MOH-tur MUS-uhl)—the arrector pili muscle.

pilomotor nerve (py-luh-MOH-tur NURV)—a nerve causing contraction of one of the arrectores pilorum muscles.

pilomotor reflex (py-luh-MOH-tur REE-fleks)—erection of hairs of the skin (gooseflesh) as a response to cold or emotional stimuli.

pilonidal (py-luh-NY-dul)—pertaining to hair growing within a cyst.

pilose (PY-lohs)—covered with soft hair; hairy.

pilosebaceous (py-luh-seh-BAY-shus)—pertaining to the hair follicles and the sebaceous glands.

pilosebaceous unit (py-luh-seh-BAY-shus YOO-knit)—the hair unit that contains the hair follicle and appendages: the hair root, bulb, dermal papilla, sebaceous appendage, and arrector pili muscle.

pilosis (py-LOH-sis)—abnormal or excessive development of hair.

pilosity (py-LAHS-ih-tee)—the state of being pilose or hairy.

pilous gland (PY-lus GLAND)—the sebaceous gland of a hair follicle.

pilus (PY-lus); pl., pilli (PY-lee)—a hair.

pilus cuniculatus (PY-lus kuh-nik-yuh-LAY-tus)—a burrowing hair.

pilus incarnatus (PY-lus in-kar-NAY-tus)—ingrown hair.

pilus incarnatus recurvus (PY-lus in-kar-NAY-tus ree-KUR-vus)—an ingrown hair caused by a curved hair reentering the skin.

pimple (PIM-pul)—also known as *papule* or *pustule*; any small, pointed elevation of the skin.

pin curl (PIN KURL)—a strand of hair, combed smooth, and wound into a circle with the ends on the inside of the curl.

pin curl base (PIN KURL BAYS)—also known as *pin curl foundation*; the area of the scalp where a pin curl is secured; the base may be sectioned into a square, a slanted oblong, an arc, or a C-shaped base.

pin curl direction (PIN KURL dih-REK-shun)—the line in which a pin curl is moved or designed to move.

pin curl foundation (PIN-kurl fown-DAY-shun)—also known as *pin curl base*; the area at the scalp where the pin curl is secured.

pin curl stem (PIN KURL STEM)—the part of the pin curl between the base and the first arc of the circle of hair.

pin curl wave (PIN KURL WAYV)—the technique of alternating the direction of the rows of pin curls to form a wave when the hair is combed.

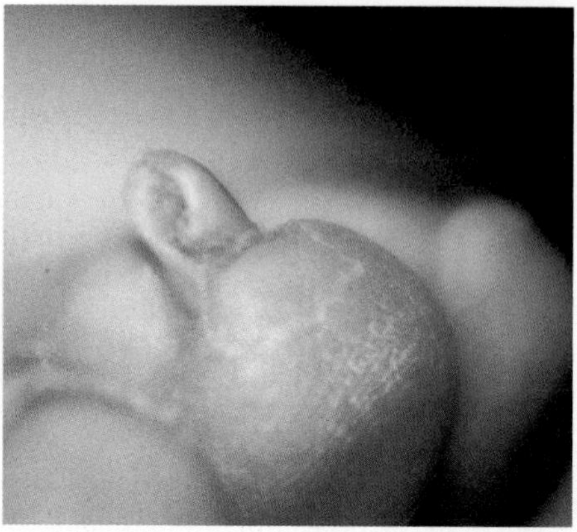

Courtesy of Godfrey F. Mix, DPM Sacramento, CA.

pincer nail

pincer nail (PIN-sir NAYL)—also known as *trumpet nail*; increased crosswise curvature throughout the nail plate caused by an increased curvature of the matrix. The edges of the nail plate may curl around to form the shape of a trumpet or sharp cone at the free edge.

pincurling (PIN-kurl-ing)—the forming of circles or ringlets by winding the hair and fastening the circles in place with clips.

pineal body (PY-nee-ul BAHD-ee)—a ductless gland attached to the brain.

pineal gland (PY-nee-ul GLAND)—plays a major role in sexual development, sleep, and metabolism.

pinkeye (PINGK-eye)—an acute, highly contagious conjunctivitis marked by redness of the eyeball.

pinna (PIN-uh)—the external ear.

pint (PYNT)—a liquid or dry measure, equal to $^{1}/_{2}$ quart or 0.47 liter.

pisiform (PY-suh-form)—pea-shaped; a bone of the wrist.

pit (PIT)—a surface depression or hollow.

pit scar (PIT SKAR)—a scar that heals with a hollow pit; usually caused by acne.

pith (PITH)—center; the marrow of the bones; the center of the hair.

pituitary gland (puh-TOO-uh-tair-ee GLAND)—the most complex organ of the endocrine system. It affects almost every physiologic process of the body: growth, blood pressure, contractions during childbirth, breast-milk production, sexual organ functions in both women and men, thyroid gland function, and the conversion of food into energy (metabolism).

pityriasis (pit-ih-RY-uh-sus)—technical term for dandruff; characterized by excessive production and accumulation of skin cells.

pityriasis capitis simplex (pit-ih-RY-uh-sus KAP-ih-tis SIM-pleks)—technical term for classic dandruff; characterized by scalp irritation, large flakes, and itchy scalp.

pityriasis pilaris (pit-ih-RY-uh-sus py-LAYR-is)—a skin disorder characterized by an eruption of papules surrounding the hair follicles; each papule is pierced by a hair and tipped with a horny plug or scale.

pityriasis steatoides (pit-ih-RY-uh-sis stee-uh-TOY-deez)—severe case of dandruff characterized by an accumulation of greasy or waxy scales, mixed with sebum, which stick to the scalp in crusts.

pityroid (PIT-ih-royd)—pertaining to a condition of the skin or scalp characterized by thin scales.

pityrosporum ovale (pit-ih-roh-SPOH-rum oh-VAY-lee)—a type of yeast sometimes associated with seborrheic dermatitis.

pivot point (PIV-ut POYNT)—pivot hair shaping; the exact point from which the hair is directed in forming a curvature or shaping.

placental extract (pluh-SEN-tul EK-strakt)—the nourishing substance surrounding an embryo or fetus; afterbirth; used in some facial preparations.

plait (PLAYT)—also known as *braiding*; to interweave strands of hair into an intricate pattern.

plankton extract (PLANGK-tun EK-strakt)—the microscopic animal and plant life found in the oceans and in fresh water; algae or seaweed; used in certain cosmetic preparations, usually in facial and body treatment preparations.

plant extracts (PLANT EK-strakts)—organic substances extracted from leaves, roots, and flowers of various plants for use in products such as perfumes and grooming aids.

planta pedis (PLAN-tuh PEE-dis)—the sole of the foot.

plantar (PLANT-ur)—pertaining to the sole of the foot.

plantar arterial arch (PLANT-ur ART-eer-ee-ul ARCH)—the arch in the sole of the foot made by the lateral plantar artery and branch of the dorsalis pedis artery.

plantar fascia (PLAN-ter FAY-she-uh)—a fibrous membrane of variable thickness, devoid of fat, which invests the muscles of the foot and heel, forms sheaths for the nerves and vessels, becomes specialized around the joints to form or strengthen ligaments, envelops various organs and glands, and binds all the structures together into a firm compact mass.

plantar fasciitis (PLAN-ter fash-EE-eye-tus)—inflammation of the plantar fascia, usually noninfectious, and often caused by overuse, elicits foot and heel pain.

plantar flexion (PLANT-ur FLEK-shun)—bending the foot or toes downward toward the sole of the foot.

plantar flexor (PLANT-ur FLEK-sur)—muscle that bends the foot downward.

plantar reflex (PLANT-ur REE-fleks)—flexing of the toes in response to stroking massage movements on the outer sides of the soles.

plasma (PLAZ-muh)—the fluid part of the blood in which the red and white blood cells and platelets flow.

plastic surgeon (PLAS-tik SUR-jun)—a surgeon who builds up or molds tissue and bones to repair physical defects.

plasticizer (PLAS-tih-sy-zur)—ingredients used to keep nail enhancement products flexible.

platelets (PLAYT-lets)—also known as *thrombocytes*; much smaller than red blood cells; contribute to the blood-clotting process, which stops bleeding.

platinum blond (PLAT-ih-num BLAHND)—very light, almost white-blond hair.

platysma muscle (plah-TIZ-muh MUS-uhl)—broad muscle extending from the chest and shoulder muscles to the side of the chin; responsible for lowering the lower jaw and lip.

platysmal bands (plah-TIZ-muhl BAHNDS)—bands found vertically in the neck which are a result of dynamic movement of the neck and jaw.

pleat (PLEET)—also known as *classic French twist*; a technique used for formal hairstyling that creates a look of folded hair.

pledget (PLEJ-et)—a compress; a small, flat mass of absorbent cotton or the like.

plexus (PLEK-sus)—a network of nerves or veins.

plicatured nail (plik-a-CHOORD NAYL)—also known as *folded nail*; a type of highly curved nail usually caused by injury to the matrix, but may be inherited.

plug (PLUG)—to stop or close such as inserting a plug; a plugged follicle. Small section of hair

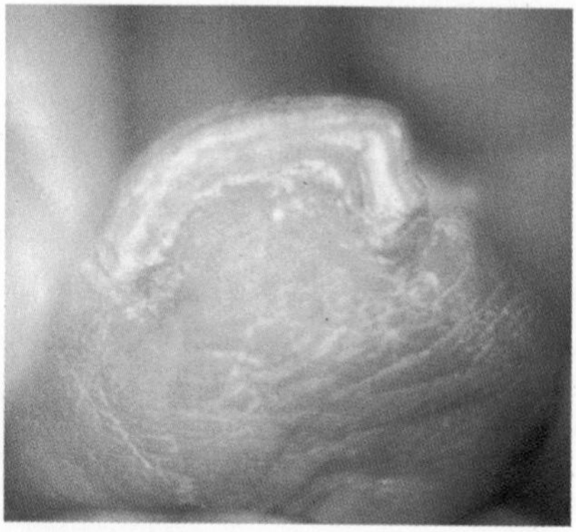

Courtesy of Godfrey F. Mix, DPM Sacramento, CA.

plicatured nail

(approximately $^{1}/_{8th}$ inch) surgically removed including follicles, papillae, and hair bulbs and reset in a bald area; two- or three-prong connector at the end of an electrical cord that connects an apparatus to an electrical outlet.

podiatrist (poh-DY-uh-trist)—one who treats diseases of the feet.

point (POYNT)—a sharp end or apex; an abscess, the wall of which becomes thin and breaks.

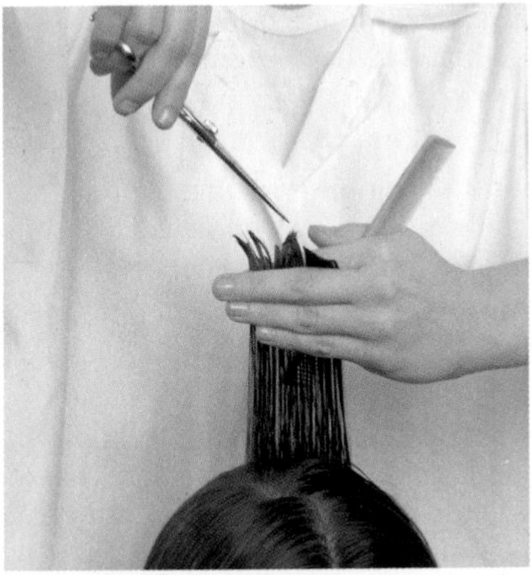

© Milady, a part of Cengage Learning. Photography by Paul Castle.

point cutting

point cutting (POYNT CUT-ing)—haircutting technique in which the tips of the shears are used to cut *points* into the ends of the hair.

point of distribution (POYNT UV dis-trih-BYOO-shun)—also known as *radial motion*; the central point from which hair is distributed in a preplanned manner.

point of origin (POYNT UV OR-ih-jen)—in hairdressing, the place where a motion starts or the beginning of a design.

pointed nail (POYNT-ed NAYL)—nail shape suited to thin hands with long fingers and narrow nail beds. The nail is tapered and longer than usual to emphasize and enhance the slender appearance of the hand.

poisoning, blood (POY-zun-ing, BLUD)—also known as *septicemia*; the invasion of pathogenic bacteria into the blood, resulting in infection.

polarity (poh-LAYR-ut-ee)—the property of having two opposite poles such as that possessed by a magnet or electric current.

polarity therapy (poh-LAYR-ut-ee THAYR-uh-pee)—therapy using massage, exercises, and thinking practices to balance the body physically and energetically.

pole (POHL)—an electrical terminal.

poliomyelitis (poh-lee-oh-my-uh-LY-tus)—a disease affecting the motor neurons and resulting in paralysis of related muscle tissue.

poliosis (poh-lee-OH-sus)—a condition characterized by absence of pigment in the hair.

P

polish (PAHL-ish)—also known as *nail polish* or *laquer*; nail enamel formulated to strengthen, protect, and beautify the nails; clear or colored lacquer.

polish dryer (PAHL-ish DRY-ur)—a chemical preparation that speeds the drying process of freshly applied nail polish.

polish remover (PAHL-ish ree-MOOV-ur)—also known as *nail polish remover*; a solution used to remove polish from the nails.

polish thinner (PAHL-ish THIN-ur)—a chemical preparation formulated to thin nail polish that has become too thick.

polychromatic (pahl-ee-kroh-MAT-ik)—having many colors.

polyglucans (POLY-glue-canz)—ingredients derived from yeast cells that help strengthen the immune system and stimulate the metabolism; they are also hydrophilic and help preserve and protect collagen and elastin.

polymer (PAHL-uh-mur)—substance formed by combining many small molecules (monomers) or oligomers, usually in extremely long, chain-like structure.

polymer powder (PAHL-uh-mur POW-dur)—in nail technology; powder in white, clear pink, and many other colors that is combined with monomer liquid to form the nail enhancement.

polymerization (PAHL-uh-mur-eye-say-shun)—also known as *curing* or *hardening*; a chemical reaction that creates polymers.

polyp (PAHL-up)—a smooth growth extending from the surface of the skin; polyps may also grow within the body.

polypeptide bonds (pahl-ee-PEP-tyd BAHNDZ)—bonds that link peptide chains together to form protein.

polypeptide chain (pahl-ee-PEP-tyd CHAYN)—long chains of amino acids joined together by peptide bonds.

polyphenols (POLY-feen-awls)—a group of chemicals that act as antioxidants.

polysaccharides (POLY-sack-uh-ridez)—carbohydrates that contain three or more simple carbohydrate molecules.

polyunsaturated (pahl-ee-un-SACH-uh-rayt-ud)—pertaining to any of a class of fats having more than two double bonds in its molecule, or to fats used in diets to reduce blood cholesterol.

polyunsaturated fatty acids (pahl-ee-un-SACH-uh-rayt-ud FADDY ASUDS)—unsaturated fatty acids that contain two or more double bonds.

pomade (poh-MAYD)—also known as *wax*; styling products that add considerable weight to the hair by causing strands to join together, showing separation in the hair.

pomphus (PAHM-fus)—also known as *wheal*; a whitish or pinkish elevation of the skin.

pons (PAHNZ)—also known as *pons varolii*; a broad band of nerve fibers that connects the cerebrum, cerebellum, and medulla oblongata.

popliteal artery (pahp-lih-TEE-ul AHR-ter-ee)—artery that supplies blood to the foot; divides into two separate arteries known as the anterior tibial artery and the posterior tibial artery.

pore (POR)—a small opening of the sweat glands of the skin.

porosity (poh-RAHS-ut-ee)—ability of the hair to absorb moisture.

porous (POHW-rus)—made or constructed of a material that has pores or openings. Porous items are absorbent.

porous hair (POHW-rus HAYR)—hair characterized by lifted cuticle scales that allow faster absorption of moisture or chemicals into the hair.

portfolio (PORT-foe-lee-oh)—a collection of photographs depicting the technician's work.

position (POH-zish-uhn)—in nail technology; the way that a brush is held to create nail art; the brush can be positioned straight up-and-down or laid flat and pulled across the nail surface.

position stop (POH-zish-uhn STOP)—the point where the free edge of the natural nail meets the nail tip.

positive pole, P or + (PAHZ-ih-tiv POHL)—the pole from which positive electricity flows.

positive skin test (PAHZ-ih-tiv SKIN TEST)—direct proof that the substance involved in a test is hostile to the body; having a reaction to a skin test for allergy; showing signs of redness, swelling, or irritation.

posterior (poh-STEER-ee-ur)—situated behind; coming after or behind.

posterior auricular artery (poh-STEER-ee-ur aw-RIK-yuh-lur AR-tuh-ree)—the artery that supplies blood to the scalp, the area behind and above the ear, and the skin behind the ear.

posterior auricular nerve (poh-STEER-ee-ur aw-rik-yuh-LAYR NURV)—affects the muscles behind the ear at the base of the skull.

posterior auricularis (poh-STEER-ee-ur aw-rik-yuh-LAYR-us)—muscle that draws the ear backward.

posterior cerebral artery (poh-STEER-ee-ur suh-REE-brul AR-tuh-ree)—artery that supplies blood to the cortex, and the temporal and occipital bones.

posterior cutaneous nerve (poh-STEER-ee-ur kyoo-TAY-nee-us NURV)—nerve that stimulates the skin of the posterior aspect of the forearm.

posterior interosseous artery (poh-STEER-ee-ur in-tur-AHS-ee-us AR--tuh-ree)—artery that supplies blood to the muscles and skin of the forearm.

posterior tibial artery (poh-STEER-ee-ur TIB-ee-ul AR--tuh-ree)—artery that supplies blood to the ankle and the back of the lower leg.

postinflammatory hyperpigmentation (POHST-in-flam-uh-tory hy-PER-pig-MEN-tay-shun)—dark melanin splotches caused by trauma to the skin; they can result from acne pimples and papules.

postnasal (pohst-NAY-zul)—situated behind the nose.

postpartum alopecia (POHST-pahr-tum al-oh-PEE-she-a)—hair loss experienced at the conclusion of pregnancy.

potassium (poh-TAS-ee-um)—an element, the salts of which are used in medicine; an essential mineral found in vegetables and fruits, and necessary to the health of the skin; potassium and sodium regulate the water balance within the body.

potassium bromate (poh-TAS-ee-um BROH-mayt)—a metallic element of the alkali group; used in medicines as a sedative.

potassium carbonate (poh-TAS-ee-um KAR-buh-nayt)—a white salt that forms a highly alkaline solution; used to make soap and other cleansing products.

potassium chloride (poh-TAS-ee-um KLOH-ryd)—a colorless, crystalline salt; used as a buffer in solid perfumes and in some eye washes.

potassium hydroxide (poh-TAS-ee-um hy-DRAHK-syd)—a powerful alkali having emulsifying abilities; prepared by electrolysis of potassium chloride; used in the manufacture of soft soaps.

potassium permanganate (poh-TAS-ee-um pur-MANG-guh-nayt)—a salt of permanganate acid; used as an antiseptic and deodorant.

potential (poh-TEN-shul)—indicating possibility of power.

potential hydrogen (pH) (poh-TEN-shul HI-dro-jemn)—the quantity of hydrogen ions in a substance.

powder (POW-dur)—a finely ground insoluble substance forming a mass of loose particles; used as a cosmetic and in some medicines.

powder bleach (POW-dur BLEECH)—a strong, fast-acting bleach in powdered form; used for off-the-scalp lightening.

powder dry shampoo (POW-dur DRY sham-POO)—a substance composed of a mixture of orris root, borax, or other such ingredients that are used to clean hair without using soap or water.

powder lightener (POW-dur LYT-un-ur)—also known as *powder bleach*; off-the-scalp lightener.

powder puff (POW-dur PUF)—a small fluffy circle or square of cotton, sponge, or silk used to apply powder.

power density (POW-uhr DEN-sity)—the rate of energy that is being delivered to tissue by a laser light source; measured in watts per square centimeter (W/cm^2).

practical exam (PRAK-tih-cul EXAM)—one of two forms of licensing tests, a hands-on test on a live model.

preauricular nodes (PRE-ORE-ick-u-lar NODES)—lymph nodes located on the face in front of the ears.

precaution (pree-KAW-shun)—a written or verbal warning with the purpose of preventing harm and ensuring safety.

precipitate (pree-SIP-ih-tayt)—in chemistry, to cause a substance in a solution to settle in solid particles; to separate from solution or suspension by chemical or physical change.

precipitation (pree-sip-ih-TAY-shun)—in chemistry, the process of separating the constituents of a solution by reagents or by mechanical means.

precision (pree-SIZH-un)—the state or quality of being accurate and precise; exactness.

predisposition (pree-dis-puh-ZISH-un)—a condition of special susceptibility to disease; allergy.

predisposition test (pree-dis-puh-ZISH-un TEST)—also known as *allergy test, skin test,* or *patch test*; skin test designed to determine an individual's oversensitivity to certain chemicals.

prelightening (pree-LYT-tin-ing)—first step of double-process haircoloring; used to lift or lighten the natural pigment before the application of toner.

premature (pree-muh-CHOOR)—happening, arriving, existing, or performed before the usual time.

premature canities (pree-muh-CHOOR KAN-ih-teez)—premature graying of the hair.

preocrus (PREE-uh-krus)—muscle that covers bridge of nose.

prescribe (pree-SKRYB)—to set or lay down a course or rule to be followed.

presenile (pree-SEN-yl)—prematurely old.

preservatives (PRE-serv-uh-tifs)—chemical agents that inhibit the growth of microorganisms in cosmetic formulations; these kill bacteria and prevent products from spoiling.

presoftener (pree-SOF-un-ur)—a chemical solution applied to the hair in order to make the penetration of additional chemicals easier.

presoftening (pree-SOF-en-ing)—process of treating gray or very resistant hair to allow for better penetration of color.

pressing (PRES-ing)—a temporary method of straightening overcurly hair with a heated comb or iron.

pressing irons (PRES-ing EYE-urns)—an implement resembling a curling iron; used to straighten hair.

pressure (PRESH-ur)—in nail technology; amount of force that an artist applies to a brush while in the stroke motion when applying nail art.

pressure receptors (PRESH-ur ree-SEP-turz)—nerves supplying the skin that register pressure or touch; nerve fibers that respond to pressure.

price (PRYS)—the monetary value applied to goods and services sold.

prickle cell layer (PRIK-ul SEL LAY-ur)—the layer of cells between the granular cell layer and the basal cell layer of the epidermis.

prickly heat (PRIK-lee HEET)—also known as *miliaria rubra*; a cutaneous eruption of red vesicles accompanied by burning and itching; usually caused by overexposure to heat.

primary colors (PRY-mayr-ee KUL-urz)—pure or fundamental colors (red, yellow, and blue) that cannot be created by combining other colors.

primary hair (PRY-mayr-ee HAYR)—the baby-fine hair that is present over almost the entire smooth skin of the body.

primary lesions (PRY-mayr-ee LEE-jhuns)—lesions that are a different color than the color of the skin, and/or lesions that are raised above the surface of the skin.

primary terminal hair (PRIH-mar-ee TER-min-uhl HAYR)—short, thick hairs that grow on the eyebrows and lashes.

primer (PRIH-mur)—substance that improves adhesion.

prioritize (PRIH-or-uh-tize)—to make a list of tasks that needs to be done in the order of most-to-least important.

prism (PRIZ-um)—a transparent glass or crystal solid with triangular ends and two converging sides; it breaks up white light into its component colors; the spectrum.

procedure (proh-SEED-jur)—a series of definite steps to follow in a certain order to achieve desired results.

procerus muscle (proh-SEE-rus MUS-uhl)—covers the bridge of the nose, lowers the eyebrows, and causes wrinkles across the bridge of the nose.

processed hair (PRAH-sest HAYR)—hair that has been chemically altered through such procedures as lightening, stripping, tinting, permanently waving, or chemically relaxing.

processing (PRAH-ses-ing)—the action of a chemical solution in permanent waving, hair straightening, or haircoloring.

processing time (PRAH-ses-ing TYM)—the time or period required for the chemical solution to act on the hair.

procrastination (PRO-crass-tin-aye-shun)—putting off until tomorrow what you can do today.

profit (PROFF-it)—amount of money available after all expenses are subtracted from all revenues.

profession (pruh-FESH-un)—an occupation that requires a liberal, scientific, or artistic education.

professional (pruh-FESH-un-ul)—one who pursues as a business or livelihood a particular occupation or vocation.

professional image (pruh-FESH-un-ul IM-aje)—the impression projected by a person engaged in any profession, consisting of outward appearance and conduct exhibited in the workplace.

profile (PROH-fyl)—the outline of a face, head, figure, or an object seen in a side view.

progesterone (proh-JES-tah-rohn)—a hormone that helps prepare the uterus for pregnancy and is an important hormone in the menstrual cycle.

progestin (PROH-JES-tin)—a synthetic version of progesterone used in mini-pills for birth control.

prognosis (prahg-NOH-sis)—the foretelling of the probable course of a disease.

progressive dye (pruh-GRES-iv DYE)—color that develops gradually; metallic dye; color products that deepen or increase absorption over a period of time during processing; a coloring system that produces increased absorption with each application.

projection angle (pruh-JEK-shun ANG-gul)—also known as *projection*; the angle at which the hair is held while cutting.

proliferate (pruh-LIF-ur-ayt)—to grow by reproduction of new parts, cells, or offspring.

proliferative phase (pruh-LIF-ur-uh-tive FAZE)—the phase of wound healing in which there is increased vascularity to supply nutrients and oxygen to the wound.

prominence (PRAHM-ih-nents)—a projection.

promissory note (PRAH-miss-or-ee NOTE)—a legal document that defines the terms of a loan agreement between two parties.

promotion (PRO-moe-sun)—the process of getting the consumer's attention, with the goal of increasing business.

promotion mix (PRO-moe-shun MIX)—the communication methods used to promote business in marketing; these include advertising, public relations, publicity, direct marketing, personal selling, and sales promotion.

pronate (PROH-nayt)—to bend forward.

pronators (proh-NAY-tohrs)—muscles that turn the hand inward so that the palm faces downward.

prong (PRAWNG)—a slender pointed or projecting part of an implement.

properties (PRAHP-ur-teez)—the identifying characteristics of a substance that are observable; a peculiar quality of anything such as color, taste, smell, and the like.

prophase (PROH-fayz)—the first stage of mitosis (cell division).

***Propionibacterium acnes (P. acnes)* (pro-PEE-ah-nee-back-tear-ee-um AK-nes)**—technical term for acne bacteria.

proportion (pruh-POR-shun)—the comparative relation of one thing to another; the harmonious relationship among parts or things.

propylparaben (proh-pil-payr-A-ben)—esters of p-hydroxybenzoate widely used in cosmetics as preservatives, and to destroy bacteria and fungus.

prosthetic makeup (pros-thet-ik MAYK-up)—the application of artificial parts that are created from a variety of material and includes products such as wax, latex, foam, gels, gypsum, silicone, and rubber.

protective cream (proh-TEK-tiv KREEM)—a base cream applied to the skin to protect it against chemicals used during a perm, color, or straightening treatment.

protectors (proh-TEKT-urs)—articles or equipment that protect a client from contamination or injury during a salon service; examples include neck strips, shampoo capes, and ear pads.

protein (PROH-teen)—a complex organic substance present in all living tissues such as skin, hair, and nails; necessary to sustain life; also used in some skin and hair conditioners.

protein conditioner (PROH-teen CON-dish-en-uhr)—product designed to penetrate the cortex and reinforce the hair shaft from within.

protein filler (PROH-teen FIL-ur)—a conditioning filler.

protein hardeners (PROH-teen HAR-den-uhrz)—in nail technology; a combination of clear polish and protein, such as collagen.

protinator (PROH-tin-ay-tur)—an agent that accelerates the release of oxygen in hair lightening.

protoplasm (PROH-toh-plaz-um)—a colorless, jelly-like substance in cells in which food elements such as protein, fats, carbohydrates, mineral salts, and water are present.

protozoa (proh-toh-ZOH-ah)—subkingdom of animals, including all the unicellular animal organisms.

proximal (PRAHK-sih-mul)—situated toward the point of origin or attachment, as in a tendon or bone.

pruritus (proo-RYT-us)—persistent itching.

pseudofolliculitis barbae (SUE-doe-foh-lick-yoo-lye-tis BAR-bee)—also known as *razor bumps*; a chronic inflammatory form of folliculitis resembling folliculitis papules and pustules; generally accepted to be caused by ingrown hair.

P

Pseudomonas aeruginosa **(SUE-duh-MOAN-us)** —one of several common bacteria that can cause nail infection.

psoriasis (suh-RY-uh-sis)—skin disease characterized by red patches covered with white-silver scales. It is caused by an overproliferation of skin cells that replicate too fast. Immune dysfunction could be the cause. Psoriasis is usually found in patches on the scalp, elbows, knees, chest, and lower back.

pterygium (teh-RIJ-ee-um)—a forward growth of the eponychium (cuticle) with adherence to the surface of the nail.

ptosis (TOE-sis)—drooping of the eyelids.

puberty (PYOO-ber-tee)—the stage of life when physical changes occur in both sexes and when sexual function of the sex glands begins to take place.

public relations (PUB-lick REE-lay-shunz)—also known as *PR*; planning and developing of relationships to achieve a certain desired behavior.

publicity (PUB-liss-it-ee)—a marketing strategy used to gain free media attention.

pull (PUL)—in nail technology, the technique of pulling a liner or other brush across the surface of the nail to create a fluid line.

pulmonary (PUL-muh-nayr-ee)—relating to the lungs.

pulmonary circulation (PUL-muh-nayr-ee sur-kyoo-LAY-shun)—sends the blood from the heart to the lungs to be purified, then back to the heart again.

pulmonary valve (PUL-muh-nayr-ee VALV)—one of the two valves that regulate the flow of blood between the ventricles and the major blood vessel to which each valve connects.

pulsate (PUL-sayt)—to move with rhythmical impulses.

pulse duration (PULZ dur-ay-shun)—also known as *pulse width*; the duration of an individual pulse of laser light; usually measured in milliseconds.

pumice (PUM-is)—also known as *pumice stone* or *pumice rock*; hardened volcanic substance, white or gray in color; used for smoothing and polishing.

punctata, acne (punk-TAH-tah, AK-nee)—a form of acne in which the lesions are pointed papules with a comedone in the center.

punctate keratitis (PUNK-shoo-ate KERA-ty-tiz)—calluses resulting from prolonged and frequent exposure to friction.

P

pungent (PUN-jent)—sharp, foul, or irritating odor.

pupil (PYOO-pul)—the small opening in the iris of the eye through which light enters.

pure substance (PYOOR SUB-stantz)—a chemical combination of matter in definite (fixed) proportions.

purpura (PUR-puh-rah)—a disease characterized by hemorrhage into the skin, resulting in the formation of purple patches on the skin and mucous membranes.

pus (PUS)—a fluid created by infection.

pusher (PUSH-ur)—a steel instrument used to loosen the cuticle from the nail.

pustular (PUS-tyuh-lur)—pertaining to or characterized by pustules.

pustule (PUS-chool)—raised, inflamed papule with a white or yellow center containing pus in the top of the lesion referred to as the head of the pimple.

pustulosa, acne (pus-tyuh-LOH-suh, AK-nee)—a form of acne characterized by pustules.

pyogenic (py-oh-JEN-ik)—pus-forming.

pyosis (py-OH-sis)—the formation of pus.

pyramidal bone (pih-RAM-ih-dul BOHN)—the wedge-shaped bone of the carpus.

pyramidalis nasi (pih-ram-ih-DAY-lis NAY-sye)—procerus; muscle of the nose.

pyogenic granuloma (py-oh-JEN-ik GRAN-yoo-low-mah)—severe inflammation of the nail in which a lump of red tissue grows up from the nail bed to the nail plate.

Q

quadrant (KWAHD-rent)—also known as *pie-shaping* or *wedge-shaping*; a quarter of a circle; anything resembling the quarter section of a circle.

quadratus (kwah-DRA-tus)—a square-shaped muscle; a muscle of the lower jaw.

quadratus labii inferioris (kwah-DRA-tus LAY-bee-eye in-feer-ee-OR-is)—a muscle surrounding the lower lip.

quadratus labii superioris (kwah-DRA-tus LAY-bee-eye soo-peer-ee-OR-is)—a muscle surrounding the upper lip.

quadriceps femoris (KWAHD-ruh-seps FEM-uh-rus)—the large extensor muscle of the thigh.

quadriplegia (kwahd-ruh-puh-LEE-jee-uh)—paralysis of the arms and legs resulting from a stroke or damage to the spinal cord.

quality of hair (KWAHL-uh-tee UV HAYR)—the form, length, elasticity, size, and texture of the hair.

quantitative analysis (KWAHN-tih-tay-tiv uh-NAL-ih-sis)—in chemistry; the process of finding the amount or percentage of an element or ingredient present in a material or compound.

quartz lamp (KWORTZ LAMP)—a glass bulb lamp used for cosmetic purposes; the cold quartz lamp produces mostly short ultraviolet rays, and the hot quartz lamp is an all-purpose lamp used for tanning and for germicidal purposes.

quaternary ammonium compounds (quats) (KWAT-ur-nayr-ee uh-MOH-nee-um KAHM-powndz)—also known as *quats*; a group of compounds of organic salts of ammonia employed effectively as disinfectants, that are very effective when used properly in the salon or spa setting.

quaternary colors (KWAT-ur-nayr-ee KUHL-urs)—all combinations that create any color not described as primary, secondary, or tertiary.

quaternium (kwah-TAYR-nee-um)—pertaining to a quaternary ammonium compound; used as an ingredient in hair conditioners.

questionnaire (KWES-shun-air)—also known as *intake form* or *client questionnaire*; form that provides the technician with a complete client profile, including important information about a client's habits and health.

quinine (KWY-nyn)—an alkaloid from cinchona bark that enters into the composition of some hair lotions and medicines.

quota (KWOAH-tuh)—a method for gauging the amount of sales and targeting production levels.

R

radial artery (RAY-dee-ul AR-tur-ee)—artery, along with numerous branches, that supplies blood to the thumb side of the arm and the back of the hand; supplies the muscles of the skin, hands, fingers, wrist, elbow, and forearm.

radial motion (RAY-dee-ul MOH-shun)—also known as *point of distribution*; the central point from which hair is distributed in a preplanned manner.

radial nerve (RAY-dee-ul NURV)—sensory-motor nerve that, with its branches, supplies the thumb side of the arm and back of the hand.

radial pulse (RAY-dee-ul PULS)—the pulse in the radial artery felt at the wrist near the base of the thumb.

radiation (ray-dee-AY-shun)—the process of giving off light or heat rays; energy radiated in the form of waves or particles.

radiation burn (ray-dee-AY-shun BURN)—a burn resulting from overexposure to radiant energy such as X-rays, radium, or strong sunlight.

radiation therapy (ray-dee-AY-shun THAYR-uh-pee)—the treatment of disease and skin conditions by any type of radiation, most commonly with ionizing radiation such as beta and gamma rays, and by X-rays.

radical (RAD-ih-kul)—extreme; in chemistry, a group of atoms passing from one compound to another, acting as a single atom.

radium (RAY-dee-um)—a radioactive metallic element; the rays from this metal are used in the treatment of some skin diseases.

radius (RAY-dee-us)—(1.) a line extending or radiating from a center point to the circumference or outer limit of a circle; (2.) smaller bone in the forearm on the same side as the thumb.

ragged (RAG-ud)—having an irregular edge or outline; uneven.

raise (RAYZ)—to make higher; to elevate or lift.

raised scar (RAYZD SKAR)—scar tissue that has healed and formed above the level of the surrounding skin.

rake (RAYK)—a high-frequency electrode used in scalp treatments.

rake comb (RAYK KOHM)—a large-toothed comb designed to remove tangles.

range of motion (RAYNJ UV MOH-shun)—the action of a joint through the entire extent of its movement.

rapport (RAP-ohr)—a close and empathetic relationship that establishes agreement and harmony between individuals.

ratio (RAY-shee-oh)—a proportion; the relationship between two items with respect to quantity, size, or amount.

rat-tail comb (RAT-tayl KOHM)—also known as *tail-comb, fantail comb*, or *teasing comb*; a comb designed with teeth on one end and a long, slender tail at the other; used to section and subsection the hair.

ratting (RAT-ing)—also known as *teasing*, *ruffing*, or *backcombing*; the technique of back-combing sections of hair from ends toward the scalp, forming a cushion or base over which longer hair is combed.

ray (RAY)—a beam of light or heat.

razor (RAY-zur)—also known as *hair shaper*; an instrument with a sharp cutting edge used for shaving and haircutting.

© Milady, a part of Cengage Learning

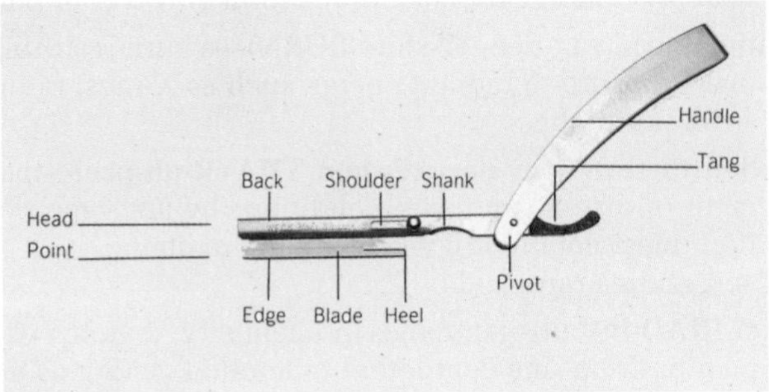

razor

razor blade (RAY-zur BLAYD)—the cutting edge of the razor; disposable blade for insertion into the back of the razor.

razor hone (RAY-zur HOHN)—a rectangular block of abrasive material such as a fine-grained hard stone used to sharpen razor blades.

razor rotation (RAY-zur row-TAY-shun)—texturizing technique similar to razor-over-comb, done with small circular motions.

razor-over-comb (RAY-zur-OH-vur-KOM)—texturizing technique in which the comb and the razor are used on the surface of the hair.

razor strop (RAY-zur STROHP)—also known as *strop*; a strap-like device made of leather and/or canvas; used to bring the razor blade to a smooth, whetted edge.

reactant (ree-AK-tant)—a substance that is affected or altered during the course of a chemical reaction.

reagent (ree-AY-jent)—a substance used in detecting, examining, or measuring other substances because of its chemical or biological activity.

rebalance (REE-bal-ans)—term often used to refer to the maintenance of a nail enhancement.

rebuild (ree-BILD)—in cosmetology, to replace damaged protein structure in the hair by conditioners.

recede (ree-SEED)—to move back; to slope backward as in a receding hairline.

receptacle (ree-SEP-tuh-kul)—a container used for storage; a basin.

receptive (ree-SEP-tiv)—able or inclined to receive; open or responsive to ideas or suggestions.

receptor (ree-SEP-tur)—nerve ending; a cell or group of cells that receive stimuli such as a pain or sensation receptor of the skin; a special protein on a cell's surface or within the cell that binds to specific ligands (special receptors).

recess (REE-ses)—a hollow, depression, or indentation.

recline (ree-KLYN)—to lie down or back; to cause to assume a recumbent position.

recondition (ree-kahn-DIH-shun)—in cosmetology, to restore the hair to its natural healthy state by conditioning.

reconditioner (ree-kahn-DIH-shun-ur)—a product formulated to improve the condition of hair by replacing lost protein, moisture, oil, or the like.

reconditioning (ree-kahn-DIH-shun-ing)—the application of a special product to the hair in order to improve its condition.

reconstructing (ree-kahn-STRUKT-ing)—in cosmetology, replacing internal and external protein structure in the hair.

reconstruction perm (ree-kahn-STRUK-shun PURM)—also known as *perm* or *Jheri Curl*; permanent wave procedure that first removes excessive curl and then reconstructs desired curl pattern.

reconstructive surgery (REE-con-struct-if SIR-JUR-ee)—restoring a bodily function; necessary surgery for accident survivors and those with congenital disfigurements or other diseases.

record card (REK-urd KARD)—card designed with a special form to keep a record of the services rendered, formulas, supplies used, and any condition pertaining to a client.

record keeping (REK-urd KEEP-ing)—maintaining accurate and complete records of all financial activities in your business.

rectifier (REK-tih-fy-ur)—an apparatus to change an alternating current (AC) to direct current (DC).

rectum (REK-tum)—the terminal portion of the digestive tube.

rectus (REK-tus)—straight; any of several straight muscles; small muscles of the eye.

rectus capitis anterior (REK-tus KAP-ih-tis an-TEER-ee-ur)—the muscle that flexes the head.

rectus capitis lateralis (REK-tus KAP-ih-tis lat-uh-RAY-lis)—muscle that assists in lateral movements of the head.

rectus capitis posterior (REK-tus KAP-ih-tus puh-STEER-ee-ur)—muscle that functions to extend the head.

red (RED)—the color of the spectrum farthest from violet; one of the primary colors; a warm hue.

red blood cells (RED BLUD SELLS)—also known as *red corpuscles* or *erythrocytes*; produced in the red bone marrow; blood cells that carry oxygen from the lungs to the body cells and transport carbon dioxide from the cells back to the lungs.

red corpuscle (RED KOR-pus-ul)—also known as *erythrocyte*; carries oxygen from the lungs to the body cells, then transports carbon dioxide from the cells back to the lungs.

red light (RED LYT)—a light-emitting diode for use on clients in the stimulation of circulation and collagen and elastin production.

redox (REE-dux)—a contraction for reduction–oxidation reaction.

redox reactions (REE-dux REE-ak-shuhns)—chemical reaction in which the oxidizing agent is reduced and the reducing agent is oxidized.

reducing agent (ree-DOOS-ing AY-jent)—a substance that adds hydrogen to a chemical compound or subtracts oxygen from the compound.

reduction (ree-DUK-shun)—the process through which oxygen is subtracted from or hydrogen is added to a substance through a chemical reaction; to make smaller; to lessen; realigning a bone that is dislocated or fractured.

reduction reaction (ree-DUK-shun ree-ACK-shun)—also known as *redox*; a chemical reaction in which oxygen is subtracted from or hydrogen is added to a substance.

reepithelialization (RE-EPP-ih-theel-ee-ahl-eye-zay-shun)—formation of new epidermis and dermis over an area of injury. The epithelial cells from the wound margin and the pilosebaceous units migrate to repair damage.

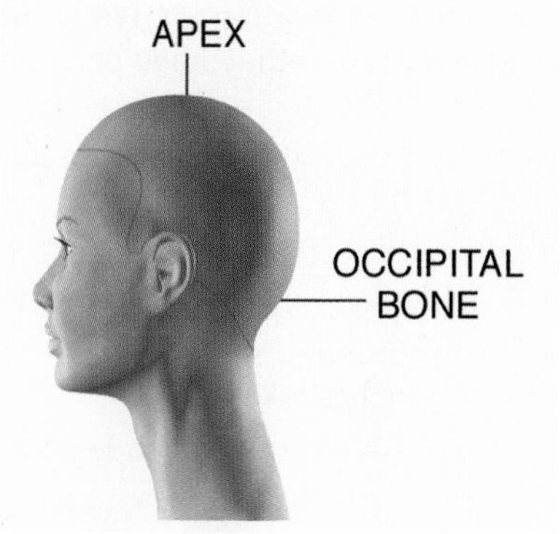

© Milady, a part of Cengage Learning
reference points

reference points (REF-err-ence POINTS)—points on the head that mark where the surface of the head changes or the behavior of the hair changes, such as ears, jaw line, occipital bone, apex, and so on; used to establish design lines that are proportionate.

refined (ree-FYND)—free from impurities; cultivated; polished. In esthetics, describes a plant extract, usually referring to a fixed oil that has gone through the process of removing colors, odors, or other naturally occurring compounds, such as a refined grapeseed oil.

refined hair (ree-FYND HAYR)—hair that has been chemically treated to make it more pliable.

reflective listening (ree-FLEKT-iv LIS-en-ing)—listening to the client and then repeating, in your own words, what you think the client is telling you.

reflex (REE-fleks)—automatic reaction to a stimulus that involves the movement of an impulse from a sensory receptor along the sensory nerve to the spinal cord. A responsive impulse is sent along a motor neuron to a muscle, causing a reaction (for example, the quick removal of the hand from a hot object). Reflexes do not have to be learned; they are automatic.

reflexology (ree-flexs-AHL-uh-jee)—a practice based on the belief that working on areas or reflex points found on the hands, feet, ears, and face can reduce tension in the body's corresponding organs and gland structures. Its origin is unknown.

reformation curls (REE-for-may-shun KURLZ)—also known as *soft-curl permanent*; combination of a thio relaxer and thio permanents whereby the hair is wrapped on perm rods; used to make existing curl larger and looser.

regimen (REJ-uh-men)—a systematic course of action; a plan to improve health; a particular condition.

regrowth (ree-GROHTH)—a new growth of hair or nail.

R

rehydration (ree-hy-DRAY-shun)—the restoration of water to the skin or other parts of the body when they have become dehydrated.

Reiki (RAY-KEE)—universal life-force energy transmitted through the palms of the hands that helps lift the spirits and provide balance to the whole self: body, mind, and spirit.

rejuvenate (ree-JOO-vuh-nayt)—to make young or vigorous again.

relapse (REE-laps)—the return of symptoms and signs of a disease or condition after apparent recovery has taken place.

relaxer (ree-LAK-sur)—a chemical applied to the hair to remove the natural curl.

relaxer testing (ree-LAK-sur TEST-ing)—also known as *strand testing*; checking the action of the relaxer in order to determine the speed at which the natural curl is being removed.

remedy (REM-uh-dee)—a medicine or treatment that relieves or cures a condition.

remover (ree-MOOV-ur)—in haircoloring, a chemical compound formulated to remove color from the hair; in tint stain remover, a product to remove tint stains from the skin; in nail care, a product formulated to remove nail polish.

renal (REE-nul)—relating to the kidney.

R

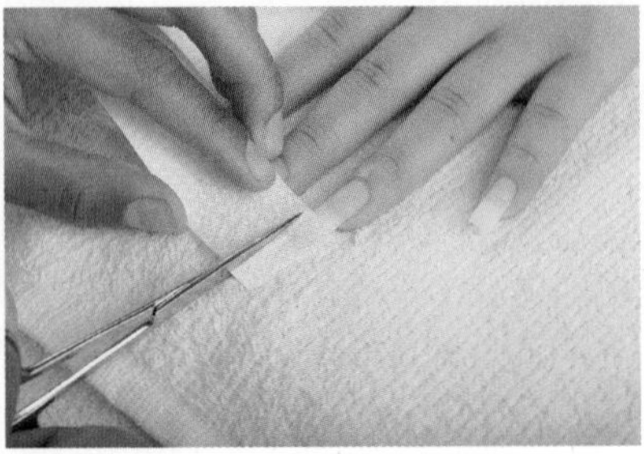

© Milady, a part of Cengage Learning. Photography by Dino Petrocelli.

repair patch

repair patch (REE-pair PATCH)—in nail technology, a piece of fabric cut to completely cover a crack or break in the nail.

repetitive motor disorder (REP-uh-tiv MOH-tur dis-OHR-dur)—another term for cumulative trauma disorder.

reprocess (ree-PRAH-ses)—to repeat a chemical service due to unsatisfactory results.

reproductive (ree-proh-DUK-tiv)—pertaining to reproduction or the process by which plants and animals produce offspring.

reproductive system (ree-proh-DUK-tiv SIS-tem)—body system that includes the ovaries, uterine tubes, uterus, and vagina in the female and the testes, prostate gland, penis, and urethra in the male. This system performs the function of producing offspring and passing on the genetic code from one generation to another.

resale tax (REE-sale TAX)—a tax imposed on those who sell retail products.

residue (REZ-ih-doo)—that which remains after a part is taken; remainder.

resilience (ree-ZIL-yence)—property of the hair enabling it to retain curl formation and spring back into curled shape after being extended; elastic.

resin (REH-zin)—mixture or organic compounds used in hair sprays and setting preparations for their holding properties.

resistance (ree-ZIST-ens)—an opposing or slowing force; the characteristics of the hair shaft that makes penetration by moisture or chemicals difficult.

resistant (ree-ZIST-ent)—hair type that is difficult for moisture or chemicals to penetrate, and thus requires a longer processing time.

resistive massage (ree-ZIS-tiv muh-SAHZH)—a massage movement to develop strength in the joints of the client's hands and wrists.

resorcinal (ruh-ZOR-sin-awl)—a chemical obtained from various resins; chiefly used as an external antiseptic in psoriasis, eczema, seborrhea, and ringworm.

respiration (res-puh-RAY-shun)—the act of breathing; the exchange of carbon dioxide and oxygen that takes place in the lungs between the blood and cells, and within the cell.

respiratory (RES-puh-rah-tor-ee)—relating to respiration.

respiratory system (RES-puh-rah-tor-ee SIS-tum)—body system consisting of the lungs and air passages; enables respiration, supplying the body with oxygen and eliminating carbon dioxide as a waste product.

restorative (ruh-STOR-ah-tiv)—to restore to an original state; repair; rebuild.

restore (ree-STOR)—to bring back to former strength; repair; rebuild; to heal or cure.

restructuring (ree-STRUK-chur-ing)—rebuilding and bringing the structural layers of the hair back into alignment.

resume (res-oo-MAY)—written summary of a person's education and work experience that highlights relevant accomplishments and achievements.

retailing (REE-tail-ing)—the act of recommending and selling products to your clients for at-home use.

retail supplies (REE-tail SUPP-lies)—items available for sale to clients.

retard (ree-TARD)—to hinder or delay.

rete (REE-tee)—a network of blood vessels or nerves.

retention (ree-TEN-shun)—keeping; maintaining.

retention hyperkeratosis (ree-TEN-shun HY-per-kera-toe-sis)—the hereditary tendency for acne-prone skin to retain dead cells in the follicle, forming an obstruction that clogs follicles and exacerbates inflammatory acne lesions such as papules and pustules.

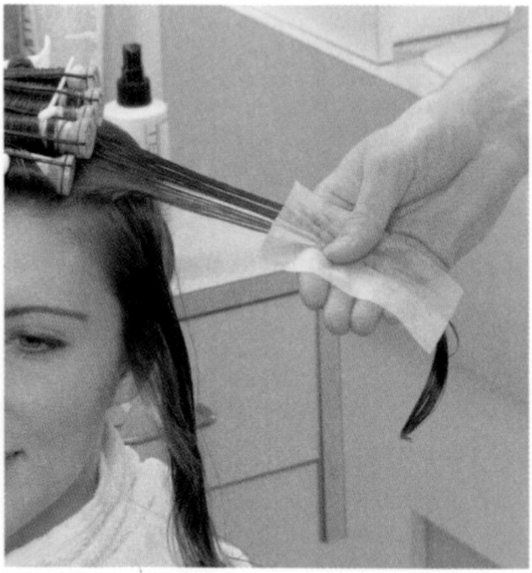

© Milady, a part of Cengage Learning. Photography by Paul Castle.

retention papers

retention papers (ree-TEN-shun PAY-purz)—also known as *end papers*; special papers used to control the ends of the hair in wrapping such as when winding hair on rods or rollers.

reticular (ruh-TIK-yuh-lur)—sponge-like structure associated with the medulla of the hair and the lower layer of the dermis.

reticular layer (ruh-TIK-yuh-lur LAY-ur)—deeper layer of the dermis that supplies the skin with oxygen and nutrients; contains fat cells, blood vessels, sudoriferous (sweat) glands, hair follicles, lymph vessels, arrector pili muscles, sebaceous (oil) glands, and nerve endings.

reticular tissue (ruh-TIK-yuh-lur TISH-yoo)—fibers that form the framework of the liver and lymphoid organs.

retina (RET-in-ah)—the sensitive membrane of the eye that receives the image from the lens.

Retin-A® (RET-in-A)—also known as *retinoic acid*; vitamin A derivative that has demonstrated an ability to alter collagen synthesis and is used to treat acne and visible signs of aging; side effects are irritation, photosensitivity, skin dryness, redness, and peeling.

retinoids (RET-in-oydz)—vitamin A derivatives, including retinoic acid, retinol, and retinyl palmitate.

retinol (RET-in-awl)—natural form of vitamin A; stimulates cell repair and helps to normalize skin cells by generating new cells.

retinyl palmitate (RET-inn-all PAL-mi-tate)—a mild retinoid.

retouch (ree-TUCH)—application of haircolor, lightener, or chemical hair relaxer to new growth of hair.

R

reusable implements (REE-use-able IMP-luh-ments)—also known as *multiuse implements*; implements that are generally stainless steel because they must be properly cleaned and disinfected between clients.

revenue (REV-uh-nu)—income generated from selling services and products, or money taken in.

reverse (ree-VURS)—to go in the opposite direction.

reverse backhand (ree-VURS BAK-HAND)—a hand position with the palm up using a downward stroke when shaving the face.

reverse backhand position/stroke (ree-VURS BAK-HAND poh-ZISH-uhn STROK)—razor position and stroke used for making the left sideburn outline and shaving the left side behind the ear during a neck shave.

reverse curl (ree-VURS KURL)—a curl formed for a style that moves hair away from the face.

reverse elevation (ree-VURS el-uh-VAYshun)—a haircut in which hair is shortest at the top of the head and longest at the lower hairline.

reverse freehand (ree-VURS FREE-HAND)—a hand position with upward palm and upward stroke; used when shaving the face.

reverse graduation (ree-VURS graj-yoo-AY-shun)—down-angle cutting of the hair.

reverse highlighting (ree-VURS HIGH-light-ing)—also known as *lowlighting*; technique of coloring strands of hair darker than the natural color.

reverse shaping (ree-VURS SHAYP-ing)—technique directing the comb downward, then immediately upward in a circular motion, away from the face.

reversible (ree-VURS-ih-bul)—capable of going through a series of changes in either direction, forward or backward as in a reversible chemical reaction.

revert (ree-VURT)—to return to a previous condition.

revolutions per minute (RPM) (REV-oh-lush-ons PER MIN-it)—in nail technology, the number of times a bit (in an electric file) turns in a complete circle in one minute.

rheostat (REE-oh-stat)—a resistance coil; an instrument used to regulate the strength of an electric current or intensity of light.

rheumatism (ROO-mah-tiz-um)—a painful disease of the muscles and joints accompanied by swelling and stiffness.

rheumatoid arthritis (ROO-muh-toyd ar-THRY-tus)—a chronic inflammatory disease in which the cartilage of joints erodes, causing them to calcify and become immovable.

rhinitis (ry-NYT-us)—inflammation of the nasal mucous membrane.

rhinokyphosis (ry-noh-ky-FOH-sus)—the condition of having an abnormal hump or bump in the bridge of the nose; a prominent bridge.

rhinoplasty (RY-noh-plas-tee)—plastic or reconstructive surgery performed on the nose to change or correct its appearance.

rhinothrix (RY-noh-thriks)—hair growth in the nostrils.

rhysema (ry-SEE-muh)—a wrinkle line or corrugation of the skin.

rhythm (RITH-um)—a regular pulsation or recurrent pattern of movement in a design.

rhytidectomy (rit-ih-DEK-tuh-mee)—a face-lift procedure that removes excess fat at the jaw line; tightens loose, atrophic muscles; and removes sagging skin.

rib cage (RIB-kayj)—the skeletal framework of the chest made up of the sternum, the ribs, and the thoracic vertebrae.

ribboning (RIB-un-ing)—hair-setting technique in which hair is forced between thumb and back of comb to create tension.

riboflavin (RY-boh-flay-vin)—the heat stable factor of the vitamin B complex; a water-soluble vitamin and essential nutrient; used in emollients and conditioning agents.

R

ribonucleic acid (RNA) (ry-boh-noo-KLEE-ik AS-ud)—a nucleic acid of high molecular weight found in the cytoplasm and nuclei of cells; aids synthesis of cell proteins.

ribosomes (RYE-bah-soms)—small, dense organelles that assemble proteins in cells.

ribs (RIBZ)—twelve pairs of bones forming the wall of the thorax.

rickettsia (rih-KEHT-si-ah)—type of pathogenic microorganism capable of producing disease such as typhus.

ridge (RIJ)—crest of a wave.

ridges (RIJ-ez)—in nail technology, vertical lines running through the length of the natural nail plate that are caused by uneven growth of the nails, usually the result of normal aging.

ridge curl (RIJ KURL)—pin curls placed immediately behind or below a ridge to form a wave.

right angle (RYT ANG-gul)—a 90° angle; an angle formed by the intersection of two perpendicular lines.

right atrium (RYT AY-tree-um)—upper-right walled chamber of the heart.

Right-to-Know Law (RITE-TO-NO LAW)—requires employers to post notices where toxic substances are present in the workplace.

right ventricle (RYT VEN-trih-kul)—lower-right thick-walled chamber of the heart.

ringed hair (RINGD HAYR)—variety of canities characterized by alternating bands of gray and pigmented hair throughout the length of the hair strand.

ringlet (RING-lut)—a small tendril, spirally curled.

rings of fire (RINGZ UV FIRE)—grooves carved into the nail caused by electric filing with bits at the incorrect angle.

ringworm (RING-wurm)—a vegetable parasitic disease of the skin and its appendages that appears in circular lesions and is contagious.

rinse (RINS)—to cleanse with a second or repeated application of water after washing; a conditioning rinse; a solution that temporarily tints or conditions the hair.

rinse, temporary (RINS, TEM-puh-rayr-ee)—an artificial coloring for the hair that coats the shaft and is removed with a single shampoo.

risk (RISK)—the chance of incurring some type of harm, damage, or loss.

risk management (RISK man-ahj-ment)—the methods used to safeguard your business against loss or damage.

risorius muscle (rih-ZOR-ee-us MUS-uhl)—muscle of the mouth that draws the corner of the mouth out and back, as in grinning.

rod (RAHD)—the round, solid prong of a curling iron; curler used for permanent waving.

rod selector chart (RAHD suh-LEK-tor CHART)—a chart designed for the selection of the proper size and circumference of permanent wave rods.

role model (ROHL MOD-uhl)—a person whose behavior and success are worthy of emulation.

rolfing (RAHLF-ing)—a method of massage manipulating connective tissue or fascia using heavy pressure from the knuckles and elbows on areas of the body; aligning the major body segments.

roll (ROHL)—to move forward on a surface by turning over and over; to form by turning over.

rolled cotton (ROHLD KAHT-un)—cotton of the absorbent type packaged in rolls for use in cosmetology service procedures.

roller (ROHL-ur)—a cylindrical object varying in diameter and length around which hair may be wound.

roller clip (ROHL-ur KLIP)—a metal pin used to secure a hair roller.

roller control (ROHL-ur kun-TROHL)—the size of the base, in relation to the diameter of the roller used, and the position of the roller to the base.

roller curl (ROHL-ur KURL)—a means of setting hair by winding a damp strand around a cylindrical object in croquignole fashion, and securing it in that position until the hair is dry.

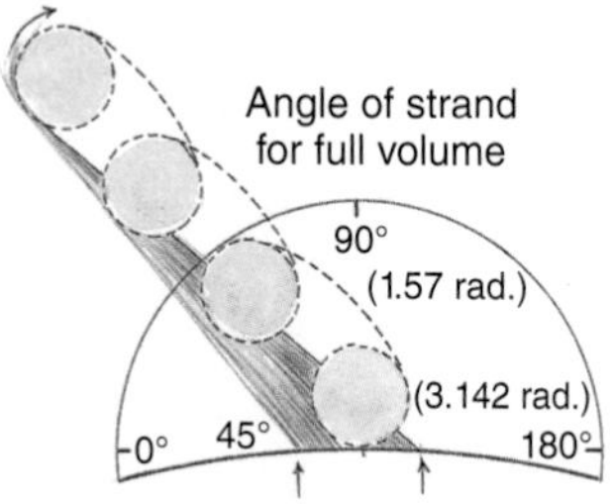

© Milady, a part of Cengage Learning
roller placement

roller direction (ROHL-ur dih-REK-shun)—the direction or line in which a roller is moved.

roller placement (ROHL-ur PLAYS-munt)—the positioning of a roller in relation to its base; one-half off or on base.

roller set (ROHL-ur SET)—setting the hair entirely with rollers.

roller tray (ROHL-ur TRAY)—an open plastic receptacle with bins or trays on different levels used to hold and store various size hair rollers.

rolling (ROHL-ing)—a massage movement in which the tissues are pressed and twisted using a fast back-and-forth movement.

rolling cream (ROHL-ing KREEM)—cleansing and exfoliating product used in facials to lift dead skin cells and dirt from the skin surface.

rolling the comb out (ROHL-ing THE KOM OUT)—a method used to put the hair into position for cutting by combing into the hair with the teeth of the comb in an upward direction.

root of hair (ROOT UV HAYR)—structure of the hair below the scalp.

root of the nail (ROOT UV THE NAYL)—base of the nail embedded underneath the skin.

root sheath (ROOT SHEETH)—the tough membrane covering the root of a hair.

root-turning (ROOT-TURN-ing)—refers to sorting the hair strands so that a cuticle points toward the hair ends in its natural direction of growth.

rope braid (ROHP BRADE)—braid created with two strands that are twisted around each other.

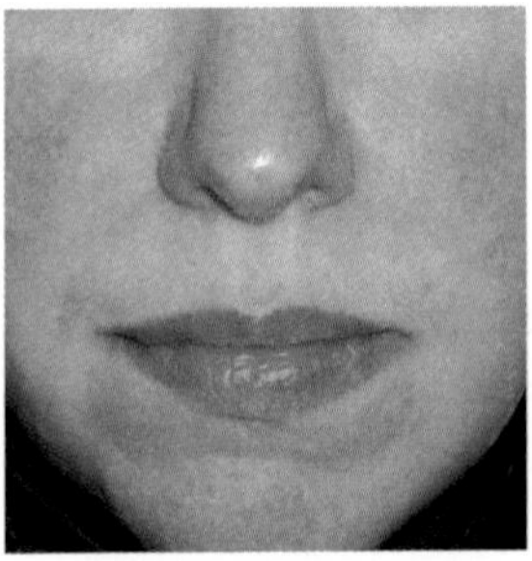

Courtesy of National Rosacea Society

rosacea

rosacea (roh-ZAY-see-uh)—chronic condition that appears primarily on the cheeks and nose, and is characterized by flushing (redness), telangiectasis (distended or dilated surface blood vessels), and, in some cases, the formation of papules and pustules.

roseola (roh-zee-OH-luh)—pertaining to a rose-colored eruption such as rubella or German measles.

rotary (ROH-tuh-ree)—turning on an axis like a wheel; moving in a circular pattern; a movement used in massage.

rotary brush (ROH-tuh-ree BRUSH)—machine used to lightly exfoliate and stimulate the skin; also helps soften excess oil, dirt, and cell buildup.

rotate (ROH-tayt)—to turn; to revolve.

rotation (roh-TAY-shun)—a massage movement for the joints using circular movements; used for fingers, hands, arms, toes, and ankles.

rouge (ROOZH)—also known as *blush* or *check color*; a cosmetic used to color the skin, especially the cheeks.

rough (RUF)—not smooth or polished; having an uneven texture; coarse.

round (ROWND)—spherical; having a contour that is circular or nearly ring-shaped; not flat or angular.

round brush (ROWND BRUSH)—a hairbrush with a circular row of bristles on a round handle, designed for styling hair with a blowdryer; styling brush. In nail technology, most common and versatile style of brush with a very good capacity for holding paint.

round nail (ROWND NAYL)—a slightly tapered nail shape; it usually extends just a bit past the fingertip.

round-shaped face (ROWND-SHAYPT FAYS)—a facial structure characterized by fullness at the cheekbones and jaw line, but shorter than an oval.

row (ROH)—an arrangement or series of items or people in a continuous line; a series of pin curls or rollers placed one after the other in a line.

rubber (RUB-ur)—a resinous, elastic material obtained from the latex of the rubber tree; used in various products such as elastic bands and fabrics.

rubbing alcohol (RUB-ing AL-kuh-hawl)—also known as *isopropyl alcohol* and *ethyl alcohol*, a preparation containing denatured ethyl alcohol or isopropyl alcohol; used as a rubefacient (dilation of the capillaries and an increase in circulation) to stimulate the tissues of the skin.

rubedo (roo-BEE-doh)—any temporary redness of the skin.

ruffing (RUF-ing)—also known as *teasing, ratting,* or *backcombing*; the technique of back-combing sections of hair from ends toward the scalp, forming a cushion or base over which longer hair is combed.

ruffle (RUF-ul)—to comb back the shortest hairs.

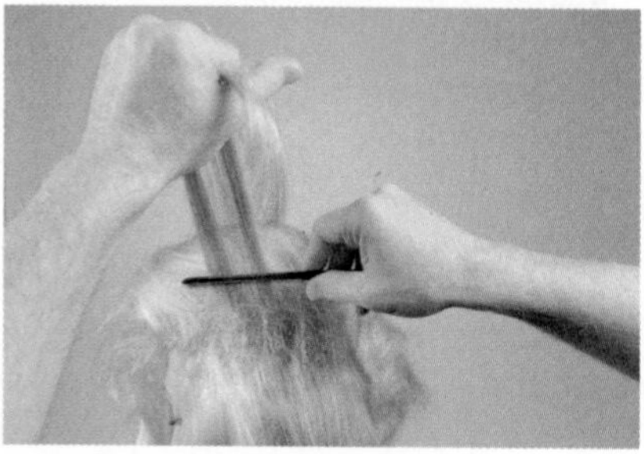

© Milady, a part of Cengage Learning. Photography by Yanik Chauvin.

ruffing

rupia (ROO-pee-ah)—thick, dark, raised crusts on the skin.

Russian strop (RUSH-an STROP)—in barbering, a type of cowhide strop that is considered to be one of the best and that requires "breaking in."

S

sable (SAY-bul)—the hair from a weasel (animal); used for fine-quality makeup and nail brushes; the color sable brown; a dark brown-black.

saccharides (SAK-uh-ridez)—also known as *carbohydrates*; any of a various group of organic compounds that contain carbon, hydrogen, and oxygen and includes cellulose, gums, sugars, and starches.

saccular (SAK-yuh-lar)—shaped like a sac.

sacrum (SAY-krum)—a triangular bone at the base of the spinal column that connects with or forms a part of the pelvis and in human beings consists of five united vertebrae.

safety razor (SAYF-tee RAY-zur)—a straight razor or shaper with a removable guard for the cutting edge of the blade.

safety plan (SAYF-tee PLAN)—a plan for avoiding potential exposure and for dealing with it should exposure occur.

sagittal plane (SAJ-ut-ul PLAYN)—an imaginary line that divides the body into left and right parts.

salary (SAL-uh-ree)—a method of compensation that specifies a certain amount of pay based on either a flat or hourly rate.

sales promotion (SAYLZ pro-MO-shun)—a marketing strategy aimed at drawing attention to your products and services with the goal of increasing the volume of business.

salicylic acid (sal-uh-SIL-ik AS-ud)—beta hydroxy acid with exfoliating and antiseptic properties; natural sources include sweet birch, willow bark, and wintergreen.

saline (SAY-leen)—salty; containing salt.

salivary gland (SAL-ih-veh-ree GLAND)—a gland in the mouth that secretes saliva.

salon (suh-LAHN)—an establishment or business devoted to a specific service or purpose as in a beauty salon.

salon operation (suh-LAHN AHP-er-ay-shun)—the ongoing, recurring processes or activities involved in the running of a business for the purpose of producing income and value.

salon policies (suh-LAHN POL-ih-sees)—the rules or regulations adopted by a salon to ensure that all clients and associates are being treated fairly and consistently.

salt (SAWLT)—in chemistry, compounds that are formed by the reaction of acids and bases.

salt bond (SAWLT BAHND)—a weak, physical, cross-link side bond between adjacent polypeptide chains.

salt and pepper (SAWLT AND PEP-ur)—a descriptive term for a mixture of pigmented and gray or white hair.

salt rub (SAWLT RUB)—a frictional application of wet salt rubbed over the skin.

salve (SAV)—a thick ointment that heals and soothes the skin.

sandpaper (SAND-pay-pur)—paper coated with fine sand; used for smoothing and polishing; used to make emery boards for manicuring.

sanitation (san-ih-TAY-shun)—also known as *sanitizing*; a chemical process of reducing the number of disease-causing germs on cleaned surfaces to a safe level.

sanitize (SAN-uh-tyz)—a chemical process for reducing the number of disease-causing germs on cleaned surfaces to a safe level.

sanitizer (SAN-ih-tyz-ur)—a chemical agent or product used to clean surface and implements to levels considered safe as determined by public health officials.

saphena (sah-FEE-nuh)—either of two large superficial veins of the leg.

saphenous nerve (sah-FEE-nus NURV)—supplies impulses to the skin of the inner side of the leg and foot.

S

saprophyte (SAP-ruh-fyt)—a nonpathogenic microorganism that normally grows on dead matter.

sarcoid (SAR-koyd)—any of various diseases characterized especially by the formation of nodules in the skin.

sarcolemma (SAR-ko-LEM-ah)—the membrane enclosing a striated muscle fiber.

sarcous (SAR-kus)—pertaining to flesh or muscle.

saturate (SACH-uh-rayt)—to cause to become soaked or completely penetrated; to absorb all that is possible to hold.

saturated solution (SACH-uh-rayt-ud suh-LOO-shun)—a solution that contains the maximum amount of substance able to be dissolved.

saturation (sach-uh-RAY-shun)—the degree of concentration or amount of pigment in a color.

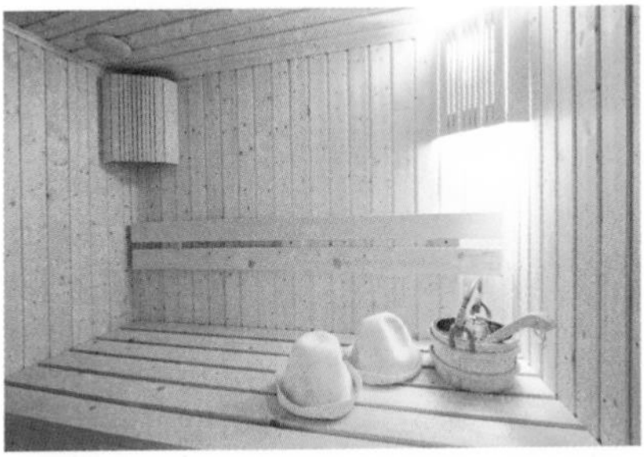
© Olena Simko/www.Shutterstock.com
sauna

sauna (SAH-nah)—vapor bath.

scab (SKAB)—a crust of hardened blood, serum, and dead cells formed over the surface of a wound.

scabies (SKAY-beez)—a contagious skin disease that is caused by the itch mite, which burrows under the skin.

scald (SKAWLD)—to burn with hot liquid or steam.

scale (SKAYL)—any thin dry or oily plate of epidermal flakes. An example is abnormal or excessive dandruff.

scaling (SKAYL-ing)—the sectioning and subsectioning of the hair to obtain the desired proportions; loss of dead epidermal cells.

scalp (SKALP)—the skin covering the cranium.

scalp antiseptic (SKALP ant-ih-SEP-tik)—a liquid used to relieve an itching scalp and arrest the growth of microorganisms.

scalp astringent lotion (SKALP UH-stinj-ent LOW-shun)—product used to remove oil accumulation from the scalp; used after a scalp treatment and before styling.

scalp conditioner (SKALP kun-DISH-un-ur)—product, usually in a cream base, used to soften and improve the health of the scalp.

scalp electrode (SKALP ee-LEK-trohd)—a rake-shaped attachment used to distribute high-frequency current in some scalp massage procedures.

scalp lotion (SKALP LOH-shun)—a liquid solution used to treat dry scalp and/or dandruff.

scalp massage (SKALP muh-SAHZH)—circular movements of the fingertips on the scalp to stimulate blood to the surface.

scalp movement (SKALP MOOV-ment)—a procedure that moves the scalp gently as part of a treatment.

scalp reduction (SKALP REE-duk-shun)—the surgical removal of the bald area, followed by the pulling together of the scalp ends.

scalp steam (SKALP STEEM)—process of using steam towels or steaming unit to soften and open scalp pores.

scalp steamer (SKALP STEEM-ur)—an apparatus used to steam the scalp.

scalp treatment (SKALP TREET-ment)—a procedure to improve the health of the scalp.

scaly (SKAY-lee)—covered with or having scales.

scaphoid bone (SKAF-oyd BOHN)—the boat-shaped bone of the tarsus and the carpus.

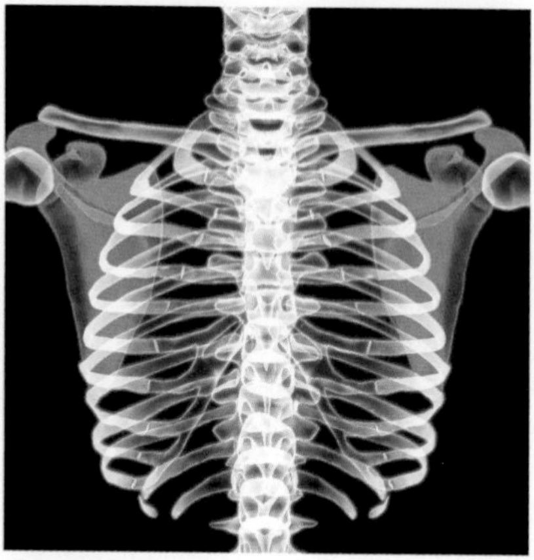

© Dim Dimich/www.Shutterstock.com

scapula

scapula (SKAP-yuh-luh)—also known as *shoulder blade*; large, flat, triangular bone of the shoulder. There are two scapulas.

scar (SKAR)—also known as *cicatrix*; light-colored, slightly raised mark on the skin formed after an injury or lesion of the skin has healed.

scarfskin (SKARF-skin)—the epidermis; especially that forming the cuticle of a nail.

sciatica (sy-AT-ik-uh)—a painful inflammation of the sciatic nerve which runs down the back of the leg; caused by injury or pressure.

sciatic nerve (sy-AT-ik NURV)—largest and longest nerve in the body.

science (SY-ens)—a body of knowledge arranged and systemized; based on observation and experiment to determine the basic nature or principles of the subject studied.

scissor-over-comb (SIS-uhr-OVER-KOM)—also known as *shear-over-comb*; haircutting technique in which the hair is held in place with the comb while the tips of the scissors are used to remove the lengths.

scissors (SIZ-urz)—also known as *shears*; a two-bladed instrument used to cut and trim.

Copyright © 2010 Shark Fin Shear Company and www.sharkfinshears.com.

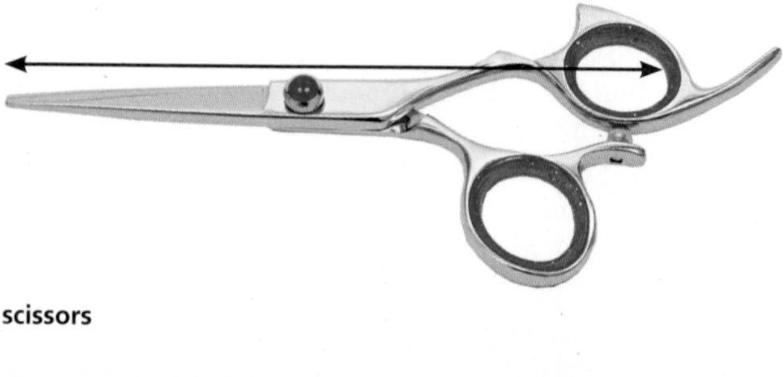

scissors

S

scleroderma (sklayr-uh-DUR-muh)—a disease of the skin characterized by hard, thick patches.

scleroid (SKLEER-oyd)—leathery or scar-like in texture.

sclerosis (skluh-ROH-sus)—pathological hardening of tissues, especially by outgrowth of fibrous tissues.

scoliosis (skoh-lee-OH-sus)—abnormal lateral curvature of the spine.

scope of practice (SOP) (SKOP UV PRAK-tis)—the list of services that you are legally allowed to perform in your specialty in your state.

S-Corp (S-korp)—business entity with features similar to a corporate structure that allows company income to be reported through the owners' personal income tax returns like a limited liability company.

Scotch hose (SKOCH HOSE)—A high-pressure hose used in water therapy that sprays the standing client (sometimes with sea water); stimulates circulation.

scratch (SKRACH)—a slight wound in the form of a tear on the surface of the skin.

scrub (SKRUB)—to rub briskly.

scrupulous (SKROO-pyoo-lus)—extremely exact; careful and painstaking.

sculpture curl (SKULP-chur KURL)—also known as *pin curl*; a curl placed close to the head to appear as if it were carved.

sculptured nails (SKULP-churd NAYLZ)—also known as *monomer liquid and polymer powder nail enhancements*; nail enhancement created by combining a liquid and powder mixture, and applying it over a nail extension, nail form, or natural nail; the hardened nail is then shaped to the desired length.

sculpturing (SKULP-chur-ing)—the formation of a hair shape and silhouette by creating volume or volume and indentation.

scurf (SKURF)—also known as *dandruff*; thin dry scales detached from the epidermis, especially in an abnormal skin condition such as dandruff.

scurvy (SKUR-vee)—a disease caused by a lack of vitamin C and characterized by spongy gums, loosening of the teeth, and a bleeding into the skin and mucous membranes.

scutula (SKUT-yoo-lah)—dry, sulfur-yellow, cup-like crusts on the scalp in tinea favosa or tinea favus.

sealer (SEEL-ur)—liquid applied over the nail polish to protect the polish and minimize chipping or cracking.

seam (SEEM)—in hairstyling, an overlapping of two ends as in a French twist.

seaweed (SEE-weed)—a plant growing in the sea; seaweed derivatives such as algae have many nourishing properties; known for its humectant and moisturizing properties, vitamin content, metabolism stimulation and detoxification, and aiding skin firmness.

seaweed wraps (SEE-weed RAPS)—wraps that include application of a seaweed mask followed by a thermal blanket to seal in heat.

sebaceous (sih-BAY-shus)—pertaining to or having the nature of oil or fat.

sebaceous cyst (sih-BAY-shus SIST)—a large protruding pocket-like lesion filled with sebum. Sebaceous cysts are frequently seen on the scalp and the back. They should be removed surgically by a dermatologist.

sebaceous filaments (sih-BAY-shus FILL-ah-mentz)—similar to open comedones, these are mainly solidified impactions of oil without the cell matter.

sebaceous gland (sih-BAY-shus GLAND)—also known as *oil glands*; protect the surface of the skin. Sebaceous glands are appendages connected to follicles.

sebaceous hyperplasia (sih-BAY-shus hy-per-PLAY-she-uh)—benign lesions frequently seen in oilier areas of the face. An overgrowth of the sebaceous gland, they appear similar to open comedones; often doughnut-shaped, with sebaceous material in the center.

seborrhea (seb-oh-REE-ah)—severe oiliness of the skin; an abnormal secretion from the sebaceous glands.

seborrhea capitis (seb-oh-REE-ah KAP-ih-tis)—seborrhea of the scalp.

S

seborrhea oleosa (seb-oh-REE-ah oh-leh-OH-sah)—excessive oiliness of the skin, especially of the forehead and nose.

seborrhea sicca (seb-oh-REE-ah SIK-ah)—an accumulation on the scalp of greasy scales or crusts due to overaction of the sebaceous glands.

seborrheic dermatitis (seb-oh-REE-ik DERMA-ty-tis)—skin condition caused by an inflammation of the sebaceous glands. It is often characterized by redness, dry or oily scaling, crusting, and/or itchiness.

seborrheic, alopecia (seb-oh-REE-ik, al-uh-PEE-she-a)—baldness caused by diseased sebaceous glands.

seborrheic keratoses (seb-oh-REE-ik kera-TOE-sis)—crusty-looking, slightly raised lesions in mature, sun-damaged skin. They often appear on the cheekbone area. They may be black, brown, gray, or sometimes flesh-toned or sallow.

sebum (SEEB-um)—a fatty or oily secretion that lubricates the skin and preserves the softness of the hair.

second-degree burn (SEK-und-duh-GREE BURN)—a burn that is deeper than a first-degree burn and has also burned the tissue of the dermis. Blisters occur with second-degree burns, and also possible scabbing. Intense redness and almost immediate swelling are characteristics of a second-degree burn, as well as considerable pain.

second-time-over shave (SEK-und-TYM-OH-ver SHAYV)—follows a regular shave to remove any rough or uneven spots using water instead of lather; may be considered a form of close shaving.

secondary color (SEK-un-deh-ree KUL-ur)—a color obtained by mixing equal parts of two primary colors; examples are green, orange, and violet.

secondary hair (SEK-un-deh-ree HAYR)—the stiff, short, coarse hair found on eyelashes, eyebrows, and within the openings or passages of the nose and ears.

secondary skin lesions (SEK-un-deh-ree SKIN LEEJ-uhns)—skin damage, developed in the later stages of disease, that changes the structure of tissues or organs, characterized by piles of material on the skin surface, such as a crust or scab, or depressions in the skin surface, such as an ulcer.

secondary terminal hair (SEK-un-deh-ree TER-min-uhl HAYR)—long hair found on the scalp, beard, chest, back, and legs.

secrete (suh-KREET)—to form and give off.

secretion (sih-KREE-shun)—the production and release of a useful substance by a gland or cell.

secretory coil (seh-KRUH-toh-ree KOYL)—coiled base of the sudoriferous (sweat) gland.

secretory nerve fibers (seh-KRUH-toh-ree NURV FY-buhrs)—fibers of the secretory nerve that are distributed to the sudoriferous glands and sebaceous glands. Secretory nerves, which are part of the autonomic nervous system (ANS), regulate the excretion of perspiration from the sweat glands, and control the flow of sebum to the surface of the skin.

secretory nerves (seh-KRUH-toh-ree NURVZ)—nerves of the sweat and oil glands, regulating perspiration and sebum excretions.

section (SEK-shun)—portion of a whole; to divide the hair by parting into uniform working areas for control.

sedentary (SED-en-teh-ree)—settled; inactive.

seep (SEEP)—to ooze out slowly.

segment (SEG-ment)—to separate into essential parts; one of the constituent parts of something.

selenium (seh-LEE-nee-um)—in nutrition, an essential trace mineral found in grains and meat; preserves tissue elasticity and aids in promotion of body growth.

selenium sulfide (seh-LEE-nee-um SUL-fyd)—a bright-orange powder used in preparations for the treatment of seborrheic dermatitis and common dandruff.

self-employment tax (SELF-em-PLOY-ment TAX)—a tax imposed on those who are self-employed, which allows them to receive retirement benefits, disability benefits, survivor benefits, and hospital insurance or Medicare, in much the same way an employee would.

self-management (SELF-MAN-aje-ment)—the ongoing process of planning, organizing, and managing one's life.

semi-hand-tied wigs (SEM-EE-hand-tyd WHIGS)—wigs constructed with a combination of synthetic hair and hand-tied human hair.

semilunar bone (sem-ee-LOO-nur BOHN)—a crescent-shaped bone of the wrist.

semilunar valve (sem-ee-LOO-nur VALV)—valve of the arteries that prevents backflow from arteries into the ventricles.

semipermanent haircolor (sem-ee-PUR-mah-nent HAYR KUL-ur)—no-lift, deposit-only, nonoxidation haircolor that is not mixed with peroxide and is formulated to last through several shampoos.

S

semipermanent rinse (sem-ee-PUR-mah-nent RINS)—a nonpermanent haircolor rinse that is removed after several shampoos.

semistandup curl (sem-ee-STAND-up KURL)— also known as *flare curl*; the placement of a curl on its base in such a manner as to allow it to partially stand away from the scalp, giving slight directed volume; used to create a transition from standup pin curls to sculptured pin curls.

senile canities (SEE-nyl kuh-NIT-eez)—grayness of the hair in elderly people.

sensation (sen-SAY-shun)—a feeling or impression arising as the result of the stimulation of an afferent nerve.

sense (SENS)—the faculty of sensation by which an individual perceives impressions such as taste, touch, smell, sight, and hearing.

sense organ (SENS OR-gun)—a living structure that receives sense impressions (the eye, ears, nose, skin, tongue, and mouth).

sensitive (SEN-sih-tiv)—easily affected by outside influences.

sensitive skin (SEN-sih-tiv SKIN)—skin that is easily damaged or reactive to substances.

sensitivity (sen-sih-TIV-ih-tee)—the state of being easily affected by certain chemicals or external conditions.

sensitization (sen-sih-TIZ-aye-shun)—allergic reaction created by repeated exposure to a chemical or a substance.

sensory (SEN-soh-ree)—relating to or pertaining to sensation.

sensory nerve (SEN-soh-ree NURV)—also known as *afferent nerves* or *sensory neuron*; carry impulses or messages from the sense organs to the brain, where sensations of touch, cold, heat, sight, hearing, taste, smell, pain, and pressure are experienced.

sensory nerve fibers (SEN-soh-ree NURV FY-buhrs)—fibers of the sensory nerves that react to heat, cold, touch, pressure, and pain. Sensory receptors that send messages to the brain.

sentient (SEN-chent)—sensitive; capable of sensation; feeling.

sepsis (SEP-sis)—also known as *blood poisoning*; the contamination of various pus-forming and other pathogenic organisms or their toxins in the blood or tissues.

septal artery (SEP-tal AR-tuh-ree)—the artery that supplies the nostrils.

septic (SEP-tik)—relating to or caused by sepsis.

septicemia (sep-tih-SEE-mee-ah)— condition that exists when pathogenic bacteria enter the bloodstream and circulate throughout the body, causing a general infection.

septum (SEP-tum)—a dividing wall; a partition, especially between bodily spaces or masses or soft tissue; separates the heart chambers.

sequence of massage (SEE-kwens UV muh-SAHZH)—the pattern or design of massage.

sequestering agent (sih-KWES-tur-ing AY-jent)—a preservative used to prevent changes in the chemical and physical composition of certain products.

serrated (sur-RAYT-ed)—having saw-like grooves along the edge.

serratus anterior (ser-RAT-us an-TEER-ee-ur)—a muscle of the chest assisting in breathing and in raising the arm.

serum (SE-rum)—concentrated liquid ingredients for the skin designed to penetrate and treat various skin conditions.

service sets (SIT-viss SETS)—sets of all the tools that will be used in a service.

set (SET)—to form and secure the hair into a pattern of curls or waves to meet the requirements of a specific hairstyle.

set of the shears (SET UV THE SHEARS)—the manner in which the blades and shanks of the shears align with each other and are joined at the tension screw or rivet.

setting (SET-ing)—an arrangement of the hair to meet the requirements of a specific hairstyle.

setting gel (SET-ing JEL)—a semisolid holding agent used to set the hair.

seventh cranial nerve (SEV-AHNTH CRAN-ee-ahl NURV)—also known as *facial nerve*; chief motor nerve of the face. Its divisions and their branches supply and control all the muscles of facial expression. It emerges near the lower part of the ear and extends to the muscles of the neck.

sexually transmitted disease (SEKS-yoo-ly TRANS-mitt-ed DIZ-eez)—also known as *venereal disease*; contagious disease (as gonorrhea or syphilis) that is typically acquired in sexual intercourse.

shade (SHAYD)—the gradation in color value by adding black to a color; a color slightly but visibly different from the one under consideration; a term used to describe a specific color.

shading (SHAYD-ing)—in haircoloring, adding depth of color to strands of hair; in makeup, shadowing a feature to create the illusion of receding or becoming less prominent.

shadow wave (SHAD-oh WAYV)—a shaping that resembles the outline of a finger wave but does not have a definite ridge and formation.

shaft (SHAFT)—slender stem-like structure; the long, slender part of the hair above the scalp.

shaking (SHAYK-ing)—in massage, a vibrating movement in which the hand is pressed on the body part and firmly moved from side to side.

shampoo (sham-POO)—to subject the scalp and hair to cleansing and massaging with some cleansing agent such as soap or detergent; a product formulated for cleansing the hair and scalp.

shampoo bowl (sham-POO BOHL)—a specially designed basin with a U-shaped construction to allow the client to lie back in a comfortable position during the shampoo service.

shampoo cape (sham-POO KAYP)—a plastic or cloth cape used to protect the client's clothing during the shampoo procedure.

shampoo molecule (sham-POO MAHL-ih-KYOOL)—large, specially treated molecules with a head and tail. The tail attracts dirt, grease, debris, and oil, but repels water. The head attracts water, but repels dirt.

shampoo station (sham-POO STAY-shun)—the area where shampoo chairs and equipment are located.

shampoo, color-enhancing (sham-POO, KUL-uhr EN-HANS-ing)—a shampoo product that cleans and adds temporary color to the hair.

shampooing (sham-POO-ing)—the act of cleaning the hair and scalp.

shape (SHAYP)—the contour of an object.

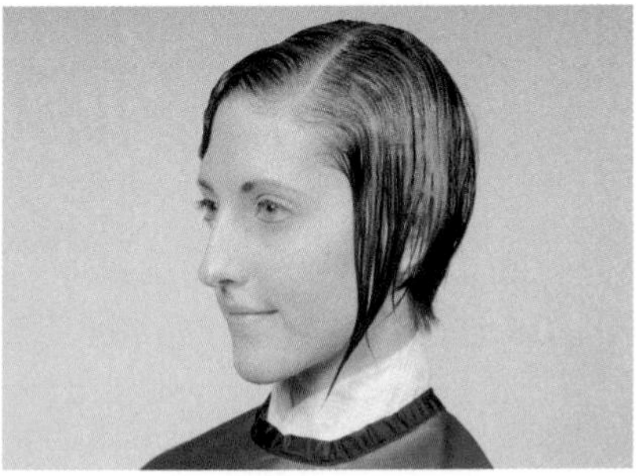

© Milady, a part of Cengage Learning. Photography by Yanik Chauvin.

shaping

shaping (SHAYP-ing)—the formation of uniform arcs or curves in wet hair, thus providing a base for various patterns in hairstyling; in haircutting, also known as *cutting, shaping,* and *trimming*; the process of shortening and thinning the hair to a particular style or to the contour of the head.

sharps container (SHARPS CON-tain-uhr)—plastic biohazard containers for disposable needles and anything sharp. The container is red and puncture-proof and must be disposed of as medical waste.

shave (SHAYV)—to cut hair or a beard close to the skin; to remove hair from an area by use of a razor.

shaving (SHAYV-ing)—the technique of removing unwanted hair from the face or other part of the body using a razor.

shaving cream (SHAYV-ing KREEM)—an emollient cream used to soften the beard before shaving.

shaving soap (SHAYV-ing SOHP)—a soap formulated to soften the beard before shaving.

shear-over-comb (SHEER-OH-ver-KOM)—haircutting technique in which the hair is held in place with the comb while the tips of the shears are used to remove the length.

shear-point tapering (SHEER-POYNT TAYP-uhr-ing)—haircutting technique used to thin out difficult areas in the haircut such as dips and hollows.

shears (SHEERZ)—also known as *scissors* or *cutting shears*; an instrument used for cutting hair.

sheath (SHEETH)—a covering enclosing or surrounding some organs.

sheen (SHEEN)—gloss; shininess.

shell (SHEL)—the clamp that presses the hair against the barrel or rod of a thermal iron.

shell strop (SHEL STROP)—a type of horsehide strop made from the muscular rump area of the horse and considered to be the best strop for use by barbers.

shiatsu massage (shee-AH-tsoo mass-AJE)—the application of pressure on acupuncture points found throughout the body to balance the body's energy flow and to promote health. It originated as a form of physical therapy in Japan.

shift (SHIFT)—to move the hair away from its natural fall position.

shin (SHIN)—also known as *shinbone*; the frontal part of a leg below the knee.

shine (SHYN)—also known as *gloss*, or *sheen*; to reflect light.

shingle (SHING-gul)—a short haircut, particularly at the nape area where the haircut starts at the hairline from zero length, becoming gradually longer toward the crown.

shingles (SHING-guls)—also known as *herpes zoster virus*; an acute inflammation of a nerve trunk by the herpes virus.

short (SHORT)—low; brief; not long.

S

short circuit (SHORT SUR-kit)—to shut or break off an electric current before it has completed its course.

shortwave (SHORT-wayv)—a form of high-frequency current used in permanent hair removal.

shoulder length (SHOHL-dur LENGTH)—the length of the hair that reaches the top part of the shoulder.

shrink (SHRINK)—to contract into a smaller area or size.

shrinkage (SHRINK-ahj)—when hair contracts or lifts through the action of moisture loss or drying.

shrivel (SHRIV-ul)—to shrink into wrinkles, especially due to loss of moisture.

siccant; siccative (SIH-kant; SIK-ah-tiv)—drying; tending to make dry.

side bonds (SYD bahnds)—also known as *cross bonds*; bonds that cross-link the polypeptide chains together and are responsible for the extreme strength and elasticity of human hair.

side height (SYD HYT)—that area of the hair from the end of the sideburns up to the point at which the vertical and horizontal bone structures meet.

side part (SYD PART)—a part in the hair that is left or right of the center, not in the center.

sideburn (SYD-burn)—continuation of the hairline in front of the ears.

sidewall (SYD-wahl)—also known as *lateral nail fold*; the area on the side of the nail plate that grows free of its attachment to the nail fold and where the extension leaves the natural nail.

silhouette (sil-oo-ET)—an outline or outer dimension.

silica (SIL-ih-kuh)—dioxide of silicon.

silicon (SIL-ih-kahn)—an abundant nonmetallic element.

silicones (SIL-ih-kohnz)—a special type of oil used in hair conditioners, water-resistant lubricants for the skin, and nail polish dryers. Oil that is chemically combined with silicon and oxygen and leaves a noncomedogenic, protective film on the surface of the skin.

silk (SILK)—a strong, glossy, tightly woven natural fiber used for nail wrapping that becomes transparent when wrap resin is applied; also used in making better quality wigs and hairpieces.

silk wraps (SILK RAPS)—made from a thin natural material with a tight weave that becomes transparent when wrap resin is applied.

silking (SILK-ing)—also known as *silking the strand*; smoothing a hot pressing iron on strands of hair before actually using the pressing iron to reduce curl.

S

silver hair (SIL-vur HAYR)—hair that has grayed and resembles the metallic white of silver metal.

silver nitrate (SIL-vur NY-trayt)—a white, crystalline salt; used as an antiseptic, germicide, and astringent in cosmetics, and as a coloring agent in hair dyes.

simple polymer chain (SIM-pul POL-ih-mur CHAYN)—result of long chain of monomers that are attached from head to tail.

simplex (SIM-pleks)—common; simple; single.

simplex, acne (SIM-pleks, AK-nee)—common pimple.

simulated (SIM-yoo-layt-ed)—fake; made to look genuine.

sinews (SIN-yoos)—fibrous cords; tendons; joins muscles together.

singe (SINJ)—in hairdressing, to burn the hair ends; to burn lightly on the surface with a lighted wax taper.

single braids (SING-gul BRAYDZ)—also known as *box braids* or *individual braids*; free-hanging braids, with or without extensions, that can be executed using either an underhand or an overhand technique.

single flat wrap (SING-gul FLAT RAP)—perm wrap that is similar to double flat wrap, but uses only one end paper, placed over the top of the strand of hair being wrapped.

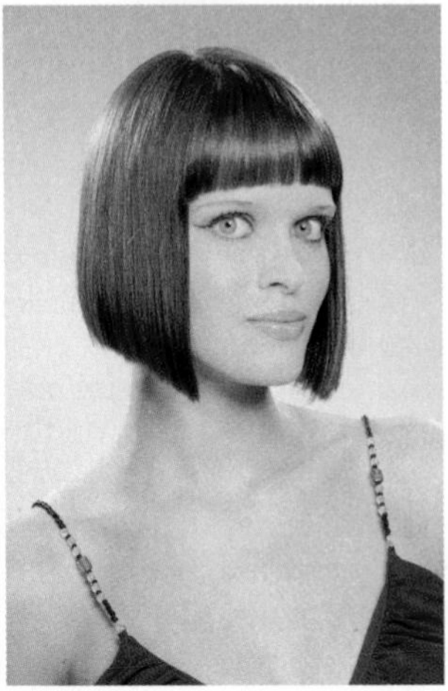

Photography by Tom Carson. Hair by Kelley Newman. Makeup by Kristi Maeger for Elon Salon, Marietta, GA

single lines

single lines (SING-gul LYNZ)—a hairstyle with only one line, such as the one-length hairstyle.

single-process haircoloring (SING-gul-PROSS-ess HAYR KULUR-ing)—also called *single process, single process application, single-process haircolor, one-process tints,* or *one-step tints*; process that lightens and deposits color in the hair in a single application.

single-prong clip (SING-gul-PRAWNG KLIP)—a clip having only one prong, designed to hold small curls on thin hair.

single-use (SING-gul USE)—also known as *disposable*; items that cannot be used more than once. These items cannot be properly cleaned so that all visible residue is removed—such as pumice stones used for pedicures—or they are damaged or contaminated by cleaning and disinfecting in exposure incident.

sink (SINK)—also known as *sinking*; the settling and flattening out of a UV gel or other product while working.

sinus (SY-nus)—a cavity or depression; a hollow in bone or other tissue.

sinusoid (SY-nuh-soyd)—resembling a sinus; a blood space in certain organs such as the liver and pancreas.

sinusoidal current (sy-nuh-SOYD-ul KUR-unt)—smooth, repetitive alternating current similar to faradic current; produces mechanical contractions and is used during scalp and facial manipulations.

skeletal membrane (SKEL-uh-tul MEM-brayn)—tissue covering the bones and cartilage.

skeletal muscles (SKEL-uh-tul MUS-uhlz)—muscles connected to the skeleton by tendons; responsible for moving the limbs, enabling facial expressions, speaking, and other voluntary movements.

skeletal system (SKEL-uh-tul SIS-tum)—forms the physical foundation of the body, composed of 206 bones that vary in size and shape and are connected by movable and immovable joints.

skeleton (SKEL-uh-tun)—the bony framework of the body.

skill (SKIL)—the mastery of an art or technique; dexterity in doing learned physical tasks.

skin (SKIN)—the external covering of the body; acts as a barrier to protect body systems from the outside elements; largest organ of the body with functions that include protection, heat regulation, secretion, excretion, sensation, absorption, and respiration.

skin abrasion peel (SKIN uh-BRAY-zhun PEEL)—a process that rubs or wears away the surface of the skin usually done with pumice stone powder; must be done only by a qualified professional person.

skin analysis (SKIN ah-NAL-ih-sis)—the examination and study of the skin to determine the appropriate treatment.

skin antiseptic (SKIN ant-ah-SEP-tik)—a liquid product formulated for the skin to retard the growth of bacteria-causing microorganisms.

skin astringent (SKIN ah-STRIN-jent)—a liquid product formulated to contract organic tissue; used to help control excessive oiliness and to invigorate the skin.

skin bleach (SKIN BLEECH)—a preparation formulated to lighten dark pigmentation spots on the skin.

skin care equipment (SKIN KAYR ee-KWIP-ment)—apparatus used during a facial treatment procedure such as lamps, atomizers, receptacles, and machines.

skin color (SKIN KUL-ur)—the color of skin as determined by melanin, hemoglobin (oxygenated and reduced), and carotenes.

skin freshener (SKIN FRESH-un-ur)—also known as *astringent* or *toner*; a liquid product used to invigorate the skin following the use of cleansing cream or lotion.

skin graft (SKIN GRAFT)—skin taken from one part of the body to replace damaged skin on another part; a service performed by a surgeon.

skin peel (SKIN PEEL)—also known as *epidermabrasion*; in mechanical skin peels, the use of rotating brushes to remove dead surface cells and debris from the skin; in product peels, a procedure using a mild product to remove dead surface cells from the skin.

skin peel product (SKIN PEEL PRAH-dukt)—a product such as vegetable enzymes in creams or lotions that give the face a mild surface peeling treatment.

skin pigmentation (SKIN pig-men-TAY-shun)—the deposition of pigment by the cells; color pigment.

skin scope (SKIN SKOHP)—also known as *magnifying lamp*; a magnifying glass and lamp combination used to analyze skin conditions..

skin tag (SKIN TAG)—small, benign outgrowths or extensions of the skin that look like flaps; common under the arms or on the neck.

skin test (SKIN TEST)—also known as *strand test*, *patch test*, *predisposition test*, or *allergy test*; a test to determine the existence or nonexistence of extreme sensitivity to certain substances such as foods or chemicals that do not adversely affect most individuals.

skin texture (SKIN TEKS-chur)—the general feel and appearance of the skin such as coarse, fine, smooth, or rough.

skin toner (SKIN TOH-nur)—a preparation that serves to freshen and tone the skin.

skin treatment (SKIN TREET-ment)—a procedure, such as a massage, to improve the health and appearance of the skin of the face and neck.

skin types (SKIN TYPEZ)—classification that describes a person's genetic skin type.

skip waving (SKIP WAYV-ing)—a setting method featuring a ridge following a shaping, against which is placed a series of overlapping pin curls, then repeating the shaping and curl placement.

skull (SKUL)—the bony case or the framework of the head divided into the cranium and facial bones.

slack (SLAK)—loose; not tight.

slant (SLANT)—at an angle or incline; in hairdressing, to make a hair parting on an angle.

slant tweezers (SLANT twee-zur)—the most common type of tweezers, and often the easiest to work with; the tip of slant tweezers is at an angle, making it easy to manipulate use.

slapping (SLAP-ing)—massage movement in which the wrists are kept flexible so that the palms come in contact with the skin in light, firm, and rapid strokes; one hand follows the other; with each slapping stroke, the flesh is lifted slightly.

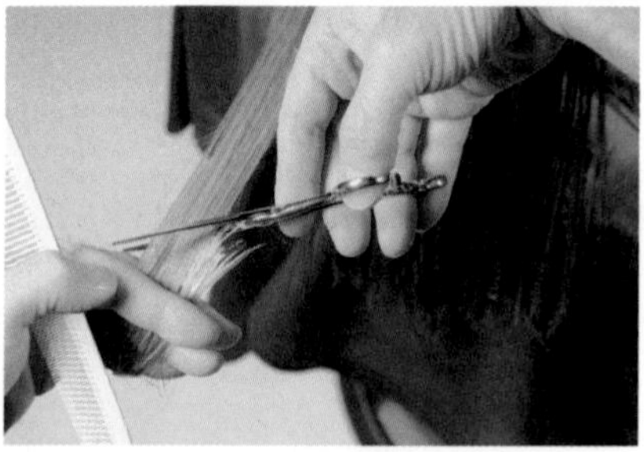
© Milady, a part of Cengage Learning. Photography by Yanik Chauvin.
slicing

slicing (SLYS-ing)—1. in hairstyling, carefully removing a section of hair from a shaping in preparation for making a pin curl (the remainder of the shaping is not disturbed). 2. In haircutting, a technique that removes bulk and adds movement through the lengths of the hair; the shears are not completely closed, and only the portion of the blades near the pivot is used. 3. In haircoloring, technique that involves taking a narrow, 1/8-inch (0.3-centimeter) section of hair by making a straight part at the scalp, positioning the hair over the foil, and applying lightener or color.

slide cutting (SLYD KUT-ting)—method of cutting or thinning the hair in which the fingers and shears glide along the edge of the hair to remove length.

slip (SLIP)—a smooth and slippery feeling.

slithering (SLITH-ur-ing)—also known as *effilating*; process of thinning the hair to graduated lengths with shears; cutting the hair with a sliding movement of the shears while keeping the blades partially opened.

slough (SLUF)—to separate dead cells from living tissue; to discard.

small intestine (SMAWL in-TES-tin)—the part of the intestine between the stomach and the colon consisting of the duodenum, jejunum, and ileum.

smaller occipital nerve (SMAWL-ur ahk-SIP-ut-ul NURV)—also known as *lesser occipital nerve*; located at the base of the skull, affects the scalp and muscles behind the ear.

smile line (SMY-uhl LYN)—in nail technology, when painting a two-color nail design, as in a French manicure, the slightly arced line of the white paint or enhancement material. Named as such because it resembles a smile.

smock (SMAHK)—a loose, lightweight garment worn to protect other clothing.

smooth face (SMOOTH FAYS)—a shaven face or face that is unblemished.

smooth muscle (SMOOTH MUS-uhl)—also known as *involuntary* or *nonstriated muscle*; muscle that functions automatically, without conscious will.

soap cap (SOHP KAP)—combination of equal parts of a prepared permanent color mixture and shampoo used the last five minutes and worked through the hair to refresh the ends.

soapless shampoo (SOHP-les sham-POO)—a shampoo made with a synthetic detergent; it can be formulated at nearly any pH but is usually slightly acidic in reaction.

sodium (SOH-dee-um)—a metallic element of the alkali metal group.

sodium bicarbonate (SOH-dee-um bye-KAR-buh-nayt)—baking soda; an alkaline inorganic salt used as a buffering agent, neutralizer, and a pH adjuster.

sodium carbonate (SOH-dee-um KAR-buh-nayt)—washing soda; used to prevent corrosion of metallic instruments when added to boiling water.

sodium chloride (SOH-dee-um KLOR-yd)—table salt (NaCL).

sodium hydroxide (SOH-dee-um hy-DRAHK-syd)—a powerful alkaline product used in some chemical hair relaxers; caustic soda; powerful alkali used in the manufacture of liquid soaps.

sodium hypochlorite (soh-DEE-um hy-puh-KLOR-yt)—common household bleach; an effective disinfectant for the salon.

sodium lauryl sulfate (soh-DEE-um LOR-ul SUL-fayt)—a metallic compound of the alkaline group; white or light yellow crystals; used in detergents; a detergent, wetting agent, and emulsifier; used in shampoos for its degreasing qualities.

sodium nitrate (SOH-dee-um NY-trayt)—a clear, odorless crystalline salt used to manufacture nitric acid; sodium nitrite; used as an oxidizing agent.

S

sodium perborate (SOH-dee-um pur-BOR-ayt)—a compound formed by treating sodium peroxide with boric acid; when dissolving the substance in water, peroxide of hydrogen is generated; used as an antiseptic and bleaching agent.

sodium sulphite (SOH-dee-um SUL-fyt)—a soft, white metallic salt of sulphurous acid; used as an antiseptic, preservative, and antioxidant in haircolor.

sodium thiosulphate (SOH-dee-um thy-uh-SUL-fayt)—a compound used in solutions for impetiginous conditions and parasitic alopecias of the beard.

soft (SAWFT)—pliable; malleable; easily worked.

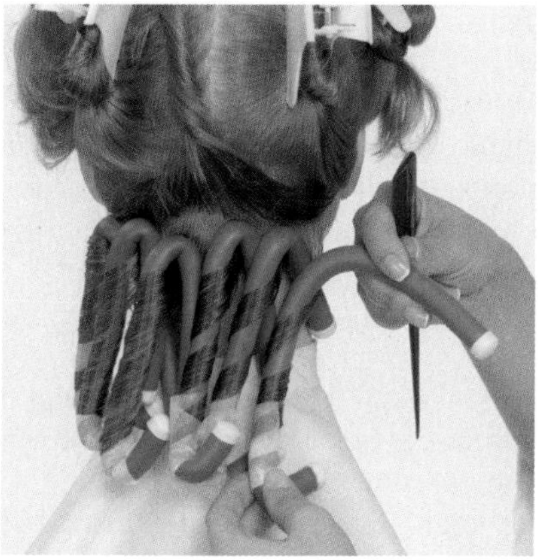

© Milady, a part of Cengage Learning. Photography by Paul Castle.

soft bender rods

soft bender rods (SAWFT ben-DUHR RAHDZ)—tool about 12 inches (30.5 centimeters) long with a uniform diameter along the entire length, around which hair is easily wound for permanent waving.

soft curl permanent (SAWFT CURL PER-man-ent)—combination of a thio relaxer and a thio permanent that is wrapped on large rods to make existing curl larger and looser.

soft press (SAWFT PRES)—technique of pressing the hair to remove 50 to 60 percent of the curl by applying the thermal pressing comb once on each side of the hair.

soft soap (SAWFT SOHP)—also known as *liquid soap*; fluid or semifluid soap.

soft UV gels (SAWFT YOU-VEE JELS)—also known as *soakable gels*; these gels are removed by soaking in acetone.

soft water (SAWFT WAW-tur)—rainwater or chemically softened water that contains only small amounts of minerals and, therefore, allows soap and shampoo to lather freely.

softener (SAWF-un-ur)—also known as *presoftener*; something that softens such as a compound added to water; in hairdressing, a term for a product applied before a permanent wave or haircolor service to lower cuticle resistance.

softening agent (SAW-fun-ing AY-gunt)—mild alkaline product applied prior to the color treatment to increase porosity, swell the cuticle layer of the hair, and increase color absorption; tint that has not been mixed with developer is frequently used.

solar (SOH-lur)—pertaining to the sun.

sole (SOHL)—single; the bottom surface of the foot.

sole proprietor (SOHL PROH-pry-eh-tohr)—individual owner and, most often, the manager of a business.

soleus (SO-lee-is)—muscle that originates at the upper portion of the fibula and bends the foot down.

solid form (SAHL-id FORM)—in hairdressing, an unbroken surface.

solubility (sahl-yuh-BIL-ih-tee)—the extent to which a substance (solute) dissolves in a liquid (solvent) to produce a homogeneous system (solution).

soluble (SAHL-yuh-bul)—capable of being dissolved.

solute (SAHL-yoot)—the substance that is dissolved in a solution.

solution (suh-LOO-shun)—a stable physical mixture of two or more substances.

solvent (SAHL-vent)—the substance that dissolves the solute and makes a solution.

spa (SPAH)—a term originally meaning "health through water." Today it most often refers to day spas or destination spas, where clients can find a wide range of treatments.

spa therapy (SPAH THAIR_uh-pee)—water treatments provided in a spa.

space (SPAYS)—the area surrounding the form or the area the hairstyle occupies.

space base (SPAYS BAYS)—an elongated stem creating a wider area between two rows of pin curls.

sparse (SPARS)—thinly diffused; not dense; consisting of a few or scattered elements; thin, irregular eyebrows or balding areas of the head.

spasm (SPAZM)—an involuntary muscular contraction.

spasmodic (spaz-MAHD-ik)—pertaining to a spasm; convulsive; intermittent.

spat (SPAT)—a slight blow or slap on the skin, used in some massage procedures.

spatula (SPACH-uh-lah)—a flexible implement with a blunt blade used for removing creams from their containers.

S

special effects haircoloring (SPESH-ahl EE-fects HAYR KUL-uhr-ing)—any technique that involves partial lightening or coloring.

specialist (SPESH-ah-list)—one who devotes himself or herself to some special branch of learning such as art, cosmetology, or business.

specialty peels (SPESH-ahl-tee PEELZ)—peels or exfoliation treatments combined with or accompanied by other performance ingredients.

spectrum (SPEK-trum)—an arrangement of rainbow colored bands produced by the passage of white light through a prism.

speed (SPEED)—a rate of motion such as fast, medium, or slow.

sphenoid bone (SFEE-noyd BOHN)—bone that joins all of the bones of the cranium together.

sphere (SFEER)—a geometric figure generated by the revolution of a semicircle around its diameter; globular.

spherical (SFEER-ih-kul)—relating to or having the shape of a sphere.

sphingolipids (SFINGO-lip-udz)—ceramides or lipid material that are a natural part of the intercellular matrix. Glycosphingolipids and phospholipids are also natural lipids found in the barrier layer.

spinal (SPY-nal)—pertaining to the spine or vertebral column.

spinal accessory (SPY-nal ak-SES-oh-ree)—also known as *accessories, accessory,* or *spinal accessory nerve;* either of a pair of motor nerves that are the eleventh cranial nerves, arise from the medulla and the upper part of the spinal cord, and supply chiefly the pharynx and muscles of the upper chest, back, and shoulders.

spinal column (SPY-nal KAHL-um)—the backbone or vertebral column.

spinal cord (SPY-nal KORD)—portion of the central nervous system that originates in the brain, extends down to the lower extremity of the trunk, and is protected by the spinal column.

spinal nerves (SPY-nul NURVZ)—the nerves arising from the spinal cord, its branches supply the muscles and scalp at the back of the head and neck.

spindle cells (SPIN-duI SELS)—alert the central nervous system to the length, stretch, and speed of the muscle; located in the belly of a muscle.

spine (SPYN)—also known as *backbone*; a short process of bone.

spiral (SPY-ral)—coil; winding around a center like a watch spring.

spiral curl (SPY-ral KURL)—method of curling the hair by winding a strand around the rod, causing the hair to spiral along the length of the rod, similar to the stripes on a candy cane.

S

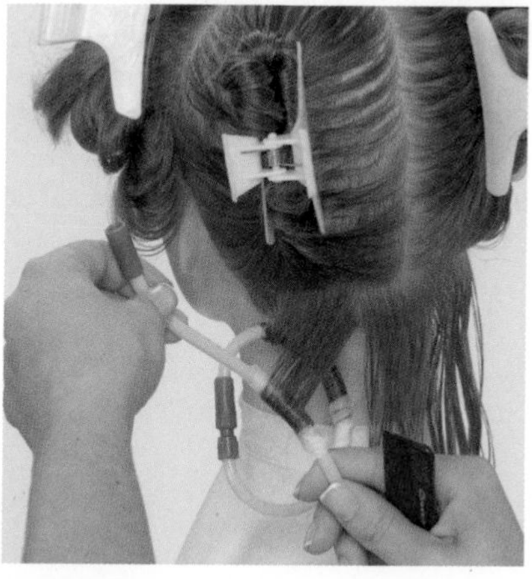

© Milady, a part of Cengage Learning. Photography by Paul Castle.

spiral perm wrap

spiral perm wrap (SPY-ral PURM RAP)—a method in permanent waving where the hair is wrapped at an angle other than perpendicular to the length of the rod, which causes the hair to spiral along the length of the rod, similar to the stripes on a candy cane.

spiral rod (SPY-ral RAHD)—a rod on which the hair is wound in a spiral manner for a permanent wave.

spirillum (spy-RIL-um); pl., spirilla (spy-RIL-ah)—spiral- or corkscrew-shaped bacterium causing diseases such as syphilis and Lyme disease.

split end (SPLIT END)—visible separation at the end of the hair due to cuticle damage.

splinter hemorrhage (SPLIN-tohr HEM-err-aje)—caused by trauma or injury to the nail bed that damage the capillaries and allows small amounts of blood flow.

sponge (SPUNJ)—an elastic, porous substance that serves as an absorbent; the skeleton of an aquatic organism cultivated for use as cosmetic and cleansing pads.

spongy hair (SPUN-jee HAYR)—hair that is overporous due to overprocessing or abuse.

spool rod (SPOOL RAHD)—a straight cold wave rod.

spore (SPOHR)—a tiny bacterial body having a protective wall to withstand unfavorable conditions.

spore-forming bacteria (SPHR-form-ing BAK-tear-ee-ah)—certain bacteria that have the ability to form protective spores to survive an inactive stage.

sports massage (SPORTS muh-SAHZH)—massage used to prepare athletes for upcoming events and to aid in body restoration following competitions.

spot bleaching or lightening (SPAHT BLEECH-ing OR LYT-un-ing)—applying bleach (lightener) to areas insufficiently lightened in order to produce even results.

spot size (SPAHT SYZ)—the diameter of the optical or laser light beam.

S

spot tinting (SPAHT TINT-ing)—applying tint to areas insufficiently colored in order to achieve even results.

spotter brush (SPOHT-ur BRUSH)—also known as *detailer*; a short, round brush, having little belly and a very fine point at the tip. This brush offers maximum control for intricate detailed work.

sprain (SPRAYN)—injury to a joint resulting in stretching or tearing of ligaments.

spray (SPRAY)—to discharge liquid in the form of a fine vapor.

spray gun (SPRAY GUN)—an applicator used to spray a fine mist.

spray machine (SPRAY muh-SHEEN)—a device employed to apply a very fine spray or mist of astringent to massage the nerve ends in the skin.

spray-on thermal protector (SPRAY-on THUR-muhl PRO-teck-tur)—product applied to hair for any thermal service to protect the hair from the harmful effects of blowdrying, thermal irons, or electric rollers.

spur (SPUR)—a pointed, horny outgrowth usually found on the feet.

squalene (SKWAY-lean)—a lubricant and perfume fixative.

squama (SKWAY-mah)—an epidermic scale made up of thin, flat cells.

squamous (SKWAY-mus)—scaly; covered with scales; thin and flat like fish scales.

squamous cell carcinoma (SKWAY-mus SELL CAR-sin-oh-muh)—type of skin cancer more serious than basal cell carcinoma; often characterized by scaly red papules or nodules.

square nail (SKWAYR-NAYL)—a nail completely straight across the free edge with no rounding at the outside edges.

square-shaped face (SKWAYR-SHAYPT FAYS)—facial structure characterized by a wide forehead and jaw; usually shorter in length than an oval.

squoval nail (SKWOVAL NAYL)—a nail with a square free edge that is rounded off at the corner edges.

stabilizer (STAY-bih-ly-zur)—also known as *fixative*; general name for an ingredient that prolongs lifetime, appearance, and performance of a product; a retarding agent or a substance that preserves a chemical equilibrium.

stack, permanent wave (STAK, PUR-mah-nent WAYV)—a wrapping technique to curl ends of long hair; wrapping begins at the hairline and progresses to the crown with sticks used to maintain an even design.

stacking (STAK-ing)—a haircutting technique using a slight gradation to achieve volume; an end permanent technique where one roller is stacked and extended above the other.

stages (STAY-jez)—the term describing the visible color changes the hair passes through during a lightening process.

stagger (STAG-ur)—to arrange rollers on rods in a zigzag order.

stain (STAYN)—brown or wine-colored discoloration with a circular and/or irregular shape. Stains occur after certain diseases, or after moles, freckles, or liver spots disappear. A port wine stain is a birthmark, which is a vascular type of nevus.

stain remover (STAYN ree-MOOV-ur)—chemical used to remove tint stains from skin.

standard precautions (SP) (STAN-dard PRUH-caw-shuns)—CDC guidelines and controls that require employers and employees to assume that all human blood and specified human body fluids are infectious for HIV, HBV, and other bloodborne pathogens. Employees should take such precautions as wearing personal protective equipment to prevent skin and mucous membrane where contact with a client's blood, body fluids, secretions (except sweat), excretions, nonintact skin, and mucous membranes.

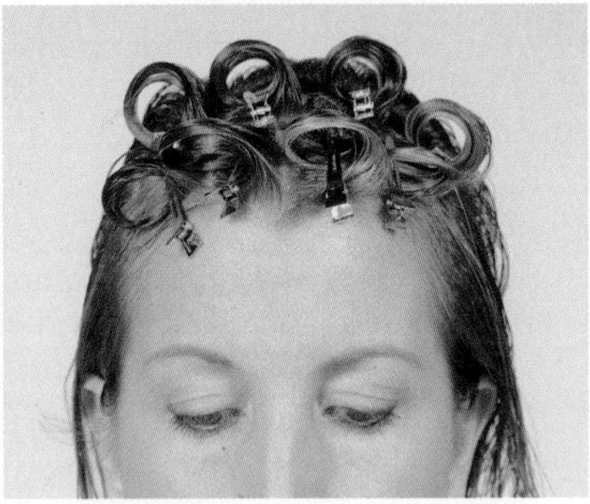

© Milady, a part of Cengage Learning. Photography by Yanik Chauvin.

standup curl

standup curl (STAND-UP KURL)—also known as *cascade curl*; forerunner of the roller; a strand of hair held directly up from the scalp and wound with a large center opening in croquignole fashion, then fastened to the scalp in a standing position.

staphylococcus (staf-uh-loh-KOK-us); pl., staphylococci (staf-uh-loh-KOKS-eye)—pus-forming bacteria that grow in clusters like a bunch of grapes. They cause abscesses, pustules, and boils.

starting knot (START-ing NAHT)—a procedure in weaving to secure the first strand of hair.

S

states of matter (STAYTS UV MATT-uhr)—the three different physical forms of matter—solid, liquid, and gas.

static electricity (STAT-ik ee-lek-TRIH-sut-ee)—a form of electricity generated by friction.

stationary design line (STAY-shun-ar-ee dih-ZYN LYN)—also known as *stationary guide*; one length; show no movement.

stationary guide (STAY-shun-ar-ee GYDE)—stable guide; in haircutting, a guideline that is one length and does not move.

staying power (STAY-ing POW-ur)—the holding ability or power of a perm or roller set.

steamer (STEEM-ur)—a facial machine that heats and produces a stream of warm steam that can be focused on the client's face or other areas of skin.

steamer, scalp (STEEM-ur, SKALP)—an apparatus used in place of hot towels for steaming the scalp.

stearic acid (stee-AYR-ik AS-ud)—a white, fatty acid occurring in solid animal fats and in some vegetable fats; used in powders, creams, lotions, and soap as a lubricant.

steatoma (stee-ah-TOH-muh)—also known as *wen*; sebaceous cyst or subcutaneous tumor filled with sebum; ranges in size from a pea to an orange. It usually appears on the scalp, neck, and back.

steatosis (stee-ah-TOH-sis)—fatty degeneration; disease of the sebaceous glands.

steep (STEEP)—to soak in a liquid to soften or cleanse.

stem (STEM)—section of the pin curl between the base and first arc (turn) of the circle that gives the circle its direction and movement; the basic question or problem.

stem cell (STEM SELL)—also known as *mother cell*; a cell capable of multiple divisions; derived from plants to protect or stimulate our own skin stem cells; for health and antiaging benefits.

stem direction (STEM dih-REK-shun)—the direction in which the stem moves from the base to the first arc.

stencil (STEN-sill)—a template that is used to prevent color from being applied beyond a certain area.

steps (STEPS)—irregular layers in a haircut.

sterile (STAIR-il)—barren; free from all living organisms.

sterilization (stayr-ih-luh-ZAY-shun)—the process that completely destroys all microbial life, including spores.

sterilize (STAYR-ih-lyz)—to make sterile or free from microorganisms, including spores.

sterilizer (STAYR-ih-ly-zur)—an apparatus used to sterilize equipment or other objects by destroying all contaminating microorganisms.

S

sternocleidomastoid artery (STUR-noh-KLEE-ih-doh-MAS-toyd AR-tuh-ree)—the artery that supplies blood to the muscles of the neck.

sternocleidomastoideus (STUR-noh-KLEE-ih-doh-mas-TOYD-ee-us)—muscle of the neck that lowers and rotates the head.

sternomastoid (stur-noh-MAS-toyd)—pertaining to the sternum and the mastoid process.

sternum (STUR-num)—also known as *breastbone*; flat bone that forms the ventral (front) support of the ribs.

steroid (STAYR-oyd)—very small hormone molecules that penetrate cell membranes.

stigma (STIG-muh)—a mark, spot, scar, or other blemish on the skin.

stimulant (STIM-yuh-lent)—an agent that arouses organic activity.

stimulus (STIM-yuh-LUS)—anything that excites or incites an organ or other part to function, become active, or respond.

stone massage (STON mass-aje)—use of hot stones and cold stones in massage or in other treatments.

stopping point (STAHP-ing POYNT)—in massage, a point on a muscle or over a pressure point where pressing movements are made during the facial or scalp massage.

straight (STRAYT)—extending in one direction without a curve or bend; not curly.

straight permanent wave rod (STRAYT PUR-mah-nent WAYV RAHD)—perm rods that are equal in diameter along their entire length or curling area.

straight profile (STRAYT PROH-fyl)—a profile that has evenly balanced facial features; being neither concave nor convex when seen in profile; considered the ideal.

straight razor (STRAYT RAY-zohr)—a hardened steel blade attached to a handle by means of a pivot.

straightening comb (STRAYT-un-ing KOHM)—also known as *pressing comb*; a comb constructed of steel or brass with a wood handle, usually heated electrically; used to remove curl from overcurly hair.

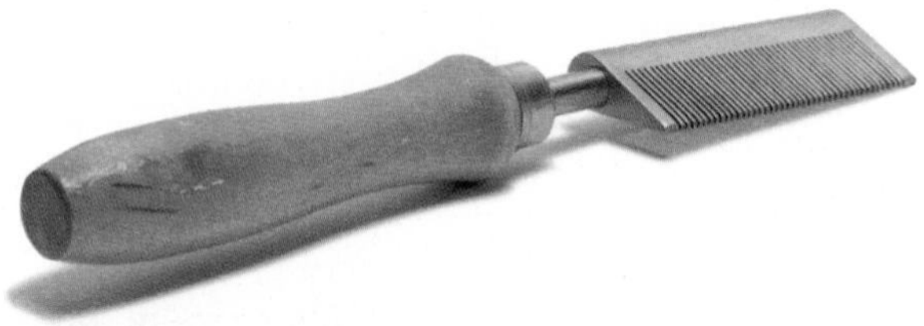

© Milady, a part of Cengage Learning. Photography by Yanik Chauvin.

straightening or pressing comb

straightening gel (STRAYT-un-ing JEL)—styling product applied to damp hair that is wavy, curly, or extremely curly, and then blown dry; relaxes the hair for a smooth, straight look.

strand (STRAND)—fibers or hairs that form a unit.

strand test (STRAND TEST)—a test given before tinting, lightening, permanent waving, or hair relaxing to determine the required developing or processing time; a test to determine the degree of porosity and elasticity of the hair, as well as the ability of the hair to withstand the effects of chemicals.

S

stratum (STRAT-um); pl., strata (STRAT-ah)—a layer as in tissue.

stratum basale (STRAT-um buh-SAY-lee)—basal layer; the cell-producing layer of the epidermis.

stratum corneum (STRAT-um KOR-nee-um)—also known as *horny layer*; outer layer of the epidermis.

stratum germinativum (STRAT-um jur-min-ah-TIV-um)—also known as *basal cell layer*; active layer of the epidermis above the papillary layer of the dermis; cell mitosis takes place here that produces new epidermal skin cells and is responsible for growth.

stratum granulosum (STRAT-um gran-yoo-LOH-sum)—also known as *granular layer*; layer of the epidermis composed of cells filled with keratin that resemble granules; replace cells shed from the stratum corneum.

stratum lucidum (STRAT-um LOO-sih-dum)—clear, transparent layer of the epidermis under the stratum corneum; thickest on the palms of hands and soles of feet.

stratum malpighian (STRAT-um mal-PIG-ee-an)—the germinative or innermost layer of the epidermis including the spinosum or spiny layer.

stratum mucosum (STRAT-um myoo-KOH-sum)—mucous or malpighian layer of the skin.

stratum spinosum (STRAT-um spy-NOH-sum)—also known as *spiny layer*; layer of the epidermis above the stratum germinativum layer containing desmosomes, the intercellular connections made of proteins.

streptococcus (strep-toh-KOK-us); pl., streptococci (strep-toh-KOK-eye)—pus-forming bacteria arranged in curved lines resembling a string of beads. They cause infections such as strep throat and blood poisoning.

stress (STRES)—a force or system of forces exerted on the body that result in strain and/or injury.

stress area (STRES AIR-ee-uh)—the part of the nail enhancement where the natural nail grows beyond the finger and becomes the free edge. This area needs strength to support the nail extension.

stress strip (STRES STRIP)—strip of fabric cut to 1/8-inch in length and applied to the weak point of the nail during the Four-Week Fabric Wrap Maintenance to repair or strengthen a weak point in a nail enhancement.

stretch wig (STRECH WIG)—a wig that has been constructed with a completely elasticized foundation that will stretch to fit a wide range of head sizes.

striated muscles (STRY-ayt-ed MUS-uhlz)—also known as *skeletal muscles*; muscles that are attached to the bones and that are voluntary or are consciously controlled.

stringy hair (STRING-ee HAYR)—limp hairs matted together forming a rope-like strand.

striper brush (STRY-per BRUSH)—an extremely long, flat brush having only a few fibers. It is incredibly efficient when creating long lines, striping effects, and animal prints.

stripping (STRIP-ing)—also known as *bleaching* or *lightening*; the removal of color from the hair shaft; bleaching; strong shampoos or soaps that remove some of the color from the hair.

stroking (STROHK-ing)—also known as *effleurage*; a gliding movement over a surface; to pass the finger or any instrument gently over a surface;.

strong hair (STRAWNG HAYR)—hair that is somewhat resistant to treatments; usually coarser than average hair.

strontium sulfide (STRAHN-chum SUL-fyd)—a light gray powder capable of liberating hydrogen sulfide in the presence of water; used as a depilatory.

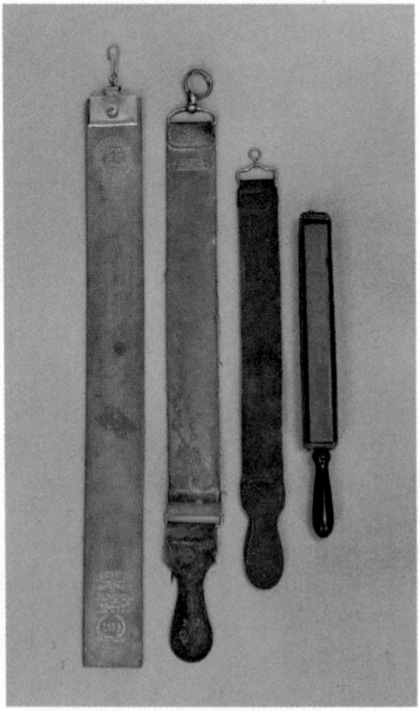

© Milady, a part of Cengage Learning. Photography by Yanik Chauvin.

strops

strop (STROP)—also known as *razor strop*; an elongated piece of leather or other materials used to smooth the edge and polish the conventional straight razor.

sty, stye (STY); pl., sties, styes (STYZ)—inflammation of one of the sebaceous glands of the eyelid.

style (STYL)—the current, fashionable mode of dress, makeup, or hair design; the specific shape, size, and placement of curls and waves of a finished hairstyle.

styling chair (STYL-ing CHAYR)—an adjustable chair, usually with a footrest, in which the client sits while the hair is being styled.

S

styling comb (STYL-ing KOHM)—a comb designed with one-half row of thin, close teeth and the other half with wider spaces between the teeth; used to aid in styling hair.

styling gel (STYL-ing JEL)—a jelly-like preparation used to aid in styling the hair and add stiffness.

styling lotion (STYL-ing LOH-shun)—a liquid preparation used to add body and staying power to the finished hairstyle.

styling station (STYL-ing STAY-shun)—a space or unit in a salon containing the furnishings, implements, and products needed to cut and style hair.

stylist (STYL-ist)—one who develops, designs, advises on, or creates styles.

stylus (STY-lus)—tool with a solid handle and a rounded ball tip on each end that can range in size. An excellent tool for marbleizing or dotting small circles of color on a nail.

styptic (STIP-tik)—an agent causing contraction of living tissue; used to stop bleeding; an astringent.

subclavian (sub-KLAY-vee-an)—lying under the clavicle such as the subclavian artery.

subcutaneous (sub-kyoo-TAY-nee-us)—also known as *hypodermis, adipose,* or *subcutis tissue*; fatty tissue found below the dermis that gives smoothness and contour to the body, contains fat for use as energy, and also acts as a protective cushion for the outer skin.

subcutaneous mycosis (sub-kyoo-TAY-nee-us MY-ko-sis)—a fungal infection occurring below the skin.

subcutis (sub-KYOO-tis)—subdermis; subcutaneous tissue; under or beneath the corium or dermis; the true skin.

subdermis (sub-DUR-mis)—subcutis or subcutaneous tissue of the skin.

subdivide (SUB-dih-vyd)—to divide a section into smaller sections.

subjective symptoms (SUB-jek-tif SYM-tumz)—symptoms that can be felt or experienced only by the person affected.

sublingual (SUB-ling-wal)—under the tongue.

submental (sub-MEN-tul)—below the mentalis, the area within the anatomic triangular margins of the mandible where the double chin resides.

submental artery (sub-MEN-tul AR-tuh-ree)—artery that supplies blood to the chin and lower lip.

suboccipital nerve (sub-ahk-SIP-ut-ul NURV)—nerve that stimulates the deep muscles of the back and the neck.

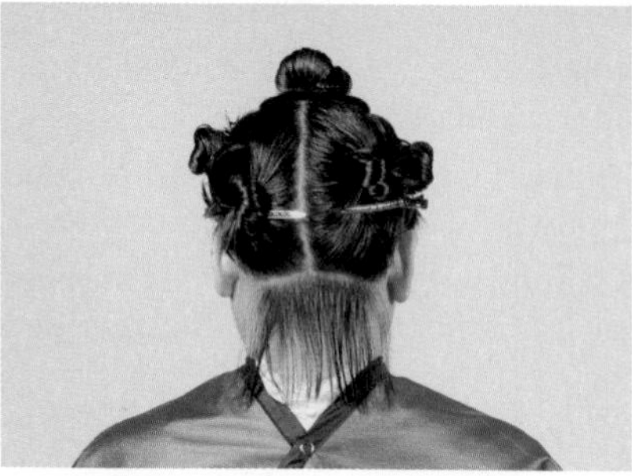

© Milady, a part of Cengage Learning. Photography by Yanik Chauvin.

subsections

subsections (SUB-sek-shunz)—smaller sections within a larger section of hair, used to maintain control of the hair while cutting.

suction machine (SUK-shun muh-SHEEN)—an apparatus used in some facial treatment procedures to dislodge debris from the follicles.

sudamen (soo-DAY-men); pl., sudamina (soo-DAM-ih-nah)—a disorder of the sweat glands with obstruction of their ducts.

sudor (SOO-dor)—sweat; perspiration.

sudoriferous (sood-uh-RIF-uh-rus)—carrying or producing sweat.

sudoriferous ducts (sood-uh-RIF-uh-rus DUKTS)—the excretory ducts of the sweat glands.

sudoriferous glands (sood-uh-RIF-uh-rus GLANDZ)—also known as *sweat glands*; excrete perspiration and detoxify the body by excreting excess salt and unwanted chemicals.

sudorific (sood-uh-RIF-ik)—causing or inducing perspiration.

sugaring (SHUH-gar-ing)—ancient method of hair removal. The original recipe is a mixture of sugar, lemon juice, and water that is heated to form syrup, molded into a ball, and pressed onto the skin and then quickly stripped away.

sulfide (SUL-fyd)—compound of sulfur and an oxide.

sulfite (SUL-fyt)—any salt or sulfurous acid.

sulfur, sulphur (SUL-fur)—a solid, nonmetallic element, usually yellow in color; it is insoluble in water. Reduces oil-gland activity and dissolves the skin's surface layer of dry, dead cells. This ingredient is commonly used in acne products.

sulfur bonds (SUL-fur BAHNDZ)—also known as *S bonds*; sulfur crossbonds formed by the attraction of opposite electric charges in the hair that hold the chains of amino acids together; position determines curl present in the hair.

sulfuric acid (sul-FYOO-rik AS-ud)—also known as *oil of vitriol*; colorless and nearly odorless, heavy, oily corrosive liquid; employed as a caustic.

sun protection factor (SPF) (SUN-proh-TEK-shun FAK-tur)—ability of a product to delay sun-induced erythema, the visible sign of sun damage. The SPF rating is based only on UVB protection, not UVA exposure.

sunburn (SUN-burn)—inflammation of the skin caused by exposure to the sun.

sunlamp (SUN-lamp)—a lamp that radiates ultraviolet rays; used in cosmetic and therapeutic face and body treatments.

suntan (SUN-tan)—deepening the pigmentation of the skin as a result of sun exposure.

superciliary (soo-pur-SIL-ee-ayr-ee)—pertaining to or referring to the region of the eyebrow.

supercilium (soo-pur-SIL-ee-um); pl., supercilia (soo-pur-SIL-ee-ah)—the eyebrow.

supercritical carbon dioxide (CO_2) (SOOP-uhr-crit-icle CAR-bun DIE-oz-eyed)—a modern method of extraction in which the plant material is placed in a high-pressure container with CO_2 that is in a state midway between being a liquid and a gas.

superficial (soo-pur-FISH-al)—pertaining to or being on the surface.

superficial cervical (soo-pur-FISH-al SUR-vih-kal)—a cranial nerve that supplies the muscle and skin of the neck.

superficial fascia (soo-pur-FISH-ul FAYSH-uh)—a sheet of subcutaneous tissue; tissue that attaches the dermis to underlying structures.

superficial mycosis (soo-pur-FISH-ul MY-coe-sis)—a skin condition that results from the introduction of vegetative matter to an open wound; infection is limited to the dermis.

superficial peroneal nerve (soo-pur-FISH-ul pare-oh-NEE-uhl NURV)—also known as *musculocutaneous* nerve; extends down the leg, just under the skin, supplying impulses to the muscles and the skin of the leg, as well as to the skin and toes on the top of the foot, where it becomes the dorsal nerve, also known as the *dorsal cutaneous nerve*.

superficial temporal artery (soo-pur-FISH-ul TEM-puh-rul AR-tuh-ree)—a continuation of the external carotid nerve artery; supplies blood to the muscles of the front, side, and top of the head.

superfluous hair (soo-PUR-floo-us HAYR)—excessive, more than is needed, unwanted hair.

superior (soo-PEER-ee-ur)—higher; upper; better; of more value.

superior auricularis (soo-PEER-ur aw-rik-yuh-LAYR-is)—the muscle that draws the ear upward.

superior labial artery (soo-PEER-ee-ur LAY-bee-ul AR-tuh-ree)—artery that supplies blood to the upper lip and region of the nose.

superior labial nerve (soo-PEER-ee-ur LAY-bee-ul NURV)—nerve that receives stimuli from the skin of the upper lip.

superior maxillary (soo-PEER-ee-ur MAK-suh-layr-ee)—the upper jawbone.

superior palpebral nerve (soo-PEER-ee-ur PAL-puh-brul NURV)—nerve that receives stimuli from the upper eyelid.

superior vena cava (soo-PEER-ee-ur VEE-nuh KAH-vuh)—the large vein that carries blood to the upper right chamber of the heart.

superioris (soo-peer-ee-OR-is)—a muscle that elevates.

supinator (SOO-puh-nayt-ur)—a muscle of the forearm that rotates the radius outward and the palm upward.

supple hair (SUP-ul HAYR)—hair that is easily managed; pliable, not stiff.

supporting curl (suh-PORT-ing KURL)—a pin curl made in the same direction as the first line of curls.

supraclavicular (soo-pruh-kluh-VIK-yoo-lar)—above the clavicle.

supraclavicular nerve, intermediate (soo-pruh-kluh-VIK-yoo-lar NURV, in-tur-MEE-dee-ut)—nerve that receives stimuli from the lower anterior aspect of the neck and interior chest wall.

supraclavicular nerve, lateral (soo-pruh-kluh-VIK-yuh-lar NURV, LAT-ur-ul)—nerve that receives stimuli from the skin of the lateral aspect of the neck and shoulder.

supraorbital (soo-pruh-OR-bih-tul)—above the orbit or eye.

supraorbital artery (soo-pruh-OR-bih-tul AR-tuh-ree)—artery that supplies blood to the upper eyelid and forehead.

S

supraorbital nerve (soo-pruh-OR-bih-tul NURV)—affects the skin of the forehead, scalp, eyebrow, and upper eyelid.

suprascapular artery (soo-pruh-SKAP-yoo-lar AR-tuh-ree)—the artery that supplies blood to the shoulder joints and muscles surrounding the area.

supratrochlear (soo-pruh-TRAHK-lee-ur)—above the trochlea or pulley of the superior oblique muscle.

supratrochlear artery (soo-pruh-TRAHK-lee-ur AR-tuh-ree)—artery that supplies blood to the anterior scalp.

supratrochlear nerve (soo-pruh-TRAHK-lee-ur NURV)— nerve that affects the skin between the eyes and upper side of the nose.

sural nerve (SOO-ral NURV)—supplies impulses to the skin on the outer side and back of the foot and leg.

surface tension (SUR-fis TEN-shun)—the tension or resistance to rupture possessed by the surface film of a liquid.

surfactant (sur-FAK-tant)— a contraction of *surface active agents*; substances that allow oil and water to mix, or emulsify.

suspensions (sus-PEN-shunz)—unstable physical mixtures of undissolved particles in a liquid.

sustainability (SUS-tane-abil-eh-tee)—meeting the needs of the present without compromising the ability of future generations to meet their needs. The three facets of sustainability are the three E's: the *Environment*, the *Economy*, and social *Equity*.

swab (SWAHB)—absorbent cotton wrapped around the end of a short, pliable stick; used for the application of solutions and for removing excess makeup.

sweat (SWET)—to exude or excrete moisture from the pores of the skin; perspire.

sweat gland (SWET GLAND)—small, convoluted tubules that secrete sweat; found in the subcutaneous tissue and ending at the opening of the pores.

Swedish massage (SWEE-dish muh-SAHZH)—a system of traditional manipulations including effleurage, petrissage, vibration, friction, and tapotement for muscles and joints.

sweep (SWEEP)—to brush or comb the hair upward, moving or extending it in a wide curve or over a wide area; upsweep.

swirl (SWURL)—formation of a wave in a diagonal direction from the back to the side of the head.

switch (SWICH)—a long length of wefted hair mounted with a loop on the end; usually constructed with three stem strands to provide flexibility in styling; a separate tress of hair or a substitute worn by women to increase the apparent mass of hair.

swivel clamp (SWIV-ul KLAMP)—a clamp used to secure a wig block or mannequin head to a tabletop.

sycosis (sy-KOH-sis)—a chronic pustular inflammation of the hair follicles.

sycosis barbae (sy-KOH-sis BAR-bee)—a chronic inflammatory disease involving the hair follicles especially of the bearded part of the face and marked by papules, pustules, and tubercles perforated by hairs with crusting.

sycosis tinea (sy-KOH-sis TIN-ee-uh)—parasitic ringworm of the beard; barber's itch.

sycosis vulgaris (sy-KOH-sis vul-GAYR-is)—a pustular, follicular lesion caused by staphylococci; nonparasitic sycosis of the beard.

symmetrical (sih-MET-rih-kal)—uniform and balanced in proportion and style.

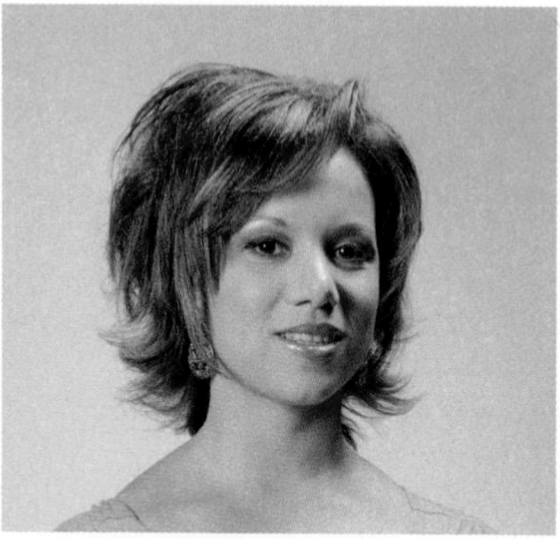

© Milady, a part of Cengage Learning. Photography by Yanik Chauvin.

symmetrical balance

symmetrical balance (sih-MET-rih-kal BAL-ans)—the same on both sides; two halves of a style; form a mirror image of one another.

symmetrical hairstyle (sih-MET-rih-kal HAYR-styl)—a hairstyle with a similar design on both sides of the face.

symmetry (SIM-ut-ree)—balanced proportions; harmony of line and form.

sympathetic division (sim-puh-THET-ik div-eh-zun)—part of the autonomic nervous system that stimulates or speeds up activity and prepares the body for stressful situations, such as in running from a dangerous situation, or competing in a sports event.

sympathetic nervous system (sim-puh-THET-ik NUR-vus SIS-tem)—that part of the autonomic nervous system concerned with mediating involuntary responses of the body such as heart rate, salivary secretion, blood pressure, digestion, and so forth.

S

symptom, objective (SIMP-tum, ahb-JEK-tiv)—a symptom that can be seen, as in pimples or pustules.

symptom, subjective (SIMP-tum, sub-JEK-tiv)—a symptom that can be felt but not seen, such as itching.

symptomatica alopecia (simp-tum-AT-ih-kuh al-uh-PEE-sha)—loss of hair due to illness.

synarthrotic joints (sin-ahr-THRAH-tik JOYNTS)—immovable joints such as the skull.

synergetic (sin-ur-JET-ik)—working together; the combined action or effect of two or more organs or agents; coordination of muscular or organ functions by the nervous system in such a way that specific movements and actions can be performed.

synovial fluid (suh-NOH-vee-uhl FLOO-id)—a transparent viscid fluid that lubricates the surfaces of joints to prevent friction.

synthetic (sin-THET-ik)—produced artificially, not naturally.

synthetic hair (sin-THET-ik HAYR)—a man-made, hairlike fiber made from nylon, dynel, rayon, or other like product, or from any combination of these fibers.

synthetic polymer conditioners (sin-THET-ik POLY-mur con-DISH-on-uhrz)—formulated to prevent breakage and correct excessive porosity on badly damaged hair.

syphilis (SIF-il-lis)—a sexually transmitted disease caused by *Treponema pallidum*.

system (SIS-tum)—a group of bodily organs acting together to perform one or more functions; an arrangement of objects that completes a unit; a procedure or established way of doing something.

systemic (sis-TEM-ik)—pertaining to a system or to the body as a whole; affecting the body generally.

systemic circulation (sis-TEM-ik sir-KYU-lay-shun)—also known as *general circulation*; carries the blood from the heart throughout the body and back to the heart.

systemic disease (sis-TEM-ik DIZ-eez)—disease that affects the body as a whole, often due to under-functioning or over-functioning of internal glands or organs. This disease is carried through the blood stream or the lymphatic system.

systemic mycosis (sis-TEM-ik MY-coe-sis)—a fungal infection that affects the internal organs.

systole (SIHS-toe-lee)—contraction of the heart (as opposed to *diastole*).

T

T pin (TEE PIN)—a pin resembling the letter T; used to secure a hairpiece to the block.

T-zone (TEE-ZOHN)—center area of the face; corresponds to the "T" shape formed by the forehead, nose, and chin.

tablespoon (TAY-bul-spoon)—abbreviation, tbsp.; a large spoon used for serving food and in measuring substances; one tablespoonful equals three teaspoons, 1/2 ounce, or 15 milliliters in metric measure.

tactile (TAK-tile)—pertaining to the sense of touch; capable of being felt.

tactile corpuscle (TAK-tile KOR-pus-ul)—small epidermal structures with nerve endings that are sensitive to touch and pressure.

tag (TAG)—also known as *skin tag*; a small appendage, flap, or polyp; cutaneous outgrowth of the skin.

tail brush (TAYL BRUSH)—also known as *color brush* or *chemical brush*; a small, flat brush with stiff bristles and a long, tapering end; used to apply a haircoloring or relaxing product to the hair.

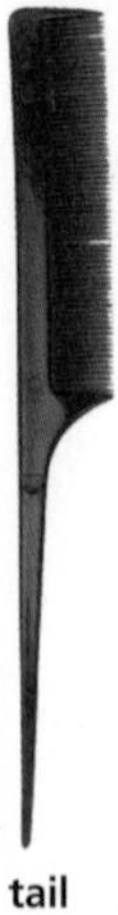

© Milady, a part of Cengage Learning. Photography by Paul Castle.

tail comb

tail comb (TAYL KOHM)—also known as *teasing comb*, *rattail comb*, or *backcombing comb*; a comb, half of which is shaped into a slender tail-like end, used for making partings and teasing the hair.

tailored neckline (TAY-lord NEK-lyn)—a hair shaping in which the hairline is low and angled in the nape area.

talcum powder (TAL-kum POW-dur)—finely powdered, purified talc used as a dusting agent for the relief of chapped skin.

talus (TAL-us)—also known as *ankle bone*; one of three bones that comprise the ankle joint. The other two bones are the tibia and fibula.

tan (TAN)— increase in pigmentation due to the melanin production that results from exposure to UV radiation; visible skin damage. Melanin is designed to help protect the skin from the sun's UV radiation.

tang (TANG)—also known as *finger tang*; a projection such as the finger rest on scissors.

tangle (TANG-gul)—a matted mass of hair; snarled hair; to become snarled.

tangled hair (TANG-guld HAYR)—also known as *trichonodosis*; fraying of the hair resulting in knots associated with breaking of the hair shaft.

tanning lotion (TAN-ing LOH-shun)—a sunscreen product, usually containing oil and other ingredients to assist in the sun tanning process; the product should include a sun protection factor (SPF) to protect skin from harmful rays while exposed to sun.

tap (TAP)—to touch or strike gently; to pat the face during the application of makeup; in massage, to strike lightly with flexed fingers.

tape (TAYP)—in hairstyling, a narrow strip of material to which adhesive is applied and used to attach false hair to the scalp or face, or to hold flat curls or bangs to the face.

taper (TAY-pur)—haircutting effect in which there is an even blend from very short at the hairline to longer lengths as you move up the head; *to taper* is to narrow progressively at one end.

taper comb (TAY-pur KOM)—a comb used for cutting or trimming hair when a gradual blending from short to longer is required within the haircut.

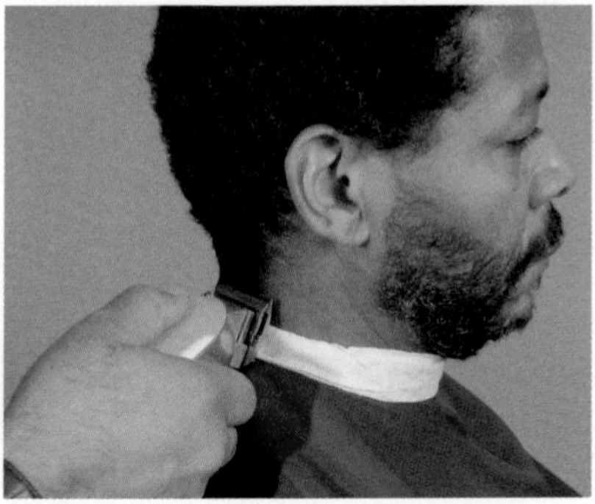

© Milady, a part of Cengage Learning. Photography by Yanik Chauvin.

tapered haircut

tapered (TAY-purd); tapering (TAY-pur-ing)—haircuts in which there is an even blend from very short at the hairline to longer lengths as you move up the head; to taper is to narrow progressively at one end.

tapering shears (TAY-pur-ing SHEERZ)—scissors designed for thinning hair and shaping blunt ends.

tapotement (tah-POT-ment)—also known as *percussion*; massage movements consisting of short quick tapping, slapping, and hacking movements.

tapping (TAP-ing)—a massage movement; striking lightly with the partly flexed fingers.

T

target market (TAR-get MAR-ket)——the group that has been identified as the desired clientele and to which marketing and advertising efforts will be directed.

tarsal artery (TAR-sul AR-tuh-ree)—artery that supplies blood to the foot and tarsal joints. There are seven bones—talus, calcaneus, navicular, three cuneiform bones, and the cuboid. The other two subdivisions are the metatarsal and the phalanges.

tarsus (TAR-sus)—the root or posterior part of the foot or instep; the seven bones of the instep.

taut (TAWT)—tightly drawn; firm; not slack.

tease (TEEZ)— also known as *backcombing, ratting, French lacing,* or *ruffing*; in hairstyling, to comb small sections of hair from the ends toward the scalp to form a cushion or base.

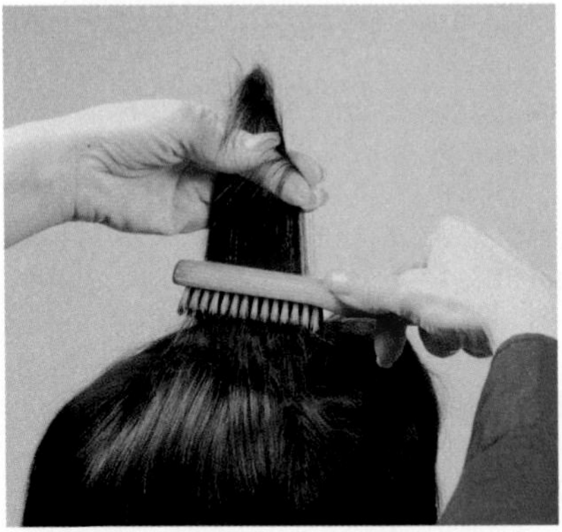

© Milady, a part of Cengage Learning. Photography by Yanik Chauvin.

teasing brush

teasing brush (TEEZ-ing BRUSH)—a small brush with short, stiff bristles and a long, thin handle; used to brush sections of hair from the ends toward the scalp.

teasing comb (TEEZ-ing KOHM)—a comb designed with alternating short and long teeth; used to comb sections of hair from the ends toward the scalp.

teaspoon (TEE-spoon)—$\frac{1}{6}$ of an ounce, $\frac{1}{3}$ of a tablespoon, 5 milliliters in metric measure.

technical (TEK-nih-kul)—relating to a technique; relating to a practical subject organized on scientific principles.

technician (tek-NIH-shun)—an individual trained and expert in a specific skill or subject.

technique (tek-NEEK)—manner of performance; a skill; a process.

telangiectasis (tel-an-jee-EK-tuh-sus)—also known as *spider vein*; distended or dilated surface blood vessels.

telogen effluvium (TEL-uh-jen ef-FLOO-vee-um)—the premature shedding of hair in the resting phase. Can result from various causes such as difficult childbirth, shock, drug intake, fever.

telogen phase (TEL-uh-jen FAYZ)—also known as *resting phase*; the final phase in the hair cycle that lasts until the fully grown hair is shed.

telophase (TEL-uh-fayz)—the final stage of cell mitosis in which the chromosomes reorganize to form an interstage nucleus.

T

temper **(TEM-pur)**—a process used to condition a new brass pressing comb so that it heats evenly.

temperature **(TEM-pur-uh-chur)**—the degree of heat or cold as measured by a thermometer.

temple **(TEM-pul)**—the flattened space on the side of the forehead.

temporal **(TEM-puh-rul)**—of or pertaining to the temple.

temporal artery **(TEM-puh-rul AR-tuh-ree)**—deep artery that supplies blood to the temporal muscle, the orbit, and skull.

temporal artery, medial **(TEM-puh-rul AR-tuh-ree, MEE-dee-ul)**—artery that supplies blood to the temporal muscle and eyelids.

temporal artery, superficial **(TEM-puh-rul AR-tuh-ree, soo-pur-FISH-ul)**—artery that supplies blood to the muscles of the head, face, and scalp.

temporal bone **(TEM-poh-rul BOHN)**—the bone forming the side of the head in the ear region.

temporal nerve **(TEM-poh-rul NURV)**—affects the muscles of the temple, side of the forehead, eyebrow, eyelid, and upper part of the cheek.

temporalis **(tem-poh-RAY-lis)**—muscles that coordinate with the masseter, medial pterygoid, and lateral pterygoid muscles to open and close the mouth and bring the jaw forward; sometimes referred to as chewing muscles.

temporary **(TEM-poh-rayr-ee)**—not permanent; lasting only for a specific time.

temporary haircolor **(TEM-puh-rayr-ee HAYR KUL-ur)**—nonpermanent color whose large pigment molecules prevent penetration of the cuticle layer, allowing only a coating action that may be removed by shampooing.

temporary rinse **(TEM-puh-rayr-ee RINS)**—a nonpermanent color rinse used to color the hair; is easily removed by shampoo.

tendon **(TEN-dun)**—fibrous cord or band connecting muscle to bone.

tendril **(TEN-drul)**—a small, wispy curl that appears to be falling downward.

tensile **(TEN-sul)**—capable of being stretched.

tensile strength **(TEN-sul STRENGTH)**—the resistance of a material to the forces of stress.

tension **(TEN-shun)**—amount of pressure applied when combing and holding a section, created by stretching or pulling the section.

tepid **(TEP-ud)**—neither hot nor cold; lukewarm.

terminal **(TUR-mih-nul)**—of or pertaining to an end or extremity; a part that forms the end.

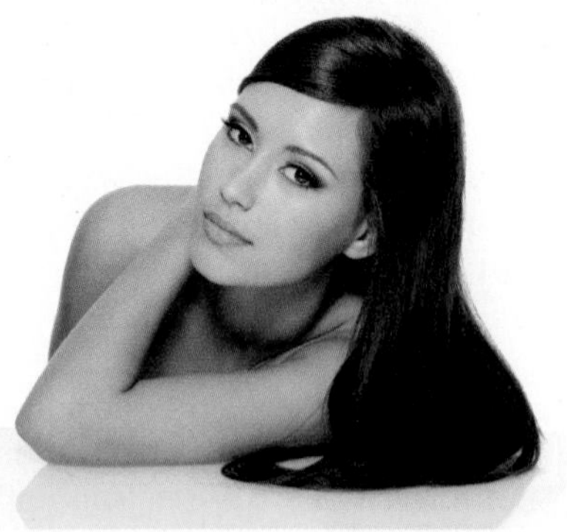
© Valua Vitaly/www.Shutterstock.com
terminal hair

terminal hair (TUR-mih-nul HAYR)—long, coarse, pigmented hair found on the scalp, legs, arms, and bodies of males and females.

terry (TAYR-ee)—a pile fabric in which the loops are uncut; a cotton fabric, very water absorbent; used for towels; terry cloth.

tertiary color (TUR-shee-ayr-ee KUL-ur)—intermediate color achieved by mixing a secondary color and its neighboring primary color on the color wheel in equal amounts.

tesla high-frequency current (TES-luh HY-FREE-quens-ee KUR-unt)—also known as *violet ray*; thermal or heat-producing current with a high rate of oscillation or vibration, commonly used for scalp and facial treatments.

Tesla, Nikola (TES-luh, nih-KOH-luh)—Croatian-American electrical engineer after whom the tesla high-frequency current is named.

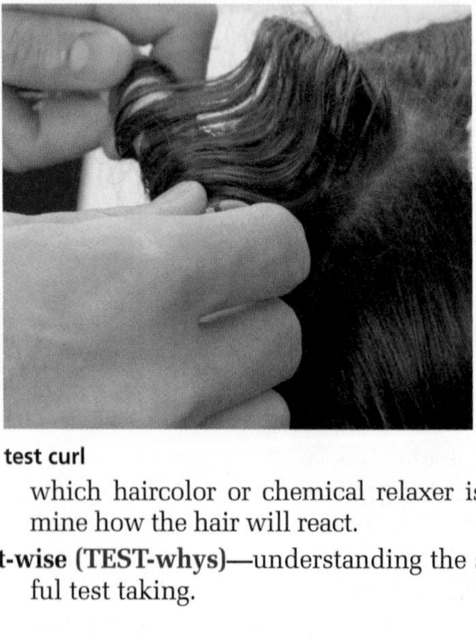
© Milady, a part of Cengage Learning. Photography by Paul Castle.
test curl

test curls (TEST KURLZ)—a method to predetermine how the client's hair will react to cold waving solution and neutralizer; process of testing the hair to determine curl for motion during the permanent wave.

test strand (TEST STRAND)—a small section of hair on which haircolor or chemical relaxer is applied to predetermine how the hair will react.

test-wise (TEST-whys)—understanding the strategies for successful test taking.

T

testes (TESS-teez)—male sexual glands that function in reproduction, as well as determining male sexual characteristics.

testosterone (TES-tos-ter-own)—the male hormone responsible for development of typical male characteristics.

tetanus (TET-un-us)—also known as *lockjaw*; an infectious disease that causes spasmodic muscle contractions of voluntary muscles.

tetter (TET-ur)—any of various vesicular skin diseases such as ringworm, eczema, and herpes.

textural combination (TEKS-chur-ul kahm-bih-NAY-shun)—a form incorporating two or more of the basic textures.

texture (TEKS-chur)—the composition or structure of a tissue or organ; the general feel or appearance of a substance.

texture, hair (TEKS-chur, HAYR)—the general quality and feel of the hair such as coarse, medium, or fine; the diameter of an individual hair strand.

texture, skin (TEKS-chur, SKIN)—the general feel and appearance of the skin such as coarse, fine, medium, thin, thick, and degree of elasticity.

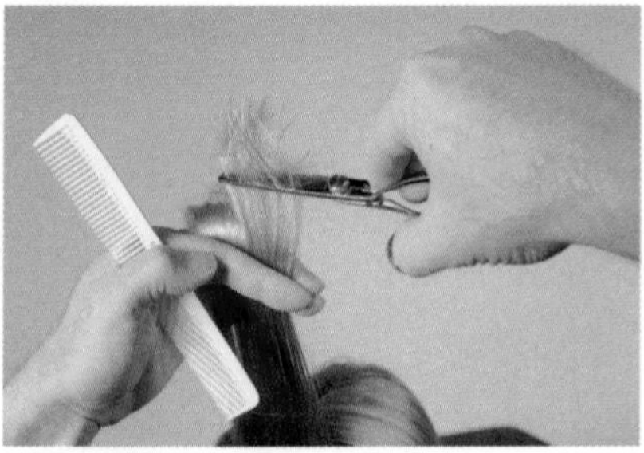

© Milady, a part of Cengage Learning. Photography by Yanik Chauvin.

texturizing

texturizing (TEKS-chur-yz-ing)—in haircutting, removing excess bulk without shortening the length; changing the appearance or behavior of the hair through specific haircutting techniques using shears, thinning shears, or a razor.

thalassemia (THAL-as-seem-ee-ah)—a condition characterized by defective hemoglobin cells, resulting in oxygen deficiency.

thalassotherapy (thai-as-oh-THAYR-uh-pee)—therapy that utilizes sea water and products from the sea.

thallium (THAL-ee-um)—a bluish-white metallic element, the salts of which have been used for epilation; thallium is highly toxic to humans.

thenar (THEE-nar)—the fleshy prominence of the palm at the base of the thumb.

theory (THEE-uh-ree)—a plan or scheme existing in the mind only; hypothesis; a reasoned and probable explanation.

therapeutic (thayr-uh-PYOOT-ik)—pertaining to the treatment of disease by remedial agents or methods.

therapeutic lamp (thayr-uh-PYOOT-ik LAMP)—an electrical apparatus producing any of the rays of the spectrum; used for skin and scalp treatments.

therapeutic treatments (thayr-uh-PYOOT-ik TREET-ments)—beneficial treatments for skin, body, or scalp.

therapeutics (thayr-uh-PYOOT-iks)—branch of medical science concerned with the treatment of disease.

therapy (THAYR-uh-pee)—the science and art of healing.

therm (THURM)—a unit of heat to which equivalents have been given; an example is a small calorie, a kilocalorie.

thermal (THUR-mul)—relating to heat.

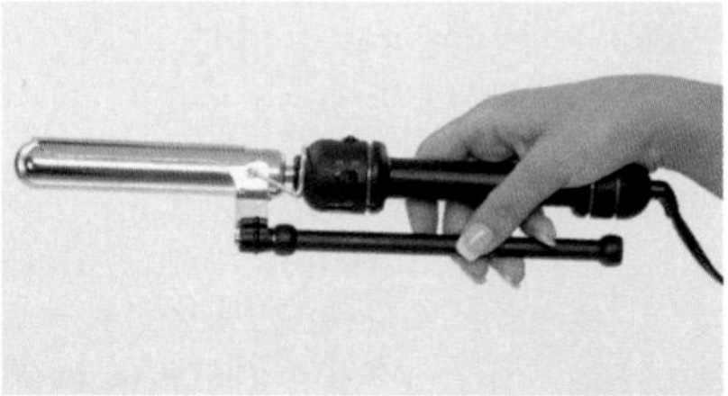

© Milady, a part of Cengage Learning. Photography by Paul Castle.

thermal iron

thermal irons (THUR-mul EYE-urnz)—implements made of quality steel that are used to curl dry hair.

thermal set (THUR-mul SET)—the technique of setting dry hair with a thermal iron or heated hair rollers.

thermal styling tools (THUR-mul STYL-ing TOOLS)—used to denote types of tools that use heat for the purpose of hairstyling.

thermal unit (THUR-mul YOO-nit)—the amount of heat required to raise the temperature of a pound of water one degree Centigrade or Fahrenheit.

thermal waving and curling (THUR-mul WAYV-ing and CURL-ing)—also known as *Marcel waving, thermal curling*; *ironing*, or *iron curling*; methods of waving and curling straight or pressed dry hair using thermal irons and special manipulative curling techniques.

thermolysis (thur-MAHL-uh-sus)—also known as *electrocoagulation*; heat effect; a high-frequency AC current that produces heat and destroys the follicle; a method of electrolysis used for permanent hair removal.

thermomassage (THUR-moh-muh-SAHZH)—massage given with the application of heat.

thermometer (thur-MAHM-ut-ur)—any device for measuring temperature.

thermostat (THUR-moh-stat)—an automatic device for regulating temperature, as in a room.

thiamine (THY-uh-min)—a water-soluble component of the vitamin B complex; primary sources are vegetables, egg yolks, organ meats, and whole grains.

thickening agent (THIK-un-ing AY-jent)—a substance that is employed to thicken watery solutions.

thinner (THIN-ur)—a product used to thin nail polish.

thinning, hair (THIN-ing, HAYR)—decreasing the thickness of the hair where it is too heavy.

thinning scissors (THIN-ing SIZ-urz)—also known as *thinning shears* or *texturizing shears*; scissors with single- or double-notched blades; used to reduce thickness or produce special texturizing effects.

thio (THY-oh)—abbreviation for ammonium thioglycolate and thioglycolic acid; used to break down cross links of the hair in chemical straightening or cold waving.

thio neutralization (THY-oh NEW-truhl-eyez-ay-shun)—a solution used to stop the action of a permanent wave solution and rebuild the hair in its new curly form.

thio relaxers (THY-oh ree-LAX-UHRS)—relaxers that use the same ammonium thioglycolate (ATG) that is used in permanent waving, but at a higher concentration and a higher pH (above 10).

thio-free waves (THY-oh FREE WAYVZ)—perms that use an ingredient other than ATG as the primary reducing agent, such as cysteamine or mercaptamine.

thioglycolic acid (thy-oh-GLY-kuh-lik AS-ud)—a colorless liquid or white crystals with a strong unpleasant odor that is used in permanent waving solutions.

third-degree burn (THURD-duh-GREE BURN)—a burn that is much deeper and more life-threatening than a second-degree burn. It may involve a deep dermal burn and may also involve burn injuries to the muscle and even the bones.

third occipital nerve (THURD ahk-SIP-ut-ul NURV)—nerve that receives stimuli from the skin of the posterior aspect of the neck and scalp.

thoracic (thuh-RAS-ik)—pertaining to the thorax.

thoracic duct (thuh-RAS-ik DUKT)—the common lymph trunk emptying into the left subclavian vein; the principle duct of the lymphatic system.

thorax (THOR-aks)—also known as *chest* or *pulmonary trunk*; consists of the sternum, ribs, and thoracic vertebrae; elastic, bony cage that serves as a protective framework for the heart, lungs, and other internal organs.

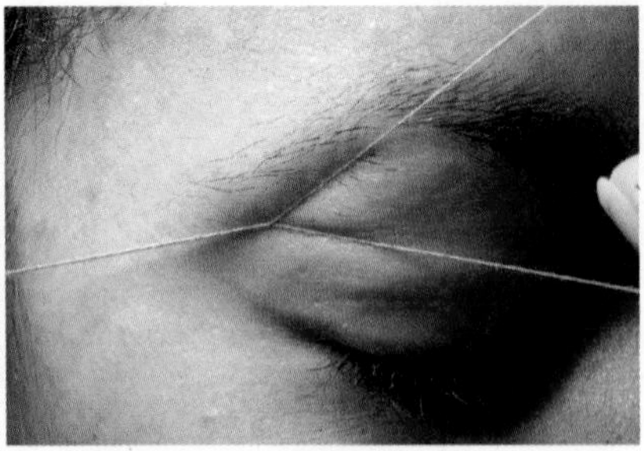
© Milady, a part of Cengage Learning. Photography by Larry Hamill.
threading

threading (THRED-ing)—also known as *banding*; method of hair removal; cotton thread is twisted and rolled along the surface of the skin, entwining hair in the thread and lifting it out of the follicle.

three-dimensional (THREE-duh-MEN-shun-ul)—having length, width, and depth.

three-dimensional shading (THREE-duh-MEN-shun-al SHAYD-ing)—a technique in which hair is bleached and toned with two shades of toner, giving a three-dimensional effect.

throat (THROHT)—the anterior aspect of the neck.

thrombocyte (THRAHM-buh-syt)—a blood platelet that aids in clotting.

thymus (THY-mus)—a ductless gland situated in lower part of the neck; the primary lymphoid organ necessary in early life for the normal development of immunologic function.

thyroid cartilage (THY-royd KART-uh-lij)—the largest cartilage of the larynx, composed of two blades that form a type of shield.

thyroid gland (THY-royd GLAND)—a large, ductless gland situated in front and on either side of the trachea; it controls how quickly the body burns energy (metabolism), makes proteins, and controls how sensitive the body should be to other hormones.

thyrotoxicosis (THY-roh-tox-eh-co-sis)—the group of clinical symptoms associated with hyperthyroidism.

T

thyroxine (thy-RAHK-seen)—a hormone secreted by the thyroid gland, the gland regulating body metabolism and weight control.

tibia (TIB-ee-ah)—also known as *shinbone*; larger of the two bones that form the leg below the knee. The tibia may be visualized as a bump on the big-toe side of the ankle.

tibial arteries (TIB-ee-ul AR-tuh-reez)—arteries that supply blood to the lower leg and foot.

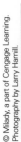

tibial nerves (TIB-ee-ul NURVZ)— a division of the sciatic nerve that passes behind the knee. It subdivides and supplies impulses to the knee, the muscles of the calf, the skin of the leg, and the sole, heel, and underside of the toes.

tibialis anterior (tib-ih-AL-is an-TEER-ih-ohr)—muscle that covers the front of the shin and bends the foot upward and inward.

ticket upgrading (TIK-it UP-grayd-ing)—also known as *upselling services*; the practice of recommending and selling additional services to your clients.

tight scalp (TYT SKALP)—a scalp that is not easily moved over the underlying structure.

tincture of benzoin (TING-chur UV BEN-zuh-wun)—a protective, antiseptic astringent used in healing skin eruptions.

tinea (TIN-ee-uh)—technical term for ringworm, a contagious condition caused by fungal infection and not a parasite; characterized by itching, scales, and, sometimes, painful lesions.

tinea barbae (TIN-ee-uh BAR-bee)—also known as *barber's itch*, a superficial fungal infection that commonly affects the skin. It is primarily limited to the bearded areas of the face and neck or around the scalp.

tinea capitis (TIN-ee-uh KAP-ih-tis)—a fungal infection of the scalp characterized by red papules, or spots, at the opening of the hair follicles.

tinea favosa (TIN-ee-uh fah-VOH-suh)—also known as *tinea favus*; fungal infection characterized by dry, sulfur-yellow, cup-like crusts on the scalp called scutula.

tinea pedis (TIN-ee-uh PED-us)—medical term for fungal infections of the feet; red, itchy rash of the skin on the bottom of the feet and/or in between the toes, usually found between the fourth and fifth toe.

tinea sycosis (TIN-ee-uh sy-KOH-sus)—ringworm of the beard.

tinea tonsurans (TIN-ee-uh TAHN-syoo-ranz)—also known as *tinea capitis*; ringworm of the scalp.

tinea unguium (TIN-ee-uh UN-gwee-um)—ringworm of the nails; a fungal disease.

tinea versicolor (TIN-ee-uh VER-suh-kul-ur)—also known as *sun spots*; a noncontagious fungal infection which is characterized by white or varicolored patches on the skin and is often found on arms and legs.

tinnitus (TIN-eye-tus)—ringing in the ears.

tint (TINT)—permanent oxidizing haircolor product having the ability to lift and deposit color in the same process; to color the hair by means of a permanent hair tint.

tint back (TINT BAK)—to return the hair to its original color.

tinting (TINT-ing)—the process of adding artificial color to hair.

tip (TIP)—also known as *chisel edge*; as in a brush, the narrow end of an object; the end of a hair, the very end of the bristles, farthest away from the handle.

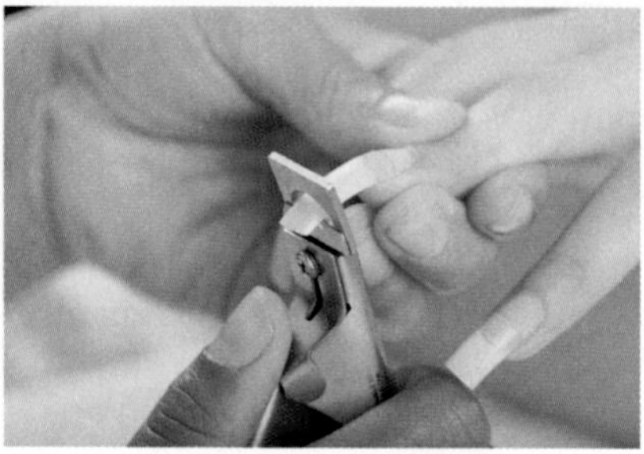

© Milady, a part of Cengage Learning. Photography by Dino Petrocelli.

tip cutter

tip cutter (TIP kut-ter)—implement similar to a nail clipper, designed especially for use on nail tips.

tipping (TIP-ing)—similar to highlighting, but the darkening or lightening is confined to small strands of hair at the front of the head; lightening the selected ends of the hair.

tissue (TISH-oo)—a collection of similar cells that perform a particular function.

tissue, connective (TISH-oo, kuh-NEK-tiv)—binding and supporting tissues.

tissue, facial (TISH-oo, FAY-shul)—soft, light absorbent papers, usually of two layers; used as a handkerchief or small towel.

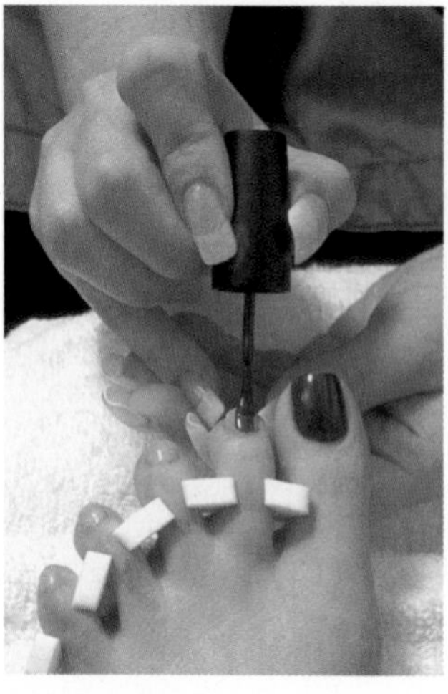

© Dusica/www.Shutterstock.com

toe separators

titanium dioxide (ty-TAYN-ee-um dy-AHK-syd)—1. inorganic physical sunscreen that reflects UV radiation; 2. key mineral ingredient with a white pigment – creates opacity and allows paste makeup to stay in place.

toe separators (TOH sep-are-ayt-ohrs)—foam rubber or cotton disposable materials used to keep toes apart while polishing the nails. A new set must be used on each client.

toenail clipper (TOH-nayl KLIP-ur)—professional implements that are larger than

T

fingernail clippers and have a curved or straight jaw, specifically designed for cutting toenails.

tocopherol (toh-KAHF-uh-rawl)—vitamin E; any of a group of four related viscous oils that constitute vitamin E; chief sources are wheat germ and cottonseed oils; used as a dietary supplement and as an antioxidant in some cosmetic preparations.

tolerance (TOL-urr-ants)—in electric nail filing, the tightness of the inside of the shank where the bit fits into the handpiece.

tone or tonality (TOHN or toh-NAL-ut-ee)—also known as *hue*; in coloring, a term used to describe the warmth or coolness of a color; in muscle tone, healthy functioning of the body or its parts.

tone on tone (TOHN awn TOHN)—a method of coloring hair in which two sections of hair are lightened and toned into two shades of the same color cast.

toner (TOHN-ur)—also known as *fresheners* or *astringents*; in haircoloring, semipermanent, demipermanent, and permanent haircolor products that are used primarily on prelightened hair to achieve pale and delicate colors; in skincare, lotions that help rebalance the pH and remove remnants of cleanser from the skin.

tonic (TAHN-ik)—also known as *toners*, *fresheners*, or *astringents*; cosmetic solution that stimulates the scalp, helps to correct a scalp condition, or is used as a grooming aid, are used after cleansing and prior to the application of a moisturizer.

tonic friction (TAHN-ik FRIK-shun)—the application of friction to the body with cold water to produce a stimulating effect.

toning (TOHN-ing)—in haircoloring, adding color to modify the end result; to tone down, to subdue a color to a softer or less emphatic shade; in muscle toning, to strengthen and/or invigorate the muscles.

tonsorial (TON-SORE-ee-ahl)—related to the cutting, clipping, or trimming of hair with shears or a razor.

tonsure (TON-shur)—a shaved patch on the head.

top coat (TAHP KOHT)—liquid, colorless nail enamel applied over polish to protect polish, prevent chipping, and impart a high gloss.

topical (TAHP-ih-kul)—pertaining to the surface; limited to a spot or part of the body.

topper (TAHP-ur)—a hairpiece, generally made on a round or oval base, and designed for use on the top of the head.

torque (TORK)—in electric filing, power of a machine or its ability to keep turning when applying pressure during filing.

touch up (TUCH UP)—also known as *retouch*; the process of coloring the new growth of tinted or lightened hair.

toupee (too-PAY)—outdated term used to describe a small hair replacement that covers the top or crown of the head.

towel blot (TOW-ul BLAHT)—the technique of gently pressing a towel over the hair to remove excess moisture or lotion.

towel dry (TOW-el DRY)—to remove excess moisture from the hair with a towel.

toxemia (tahk-SEE-mee-uh)—form of blood poisoning.

toxic (TAHK-sik)—due to, or of the nature of poison; poisonous.

toxicoderma (tahk-sih-koh-DUR-muh)—disease of the skin due to poison.

toxin (TAHK-sin)—various poisonous substance produced by some microorganisms (bacteria and viruses).

trachea (TRAY-kee-uh)—windpipe; air passage from the larynx to the bronchi and the lungs.

trachoma (truh-KOH-muh)—a contagious disease of the inner eyelids and cornea characterized by scar formation and granulation.

traction alopecia (TRAH-shun al-uh-PEE-shuh)—traumatic alopecia due to repetitive traction or twisting of hair.

transepidermal water loss (TRANS-ep-uh-der-muhl WAH-tur LOSS)—abbreviated TEWL; water loss caused by evaporation on the skin's surface.

transferable skills (TRANZ-fur-able SKILLZ)—skills mastered at other jobs that can be put to use in a new position.

transformer (tranz-FOR-mer)—a device used for increasing or decreasing the voltage of the current used; it can only be used on an alternating current.

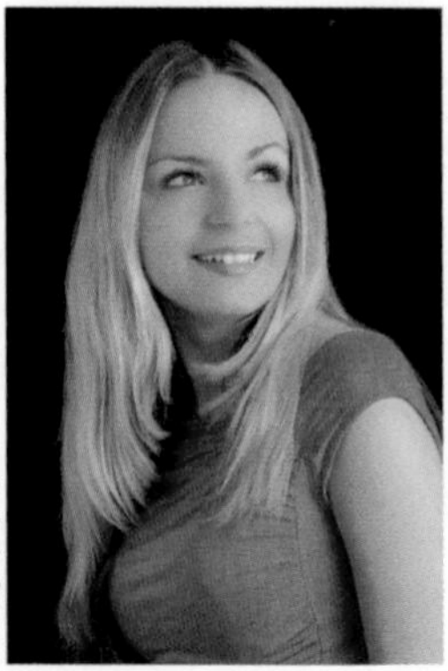
© Milady, a part of Cengage Learning. Photography by Dino Petrocelli.

transitional lines

transient erythema (TRANZ-ee-ant ah-RYTH-mee-uh)—redness that comes and goes.

transient microorganisms (TRANZ-ee-ant MY-crow-org-an-ismz)—microorganisms that travel easily on hands, clothing, or inanimate objects. They are removed through hand washing and proper cleaning and disinfection of work areas.

transitional lines (TRANS-ish-on-ahl LYNZ)—usually curved lines that are used to blend and soften horizontal or vertical lines.

T

translucent powder (tranz-LOO-sent POW-dur)—a somewhat transparent powder containing the same ingredients as other face powders but to which more titanium dioxide has been added to give the powder an opaque, colorless quality.

transplant (TRANZ-plant)—removal of hair from a part of the body or head by surgical means and affixing it to a bald area of the scalp; to transfer tissue or organ from one part of the body to another; graft.

transverse (tranz-VURS)—lying or being across; crosswise.

transverse abdominals (tranz-VURS UB-dom-in-ahlz)—the deepest of the abdominal muscles, lying under the internal obliques.

transverse facial artery (tranz-VURS FAY-shul AR-tuh-ree)—artery that supplies blood to the skin and masseter muscle.

transverse nerve (tranz-VURS NURV)—nerve that receives stimuli from the skin of the neck.

transverse plane (tranz-VURS PLAYN)—imaginary line dividing the body horizontally into upper and lower portions.

trapezius (truh-PEE-zee-us)—muscle that covers the back of the neck and upper and middle region of the back; rotates and controls swinging movements of the arm.

trapezoid (TRAP-uh-zoyd)—a small bone in the second row of the corpus.

trauma (TRAW-muh)—a wound or injury.

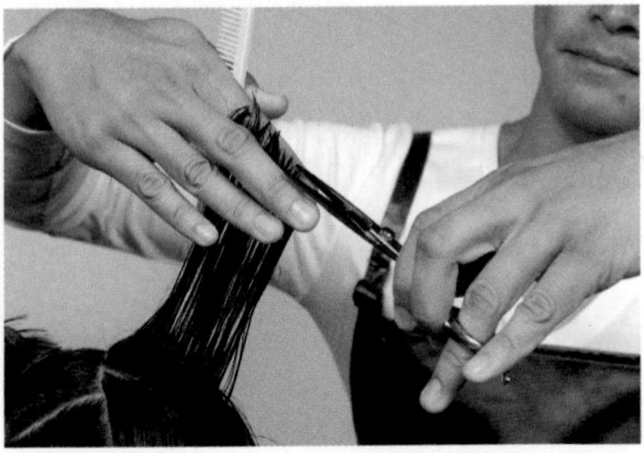

© Milady, a part of Cengage Learning. Photography by Yanik Chauvin.

traveling guide

traveling guideline (TRAV-ell-ing GUYD-line)—also known as *movable guideline*; guideline that moves as the haircutting progresses, used often when creating layers or graduation.

treatment (TREET-ment)—a substance, technique, or regimen used in therapeutic practices.

treatment cream (TREET-ment KREEM)—a specialty product designed to facilitate change in the skin's appearance.

tremor (TREM-ur)—an involuntary trembling or quivering.

treponema pallidum (trip-uh-NEE-muh PAL-ih-dum)—spirilla bacteria causing syphilis.

tress (TRES)—a lock or ringlet of hair.

tressed (TREST)—hair arranged in braids; long hair.

tretinoin (TRET-ih-no-in)—transretinoic acid; a derivative of Vitamin A used for collagen synthesis, hyperpigmentation, and for acne.

triangularis muscle (try-ang-gyuh-LAY-rus MUS-uhl)—muscle extending alongside the chin that pulls down the corner of the mouth.

triangular-shaped face (try-ANG-gyuh-lur-SHAYPT FAYS)—a face with a narrow forehead and greater width at the jawline.

triceps (TRY-seps)—large muscle that covers the entire back of the upper arm and extends the forearm.

trichiasis (trik-EYE-uh-sus)—a condition in which hairs, especially the eyelashes, turn inward, causing irritation of the eyeball.

trichloroacetic acid (TCA) peels (TRY-klor-oh-AH-seed-ick ASUD PEEL)—a strong peel used to diminish sun damage and wrinkles.

trichology (trih-KAHL-uh-jee)—scientific study of hair and its diseases and care.

trichomadesis (trik-uh-muh-DEE-sus)—abnormal hair loss.

trichonosis (trik-uh-NOH-sis)—any disease of the hair.

trichopathy (trih-KAHP-uh-thee)—pertaining to any disease of the hair.

trichophytina (trik-oh-fih-TEE-nuh)—a fungus that thrives in the hair follicles, causing tinea.

trichophyton (try-KAWF-ih-tahn)—a fungus that attacks the hair, skin, and nails, causing dermatophytosis.

trichophytosis (trih-KAWF-ih-TOH-sus)—ringworm of the skin and scalp due to invasion by fungus.

trichoptilosis (trih-kahp-tih-LOH-sus)—technical term for split ends.

trichorrhea (trik-uh-REE-uh)—a rapid loss of hair.

trichorrhexis (trik-uh-REK-sis)—brittleness of the hair.

trichorrhexis nodosa (trik-uh-REK-sis nuh-DOH-suh)—technical term for knotted hair; it is characterized by brittleness and the formation of nodular swellings along the hair shaft.

T

trichosiderin (trih-kuh-SID-ur-un)—a pigment containing iron found in human red hair.

trichosis (trih-KOH-sus)—any diseased condition of the hair.

tricuspid (try-KUS-pid)—having three points such as the right auriculoventricular valve of the heart.

tricuspid valve (try-KUS-pid VALV)—valve between the right atrium and right ventricle of the heart.

trifacial nerve (try-FAY-shul NURV)—the fifth cranial nerve; chief sensory nerve of the face; receives stimuli from the face and scalp.

trigeminal nerve (try-JEM-un-ul)—the main sensory nerve of the face; it has three major branches.: mandibular, maxillary, and ophthalmic.

triggers (TRIG-uhrs)—activities that cause flushing or flares in people with rosacea.

triglyceride (try-GLIS-ur-yd)—a fat found in adipose cells; a compound consisting of three molecules of fatty acid linked to glycerol.

trim (TRIM)—a haircut in which the hair is cut without altering the shape of the existing lines; to remove a small amount of hair from the ends.

trimmers (TRIM-uhrz)—small clippers, also known as outliners and edgers, used for detail, precision design, and fine finish work after a haircut or beard trim.

triphase (TRY-fayz)—a method of color application, first to the mid-shaft, then to ends of hair, and finally to the hair nearest the scalp.

trochlea (TRAHK-lee-uh)—a pulley-like process; a smooth articular surface of bone on which another glides.

trochlea muscularis (TRAHK-lee-uh mus-kyuh-LAYR-us)—an attachment that changes the direction of the pull of a muscle.

trochlear nerve (TRAHK-lee-ur NURV)—the fourth cranial nerve, motor nerve that controls the motion of the eye.

trophedema (troh-fuh-DEE-muh)—chronic edema of the feet or legs due to damage to nerves or blood supplying vessels in the area.

trophic (TROH-fik)—pertaining to nutrition and its processes.

trophic hormones (TROH-fik HOR-moanz)—chemicals that cause glands to make hormones.

trophology (troh-FAHL-uh-jee)—the science of nutrition.

trophopathy (troh-FAHP-uh-thee)—a disorder caused by improper or inadequate nutrition such as a vitamin or mineral deficiency.

trough (TRAWF)—the semicircular area of a wave between two ridges.

true acid waves (TROO AS-ud WAYV)—permanent wave solutions that have a pH between 4.5 and 7.0 and require heat to process; they process more slowly than alkaline waves, and do not usually produce as firm a curl as alkaline waves.

true fixative (TROO FIKS-uh-tiv)—a substance that makes something permanent; holds back evaporation of other materials.

true skin (TROO SKIN)—the corium; dermis; the underlying or inner layer of the skin.

trunk (TRUNK)—the human body exclusive of the extremities (arms, legs, neck, and head).

trumpet nail (TRUM-pet NAYL)—disorder in which the edges of the nail plate curl around to form the shape of a trumpet or sharp cone at the free edge.

tyrosinase (TAH-roz-in-ays)—the enzyme that stimulates melanocytes and thus produces melanin.

trypsin (TRIP-sun)—an enzyme found in the small intestine; trypsin changes proteins into peptones.

tryptophan (TRIP-tuh-fan)—an amino acid existing in proteins; essential in human nutrition.

tubercle (TOO-bur-kul)—an abnormal rounded, solid lump above, within, or under the skin; larger than a papule.

tuberculocidal disinfectants (tuh-bur-kyoo-LOH-syd-ahl dis-in-FEK-tant)—disinfectants that kill the bacteria that causes tuberculosis.

tuberculosis (tuh-bur-kyoo-LOH-sus)—a disease caused by bacteria that are transmitted through coughing or sneezing.

tuberculosis cutis (tuh-bur-kyoo-LOH-sis KYOO-tis)—tuberculosis of the skin.

tubular (TOOB-yuh-lur)—tube-shaped; resembling a long, hollow, cylindrical body.

tumid (TOO-mud)—swollen; enlarged; puffy.

tumor (TOO-mur)—a swelling; an abnormal cell mass resulting from excessive multiplication of cells varying in size, shape, and color.

turbinal; turbinate (TUR-buh-nul; TUR-buh-nayt)—thin layers of spongy bone on either of the outer walls of the nasal depression; turbinated body.

turbinated (TUR-buh-nayt-ud)—shaped like a top; scroll-shaped.

turgor (tur-ger)—the amount of elasticity in the skin; it can be assessed by touch.

turned hair (TURN-ed HAYR)—also known as *Remi hair*, the root end of every single strand is sewn into the base (of a wig), so that the cuticles of all hair strands move in the same direction: down.

tweezers (TWEEZ-urz)—a pair of small forceps to remove hair.

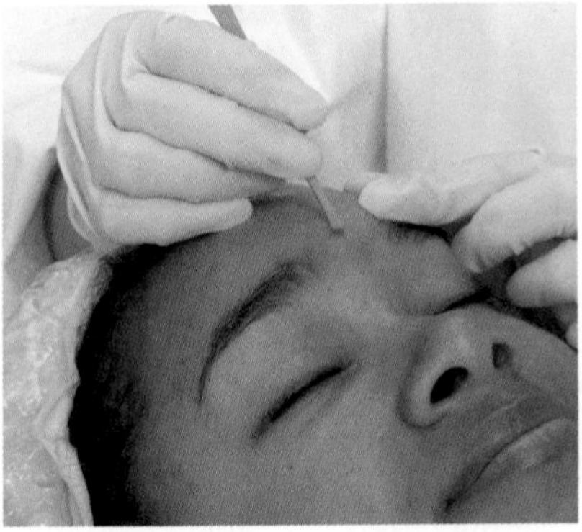

© Milady, a part of Cengage Learning. Photography by Paul Castle.

tweezing

tweezing (TWEEZ-ing)—using tweezers to remove hairs.

twine (TWYN)—to form a coil of hair; to interlace.

twist (TWIST)—also known as *French Twist*; a technique used for formal hairstyling that creates a look of conical shape.

twisting (TWIST-ing)—overlapping two strands to form a candy cane effect.

two-color method (TOO-KULUR METH-id)—in nail technology; two different colors of nail enhancement product are applied to the surface of the nail, in different places, as in a French manicure.

two-dimensional (TOO-duh-MEN-shun-ul)—having length and width.

two-dimensional shading (TOO-duh-MENshun-ul SHAYD-ing)—a haircoloring effect using two colors to add dimension or accentuate a style.

tyrosinase (TY-ruh-sin-ays)—the enzyme that reacts together with the amino acid tyrosine to form the hair's natural melanin pigment.

tyrosine (TY-ruh-seen)—an amino acid widely distributed in proteins, particularly in casein. Reacts together with the enzyme tyrosinase to form hair's natural melanin pigment.

U

ulcer (UL-sur)—open lesion on the skin or mucous membrane of the body, accompanied by pus and loss of skin depth and possibly weeping fluids or pus.

ulceroglandular (ul-sur-uh-GLAN-dyuh-lur)—pertaining to ulcers involving lymph nodes.

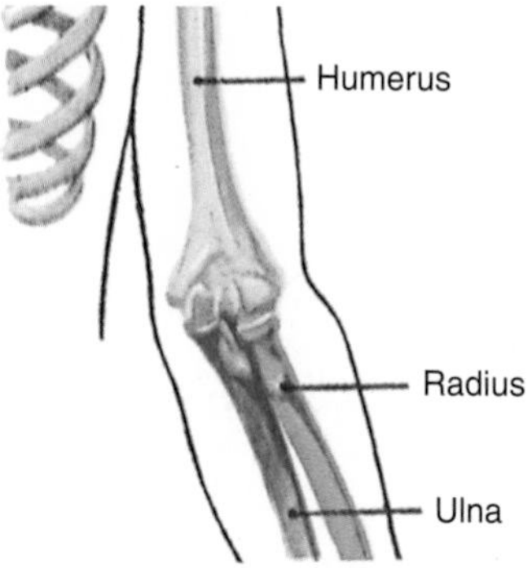

© Milady, a part of Cengage Learning
ulna

ulna (UL-nuh)—inner and larger bone in the forearm (lower arm), attached to the wrist and located on the side of the little finger.

ulnar (UL-nur)—pertaining to the ulna or to the medial aspect of the arm, as compared to the radial (lateral) aspect.

ulnar artery (UL-nur AR-tuh-ree)—along with numerous branches, this artery supplies blood to the muscle of the little-finger side of the arm and palm of the hand.

ulnar nerve (UL-nur NURV)—sensory-motor nerve that, with its branches, affects the little-finger side of the arm and palm of the hand.

ultrasonic (ULL-trah-son-ik)—frequency above the range of sound audible to the human ear; vibrations, created through a water medium, help cleanse and exfoliate the skin by removing dead skin cells; contraindications include epilepsy, pregnancy, and cancerous lesions; synonymous with ultrasound.

ultraviolet light (ul-truh-VY-uh-let LYT)—also known as *UV light, cold light,* or *actinic light*; invisible light that has a short wavelength (giving it higher energy), is less penetrating than visible light, causes chemical reactions to happen more quickly than visible light, produces less heat than visible light, and kills germs.

ultraviolet-ray sanitizer (ul-truh-VY-uh-let ray SAN-eh-tiz-uhr)—metal cabinets with ultraviolet lamps or bulbs used to store clean and disinfected tools and implements.

ultraviolet (UV) radiation (ul-truh-VY-uh-let ray-DEE-aye-shun)—invisible rays that have short wavelengths, are the least penetrating rays, produce chemical effects, and kill germs.

unadulterated (un-uh-DUL-tur-ayt-ud)—pure, unmixed.

unciform (UN-sih-form)—hook-shaped; the bone on the inner side of the second row of the carpus.

unctuous (UNG-chuh-wus)—greasy; oily.

undercutting (UN-dur-ku-ting)—cutting the hair with the head held in a forward position so that each parting is cut slightly longer than the previous parting to encourage the hair to curl under.

underdirected (un-dur-dih-REK-tud)—having less than the usual or normal amount of direction.

underelevation (un-dur-el-uh-VAY-shun)—haircutting technique in which hair is cut longer at the crown, then progressively shorter to create overlapping.

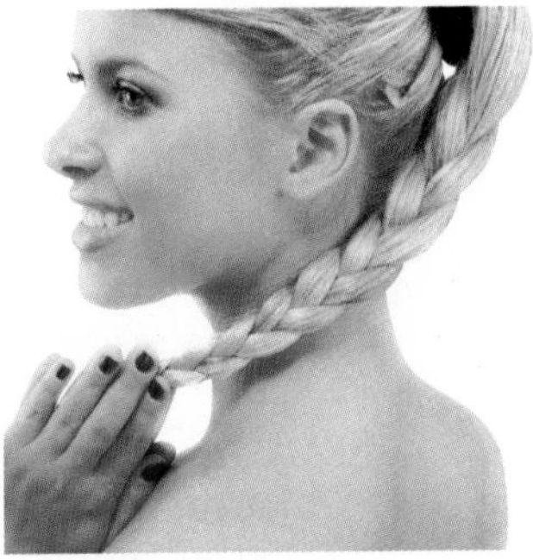

© Eduard Titov/www.Shutterstock.com

underhand technique

underhand technique (un-dur-hand TEK-neek)—also known as *plaiting*; in braiding, a technique in which the left section goes under the middle strand, then the right section goes under the middle strand.

underprocessing (un-dur-PRAH-ses-ing)—insufficient exposure of the hair to the chemical action of the waving solution or haircolor solution, resulting in little or no change in hair structure and condition, or off-toned haircolor.

undertone (UN-dur-tohn)—also known as *contributing pigment*; a subdued shade of a color; a color on which another color has been imposed and which can be seen through the other color; the underlying color that emerges during the lifting process of melanin that contributes to the end result.

undulation (un-juh-LAY-shun)—a wave-like movement or shape.

unguis (UN-gwis)—the nail of a finger or toe.

unguis incarnatus (UN-gwis in-kar-NAY-tus)—ingrown fingernails or toenails.

unguium, tinea (UN-gwee-um, TIN-ee-uh)—ringworm of the nails.

unidirectional (yoo-nih-dih-REK-shun-ul)—moving in one direction.

unidirectional current (yoo-nih-dih-REK-shun-ul KUR-rent)—also known as *direct current*; an electric current of uniform direction.

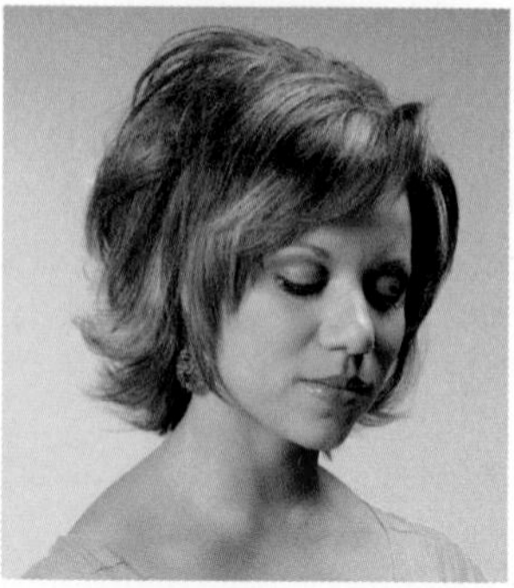

© Milady, a part of Cengage Learning. Photography by Yanik Chauvin.

uniform layers

uniform layers (YOO-nih-form LAY-urz)—haircutting technique in which hair is elevated to 90 degrees from the scalp and cut at the same length.

unipolar (yoo-nih-POH-lur)—having or acting by a single magnetic pole; the application of one electrode of a direct current to the body during a treatment.

unisex (YOO-nih-seks)—suitable for both men and women.

unit (YOO-nit)—a single thing or value.

unit wattage (YOO-nit WHAT-ahj)—the measure of how much electricity the UV lamp consumes.

United States Pharmacopeia (USP) (yoo-NYT-ud STAYTS far-muh-kuh-PEE-uh)—a scientific nonprofit organization that sets standards for the quality, purity, identity, and strength of medicines, food ingredients, and dietary supplements manufactured, distributed, and consumed worldwide.

universal precautions (YOO-nah-ver-sal PRE-caw-shuns)—a set of guidelines published by OSHA that require the employer and the employee to assume that all human blood and body fluids are infectious for bloodborne pathogens.

unpigmented hair (un-PIG-mun-ted HAYR)—hair that is lacking melanin in the cortex, primarily associated with aging and heredity.

unprofessional (un-pruh-FESH-un-ul)—in violation of ethical codes and standards of conduct of a profession.

unsaturated fatty acids (UN-sat-uhr-ated fat-tee assidz)—fatty acids that contain at least one double bond.

unstable (un-STAY-bul)—not firm; not constant; readily decomposing or changing in chemical composition or biological activity.

unwind (un-WYND)—to unwrap hair from a permanent wave or hair-setting rod.

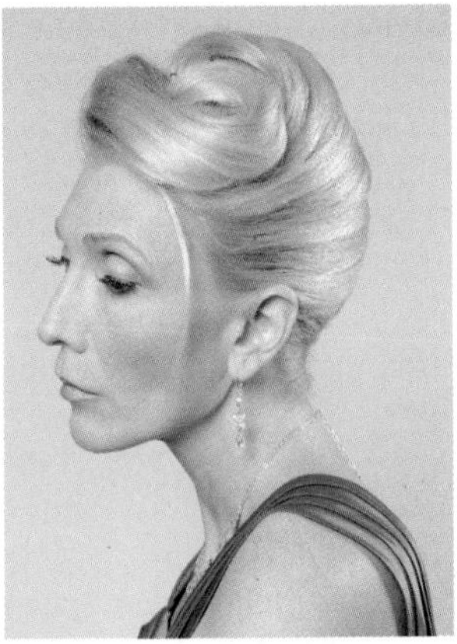
© Milady, a part of Cengage Learning. Photography by Yanik Chauvin.
updo

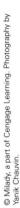

updo (UP-do)—hairstyle in which the hair is arranged up and off the shoulders.

upselling services (UP-sell-ing SER-vis-es)—also known as *upserving*; the practice of recommending or selling additional services to clients that may be performed by you or other practitioners in the salon.

upstroke (UP-strohk)—stroking upward as in shaving.

upsweep (UP-sweep)—also known as *updo*; hairstyle in which the hair is arranged up and off the shoulders.

urea (yoo-REE-uh)—a colorless crystalline compound; the chief solid component of urine and an end product of protein metabolism; properties include enhancing the penetration abilities of other substances; anti-inflammatory, antiseptic, and deodorizing action that protects the skin's surface and helps maintain healthy skin.

urethane acrylate (YUR-ah-thane AK-ri-layt)—a main ingredient used to create UV gel nail enhancements.

urethane methacrylate (YUR-ah-thane meth-AK-ri-layt)—a main ingredient used to create UV gel nail enhancements.

urethra (yoo-re-thra)—conveys urine from the bladder and carries reproductive cells and secretions out of the body.

uric acid (YOO-rik AS-ud)—a crystalline acid contained in urine; a product of protein metabolism.

uridrosis, urhidrosis (yoo-ry-DROH-sis, yur-hy-DROH-sis)—the presence of urea in the sweat in excess of normal.

urinary system (YOO-ran-aree SIS-tum)—includes the kidneys, ureters, bladder, and the urethra.

urticaria (ur-tuh-l-AYR-ee-ah)—also known as *hives*; red, raised lesions or wheals that itch severely; caused by an allergic or emotional reaction.

urticaria medicamentosa (ur-tih-l-AYR-ee-ah med-ih-kuh-ment-TOH-sah)—skin eruptions or hives due to the ingestion of a drug to which the individual is allergic.

urticaria papular (ur-tih-l-AYR-ee-ah pap-yoo-LAHR)—a hypersensitivity reaction to insect bites, manifested by crops of small papules and wheals, which may become infected because of rubbing and scratching.

uterus (YOO-ter-us)—pear-shaped, muscular organ that expands during pregnancy to accommodate the fetus.

UV bonding gels (YOO-VEE bahn-ding jelz)—gels used to increase adhesion to the natural nail plate.

UV building gels (YOO-VEE BILD-ing JELZ)—any thick-viscosity adhesive resin that is used to build an arch and curve to the fingernail.

UV gel (YOO-VEE JEL)—type of nail enhancement product that hardens when exposed to a UV light.

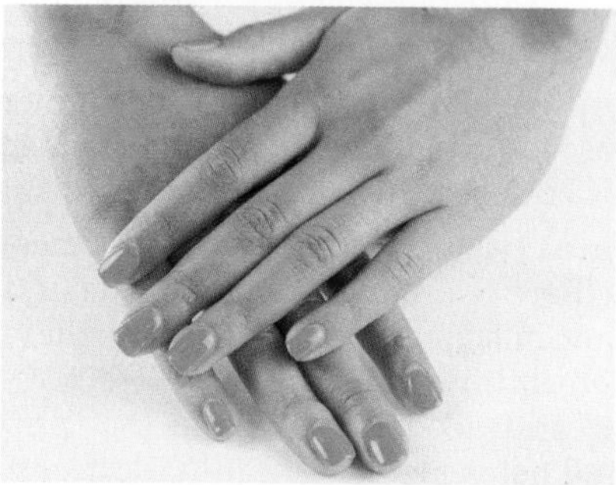

© Milady, a part of Cengage Learning. Photography by Dino Petrocelli.

UV gel nails

UV gel polish (YOO-VEE JEL POL-ish)—a very thin-viscosity UV gel that is usually pigmented and packaged in a pot or a polish bottle and used as an alternative to traditional nail lacquers.

UV gloss gel (YOO-VEE GLOS JEL)—also known as *sealing gel*, *finishing gel*, or *shine gel*; these gels are used over the finished UV gel application to create a high shine.

UV lamp (YOO-VEE LAMP)—also known as *UV light bulb*; special bulb that emits UV light to cure UV gel nail enhancements.

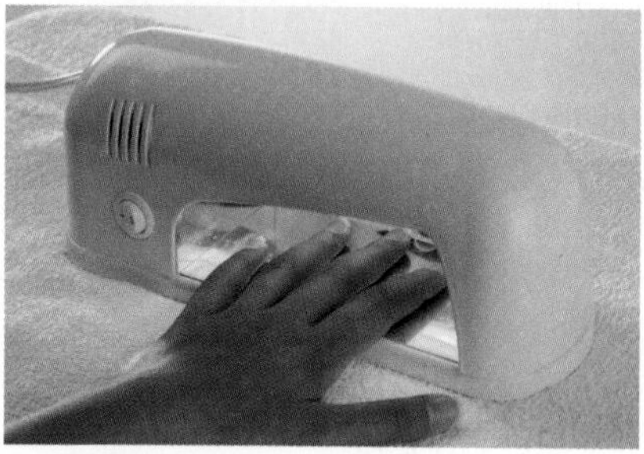

© Milady, a part of Cengage Learning. Photography by Dino Petrocelli.

UV light unit

UV light unit (YOO-VEE LYT YOO-nit)—also known as *UV light*; specialized electronic device that powers and controls UV lamps to cure UV gel nail enhancements.

UV self-leveling gels (YOO-VEE self-lev-elle-ing jel)—gels that are thinner in consistency than building gels, allowing them to settle and level during application.

UV stabilizers (YOO-VEE stay-buhl-eyes-urhs)—ingredients that control color stability and prevent sunlight from causing fading or discoloration.

U

UVA radiation (YOO-VEE-AYE ray-dih-aye-shun)—also known as *aging rays*; longer wavelengths ranging between 320 and 400 nanometers that penetrate deeper into the skin than UVB and cause genetic damage and cell death. UVA rays contribute up to 95 percent of the sun's ultraviolet radiation.

UVB radiation (YOO-VEE-BEE ray-dih-aye-shun)—also known as *burning rays*; UVB wavelengths range between 290 and 320 nanometers. UVB rays have shorter, burning wavelengths that are stronger and more damaging than UVA rays. UVB rays cause burning of the skin as well as tanning, skin aging, and cancer.

V

vaccination (vak-sih-NAY-shun)—inoculation; administration of any vaccine.

vaccine (vak-SEEN)—any preparation of microorganisms (dead, living weakened, or altered forms of a live infectious organism) that stimulates an immune response without causing illness by forming antibodies.

vacuoles (VAK-yoo-olz)—membrane-bound compartments within some eukaryotic cells that can serve a variety of secretory, excretory, and storage functions.

vacuum machine (VAK-yoom muh-sheen)—also known as *suction machine*; device that vacuums/suctions the skin to remove impurities and stimulate circulation.

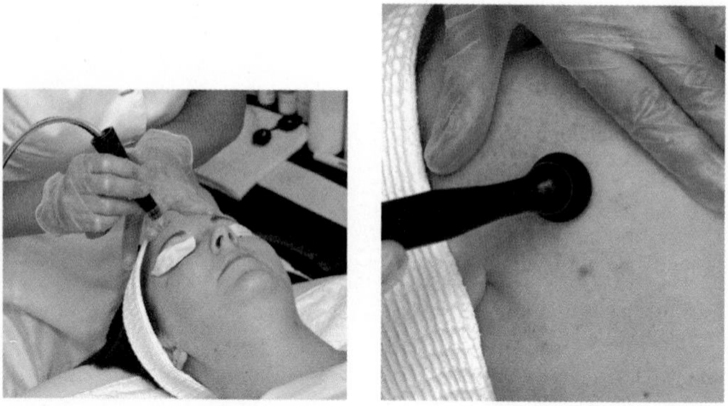

© Milady, a part of Cengage Learning. Photography by Rob Werfel.

vacuum machine

vacuum procedure (VAK-yoom proh-SEED-jur)—the use of a suction-type apparatus to cleanse the pores during a facial treatment.

vagus (VAY-gus)—pneumogastric nerve; tenth cranial nerve. Sensory-motor nerve that controls motion and sensations of the ear, pharynx, larynx, heart, lungs, and esophagus.

valine (VAL-een)—amino acid essential in human nutrition.

value (VAL-yoo)—also known as *level* or *depth* (as in hair color); fair return or equivalent in goods, services, or money for something exchanged.

values (VAL-yooz)—the deepest feelings and thoughts we have about ourselves and about life.

valve (VALV)—a structure that temporarily closes a passage or permits blood flow in only one direction.

vanishing cream (VAN-ish-ing KREEM)—a skin cream formulated to leave no oily residue on the surface of the skin.

vapor (VAY-pur)—a gas; the gaseous state of a substance that at ordinary temperature is liquid or solid.

vaporization (vay-por-ih-ZAY-shun)—act or process of converting a solid or liquid into a vapor.

vaporizer (VAY-por-eye-zur)—an apparatus designed to turn water or another substance into vapor; used in hair and skin treatments; a vaporizing machine.

variable (VAYR-ee-uh-bul)—changeable; subject to variations or changes.

variable costs (VAYR-ee-uh-bul KOSTZ)—business expenses that fluctuate, such as utilities, supplies, and advertising.

varicolored (VAYR-ee-kul-urd)—having various or several colors.

varicophlebitis (vayr-ih-koh-fluh-BY-tis)—inflammation of a varicose vein or veins.

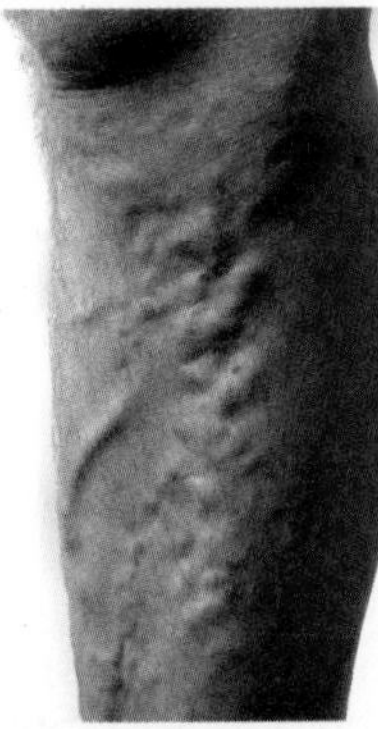

© Audie/www.Shutterstock.com

varicose veins

varicose veins (VAYR-ih-kohs VAYNZ)—vascular lesions; dilated and twisted veins, most commonly in the legs.

varnish (VAR-nish)—also known as *nail lacquer* or *nail polish*; a product used to give nails a smooth, glossy appearance.

vasa lymphatica profunda (VAY-suh lim-FAT-ih-kuh proh-FUN-duh)—the deep lymphatic vessels.

vasa lymphatica superficialia (VAY-suh lim-FAT-ih-kuh soo-pur-FISH-ee-AY-lee-uh)—the superficial lymphatic vessels.

vascular (VAS-kyoo-lur)—supplied with small blood vessels; pertaining to a vessel for the conveyance of a fluid such as blood or lymph.

vascular system (VAS-kyoo-lar SIS-tum)—body system consisting of the heart, arteries, veins, and capillaries for the distribution of blood throughout the body.

vascularization (vas-kyuh-lar-ih-ZAY-shun)—the formation of capillaries; the process of becoming vascular.

vasoconstrictor (vay-zoh-kun-STRIK-tur)—a nerve or agent that causes narrowing of blood vessels.

vasodilator (vas-oh-dih-LAY-tur)—a nerve or agent that induces expansion of the blood vessels.

vegetable dye (VEJ-tuh-bul DYE)—also known as *vegetable tints*; color; a natural organic coloring obtained from the leaves or bark of plants; examples are henna and chamomile which are used to tint hair.

vegetable facial mask (VEJ-tuh-bul FAY-shul MASK)—a mask made of fresh vegetables such as cucumber or avocado; used on the face for their beneficial enzyme action.

vegetable peel (VEJ-tuh-bul PEEL)—a mild skin peeling process using creams or lotions containing vegetable enzymes.

vegetable tints (VEJ-tuh-bul TINTS)—also known as *vegetable dye*; haircoloring products made from various plants such as Egyptian henna, indigo, or chamomile; used as hair tints or hair rinses.

vehicles (VEE-hik-uhls)—spreading agents and ingredients that carry or deliver other ingredients into the skin and make them more effective.

veins; vena (VAYNS; VEE-nuh)—thin-walled blood vessels that are less elastic than arteries; they contain cuplike valves to prevent backflow and carry impure blood from the various capillaries back to the heart and lungs.

vellus hair (VEL-us HAYR)—also known as *lanugo hair*; short, fine, unpigmented downy hair that appears on the body, with the exception of the palms of the hands and the soles of the feet.

vena cava (VEE-nuh KAY-vuh)—one of the two large veins that carry the blood to the right auricle of the heart.

vena cutanea (VEE-nuh kyoo-TAY-nee-uh)—a cutaneous vein.

venenata, dermatitis (VEN-uh-nah-tuh dur-muh-TY-tus)—inflammation produced by local action of irritating substances.

ventilate (VEN-tuh-layt)—to renew the air in a place; to oxygenate the blood in the capillaries of the lungs.

ventricle (VEN-truh-kuhl)—a thick-walled, lower chamber of the heart that receives blood pumped from the atrium. There is a right ventricle and a left ventricle.

venture capitalist(s) (VEN-shure CAP-eh-tal-ist)—a private individual (or group of individuals) who invest in businesses with the goal of gaining a return on their investment or profit.

venule (VEEN-yool)—small vessels that connect the capillaries to the veins. They collect blood from the capillaries and drain it into veins.

vermin (VUR-min)—parasitic insects such as lice and bed bugs.

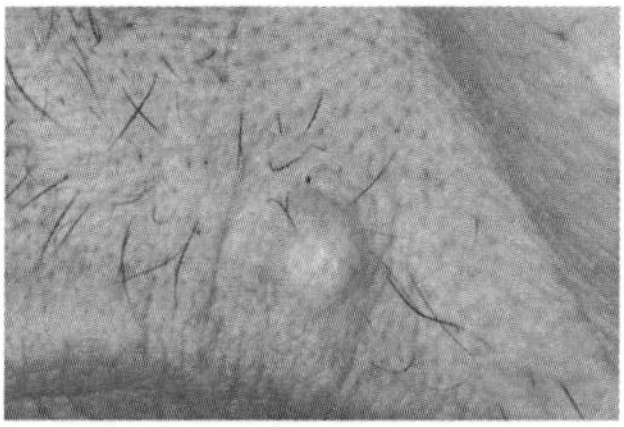

© Henrik Larsson/www.Shutterstock.com

verruca

verruca (vuh-ROO-kuh)—also known as *wart*; hypertrophy of the papillae and epidermis.

verrucose; verrucous (VUR-oo-kohs, vur-OO-kohs—warty; presenting wart-like elevations.

versican sulfate (VER-sih-can SUL-fayt)—a proteoglycan found in the dermis; it provides turgor and tautness to the skin by interacting with elastin and hyaluronic acid.

vertebra (VUR-tuh-brah); pl., vertebrae (VUR-tuh-bray)—the bony segment of the spinal column.

vertebral artery (VUR-tuh-bruhl AR-tuh-ree)—artery that supplies blood to the muscles of the neck.

vertical base (VUR-tih-kuhl BAYS)—a vertical section of a hair form used in practical exercises.

vertical lines (VUR-tih-kuhl LYNZ)—lines that are straight up and down; create length and height in hair design.

vesicant (VES-ih-kent)—an agent that produces blisters on the skin.

vesicular (vuh-SIK-yuh-lur)—relating to or containing vesicles.

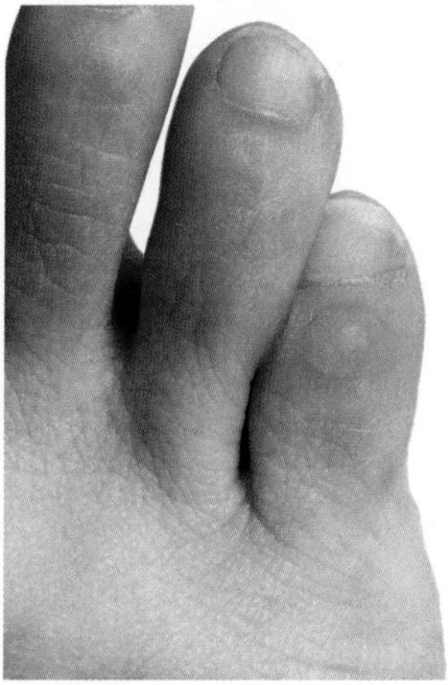

© Susan Montgomery/www.Shutterstock.com

vesicle

vesicle (VES-ih-kuhl)—small blister or sac containing clear fluid, lying within or just beneath the epidermis.

vesicle bulla (VES-ih-kuhl BOOL-ah)—a large blister.

vesiculopapular (veh-sik-yuh-loh-PAP-yuh-lur)—consisting of both vesicles and papules.

vesiculopustular (vuh-sik-yuh-loh-PUS-tyoo-lur)—consisting of both vesicles and pustules.

vessel (VES-uhl)—tube or canal in which blood, lymph, or other fluid is contained, conveyed, or circulated.

vibrate (VY-brayt)—to swing; to mark or to measure by oscillation.

vibration (vy-BRAY-shun)—in massage, the rapid shaking of the body part while the balls of the fingertips are pressed firmly on the point of application.

vibration treatment (vy-BRAY-shun TREET-ment)—massage by rapid shaking of the body part while the balls of the fingertips are pressed firmly on the point of application; given by hand, machine, or oscillator.

V

vibrator (VY-bray-tur)—an electrically driven apparatus used in some massage procedures producing stimulating impulses.

vibrator scalp treatment (VY-bray-tur SKALP TREET-ment)—massage for the scalp given with the aid of a hand vibrator.

vibratory (VY-bruh-toh-ree)—vibrations of light, rapid percussion.

vibrissa (vy-BRIS-uh); pl., vibrissae (vy-BRIS-eye)—stiff hairs in the nostrils.

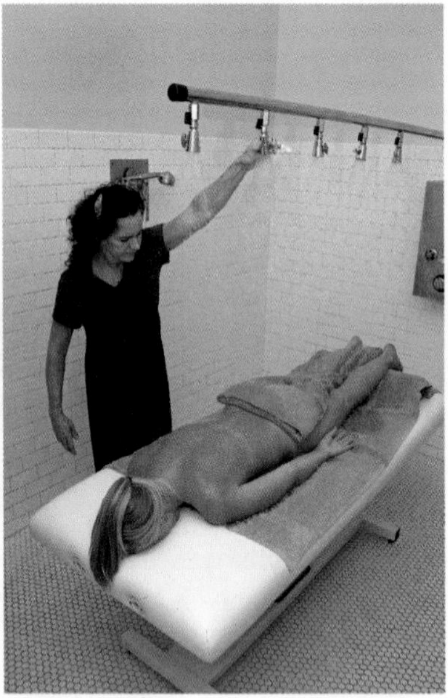

© Milady, a part of Cengage Learning. Photography by Rob Werfel.

Vichy shower

Vichy shower (VISHEE show-uhr)—an overhead shower with adjustable water pressure used in body treatments.

violet ray (VY-uh-let RAY)—also known as *high frequency*; an electric current of medium voltage and medium amperage; also called *tesla current*.

virgin application (VUR-jin APP-lih-kay-shun)—also known as *virgin tint*; first time the hair is colored.

virgin bleaching (VUR-jin BLEECH-ing)—first bleaching (lightening) of the hair.

virgin hair (VUR-jin HAYR)—natural hair that has had no previous bleaching or tinting treatments, chemicals, or physical abuse.

virgin tint (VUR-jin TINT)—also known as *virgin application*; first time the hair has been tinted.

virucidal (VI-ra-syd-uhl)—capable of destroying viruses.

virulent (VEER-yuh-lent)—extremely poisonous; marked by a rapid, severe course such as an infection; able to overcome bodily defense mechanisms.

virus (VY-rus)—a parasitic submicroscopic particle that infects and resides in cells of biological organisms. A virus is capable of replication only through taking over the host cell's reproductive function.

viscera (VIS-uh-rah)—the organs of the cranium, thorax, abdomen, or pelvis, especially the organs within the abdominal cavity.

visceral cranium (VIS-ur-ul KRAY-nee-um)—the part of the skull that forms the face and jaws.

viscosity (vis-KAHS-ut-ee)—the degree of density, thickness, stickiness, and adhesiveness of a substance that affects how the fluid flows; resistance to change of form; the resistance to flow that a liquid exhibits.

viscus (VIS-kus)—an internal organ located in the cavity of the trunk or in the thorax, cranium, or pelvis.

visible braid (VIZ-uh-buhl BRAYD)—three-strand braid that is created using an underhand technique.

visible light (VIZ-uh-buhl LYT)—the primary source of light used in facial and scalp treatments.

visible rays (VIZ-uh-buhl RAYZ)—light rays that can be seen.

visible spectrum of light (VIZ-uh-buhl SPEK-trum UV LYT)—the part of the electromagnetic spectrum that can be seen. Visible light makes up only 35 percent of natural sunlight.

vision statement (VIZ-uhn state-ment)—a long-term picture of what the business is to become and what it will look like when it gets there.

vitality (vy-TAL-ut-ee)—vigor; to grow, develop, and perform the functions of a living being.

vitamin (VY-tuh-min)—one of a group of organic substances found in minute quantities in natural food stuffs, essential to normal metabolism and the lack of which causes deficiency diseases.

vitamin A (VY-tuh-min AYE)—also known as *retinol*; an antioxidant that aids in the functioning and repair of skin cells.

vitamin C (VY-tuh-min SEE)—also known as *ascorbic acid*; an antioxidant vitamin needed for proper repair of the skin and tissues; promotes the production of collagen in the skin's dermal tissues; aids in and promotes the skin's healing process.

V

vitamin D (VY-tuh-min DEE)—fat-soluble vitamin sometimes called the *sunshine vitamin* because the skin synthesizes vitamin D from cholesterol when exposed to sunlight; essential for growth and development.

vitamin E (VY-tuh-min EE)—also known as *tocopherol*; primarily an antioxidant; helps protect the skin from the harmful effects of the sun's rays.

vitamin K (VY-tuh-min KAY)—vitamin responsible for the synthesis of factors necessary for blood coagulation.

vitiligo (vih-til-EYE-goh); pl., vitiligines (vit-ih-LIH-jih-neez)—hereditary condition that causes hypopigmented spots and splotches on the skin; may be related to thyroid conditions.

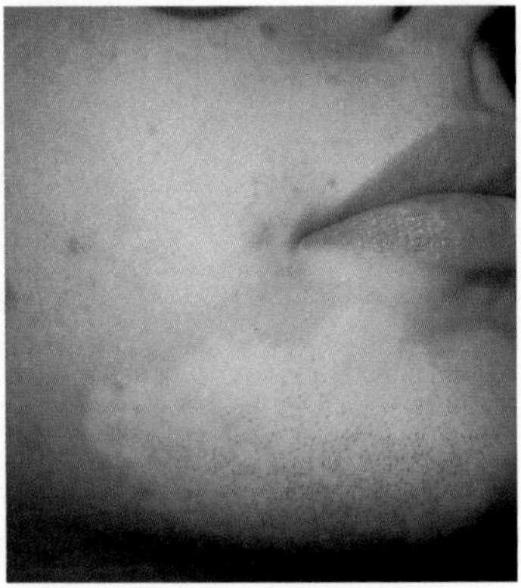

Courtesy of www.dermnet.com

vitiligo

volatile (VAHL-uh-tuhl)—easily evaporating; diffusing freely; explosive.

volatile alcohols (VAHL-uh-tuhl AL-cah-hallz)—alcohols that evaporate easily.

volatile organic compounds (VOCs) (VAHL-uh-tu ORR-gan-ik kom-poundz)—compounds that contain carbon (organic) and evaporate very easily (volatile).

volt (V) (VOLT)—also known as *voltage*; unit that measures the pressure or force that pushes electric current forward through a conductor.

voltage drop (VOL-tij DRAHP)—the decrease in the potential energy in an electric circuit due to the resistance of the conductor.

voltaic cell (vohl-TAY-ik SEL)—a receptacle for producing direct electric current by chemical action.

voltmeter (VOHLT-mee-tur)—an instrument used for measuring (in volts) the differences of potential between different points of an electrical circuit.

volume (VAHL-yoom)—amount; bulk or mass; quantity; space occupied as that which is measured in cubic units; in haircutting, the lift, elevation, and height created by the formation of curls or waves in the hair; in haircoloring, the measure of potential oxidation of varying strengths of hydrogen peroxide expressed as volumes of oxygen liberated per volume of solution.

volume-base curls (VAHL-yoom BAYS KURLZ)—a pin curl, roller placement or thermal curl placed very high on its base, providing maximum lift or volume.

volumizer (VAHL-yoo-miz-uhr)—styling product that adds volume, especially at the base, when wet hair is blown dry.

voluntary muscle (VAHL-un-tayr-ee MUS-uhl)—striated muscle under the control of the will.

vomer bone (VOH-mur BOHN)—flat, thin bone that forms part of the nasal septum.

vortices pilorum (VORT-uh-seez py-LOH-rum)—also known as *cowlick*; hair whorls.

vulgaris, acne (vul-GAYR-is AK-nee)—common pimple condition.

W

wall plate (WAWL PLAYT)—also known as *facial stimulator*; instrument that plugs into an ordinary wall outlet and produces various types of electric currents that are used for facial and scalp treatments.

wall socket (WAWL SAHK-ut)—a wall receptacle into which the plug of an electrical appliance is fitted.

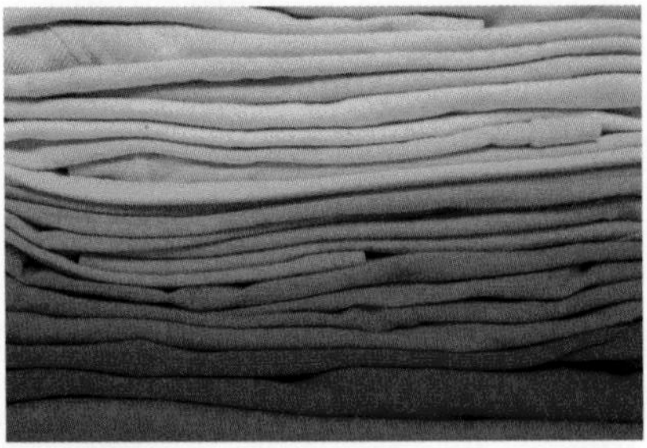

© GoodMood Photo/www.Shutterstock.com

warm colors

warm colors (WORM KUL-UHRS)—range of colors from yellow and gold through oranges, red-oranges, most reds, and even some yellow-greens.

water (WAW-tur)—most abundant of all substances, comprising about 75 percent of the Earth's surface and about 65 percent of the human body.

water-based makeup (WAW-tur BAYST MAYK-up)—a liquid makeup comprised of primary ingredients such as water, humectants, vitamins, oil absorbers, and color pigments.

water blister (WAW-tur BLIS-tur)—a blister with watery contents.

water, hard (WAW-tur, HARD)—water containing certain minerals; does not lather well with soap.

water-in-oil (W/O) (WAW-tur in oyl)—emulsions formed with drops of water that are suspended in an oil base.

water-in-oil emulsion (WAW-tur-IN-OYL EE-mull-shun)—water droplets dispersed in oil.

water, soft (WAW-tur, SAWFT)—water that lathers easily with soap and is relatively free of minerals.

water softener (WAW-tur SAWF-un-ur)—certain chemicals, such as the carbonate or phosphate of sodium that are used to soften hard water to permit the lathering of soap.

water soluble (WAW-tur SAHL-yoo-buhl)—able to dissolve or mix in water.

water vapor (WAW-tur VAY-pur)—water diffused in a vaporous form; used in some facial treatments.

watt (WAHT)—abbreviated as W; unit that measures how much electric energy is being used in one second.

wattage (WAHT-ij)—amount of electric power expressed in watts.

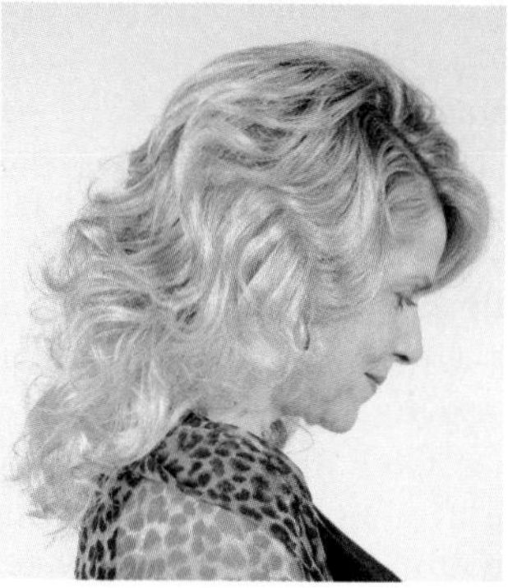

© Milady, a part of Cengage Learning. Photography by Yanik Chauvin.

wave

wave (WAYV)—two connecting C shapings placed in alternating directions.

wave clip (WAYV KLIP)—a clamp-like device with rows of small teeth used to hold a wave in place while the hair dries.

wave, cold (WAYV, KOHLD)—a method of permanent waving using chemicals instead of heat.

wave, croquignole (WAYV, KROH-ken-yohl-mar-SEL)—a wave produced with the Marcel iron using the croquignole winding.

wave, Marcel (WAYV, mar-SEL)—a wave that resembles a perfect natural wave; produced by means of heated irons.

wave pattern (WAYV PAT-URN)—the shape of the hair strands; described as straight, wavy, curly, and extremely curly.

wave, shadow (WAYV SHAD-oh)—a wave with low ridges and shallow waves.

waveform (WAYV FORM)—measurement of the distance between two wavelengths.

wavelength (WAYV-length)—distance between successive peaks of electromagnetic waves.

waves (WAYVZ)—hair formation resulting in a side-by-side series of S-like movements or half-circles going in opposite directions.

waving lotion (WAYV-ing LOW-shun)—type of hair gel that makes the hair pliable enough to keep it in place during the finger-waving procedure.

wax (WAKS)—any of numerous substances of plant or animal origin that differ from fats in being less greasy, harder, and more brittle and in containing principally compounds of high molecular weight (as fatty acids, alcohols, and saturated hydrocarbons); in cosmetology, waxes are used for facial masks and as an aid to removing superfluous hair.

wax, depilatory (WAKS, dih-PIL-uh-tor-ee)—a soft wax applied to remove superfluous hair.

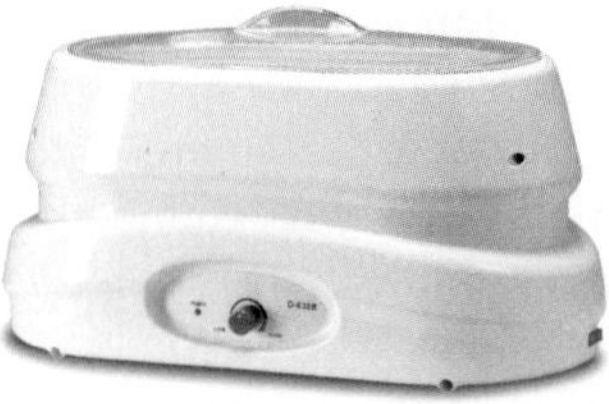
Courtesy of European Touch
wax heater

wax heater (WAKS HEET-ur)—also known as *bath*; a thermostatically controlled heating pot used to warm wax for a facial or depilatory treatment.

wax mask (WAKS MASK)—a special mixture of oils and waxes used to form a facial mask for facial treatments; these waxes may be combinations of beeswax, mineral oil, and similar oils and waxes.

W

weave technique (WEEV tek-neek)—wrapping technique that uses zigzag partings to divide base areas.

weaving (WEEV-ing)—interweaving a weft or faux hair with natural hair; coloring technique in which selected strands are picked up from a narrow section of hair with a zigzag motion of the comb, and lightener or color is applied only to these strands.

wedged parting (WEJD PART-ing)—also known as *pie-shaped parting*; a triangular sectioning pattern used as a base for a standup curl.

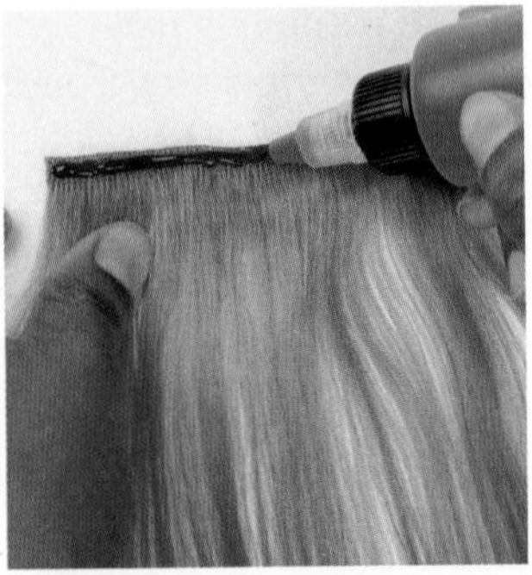
© Milady, a part of Cengage Learning. Photography by Paul Castle.
weft

weft (WEFT)—long strips of human or artificial hair with a threaded edge.

weight (WAYT)—mass in form and space; the length concentration in a hair design.

weight line (WAYT LYN)—level at which a blunt curl falls; where the ends of the hair hang together; the line of maximum length within the weight area; the heaviest perimeter area of a 0-degree or 45-degree cut.

welt (WELT)—a ridge or lump usually on the scalp.

wen (WEN)—an abnormal growth or a cyst protruding from a surface especially of the skin.

wet room (WET ROOM)—a room lined with tile or other water-impervious material and drains to service water treatments such as a Vichy shower.

wet pack **(WET PAK)**—packing the body or a part in towels that have been saturated in water or other fluids for therapeutic purposes.

wet shaping **(WET SHAY-ping)**—styling or molding the hair immediately after shampooing.

wetting agent **(WET-ing AY-jent)**—a substance that causes a liquid to spread more readily on a solid surface, chiefly through a reduction of surface tension.

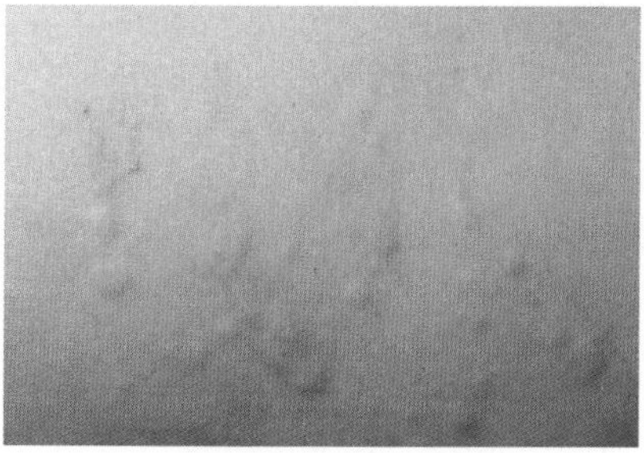

Rob Byron/www.Shutterstock.com

wheal

wheal **(WHEEL)**—itchy, swollen lesion that lasts only a few hours; caused by a blow or scratch, the bite of an insect, urticaria (skin allergy), or the sting of a nettle. Examples include hives and mosquito bites.

whirlpool **(WHURL-pool)**—a tub equipped with jets or agitators that cause the water to flow in different directions.

white blood cells **(WHYT BLUD sellz)**—also known as *white corpuscles* or *leukocytes*; blood cells that perform the function of destroying disease-causing bacteria.

white corpuscle **(WHYT KOR-pus-ul)**—also known as *white blood cell* or *leukocyte*; cell in the blood whose function is to destroy disease pathogens.

white light **(WHYT LIYT)**—referred to as *combination light* because it is a combination of all the visible rays of the spectrum.

white UV gels **(WHYT YOO-VEE JELZ)**—also known as *pigmented gels*; building gels, used early in the service, or self-leveling gels, used near the final contouring procedure.

whitehead **(WHYT-hed)**—also known as *milium* or *closed comedone*; common skin disorder caused by the formation of sebaceous matter within or under the skin.

whorl **(WHORL)**—hair that forms in a circular pattern on the crown of the head.

widow's peak **(WIH-dohz PEEK)**—a V-shaped growth of hair at the center of the forehead.

wig **(WIG)**—artificial covering for the head consisting of a network of interwoven hair.

wig block (WIG BLAHK)—a head-shaped block that may be constructed of wood, cork-filled cloth, plastic, or other materials on which hairpieces and wigs are formed or dressed.

wig cleaner (WIG KLEEN-ur)—any type of dry-cleaning fluid used to clean wigs and hairpieces.

wig conditioner (WIG kuh-DIH-shun-ur)—a product, in cream, lotion, or spray form, used to restore life and add luster to wigs or hairpieces.

wig stand (WIG STAND)—a head-shaped stand designed for keeping wigs in the proper shape when not being worn.

wiglet (WIG-lut)—a hairpiece with a flat base used on special areas of the head.

W

winding, croquignole (WYND-ing, KROH-ken-yohl)—winding the hair from the hair ends toward the scalp.

windpipe (WIND-pyp)—the trachea.

wiry hair (WYR-ee HAYR)—a hair fiber that is strong and resilient, difficult to form into a curl, and which has a smooth, hard, glossy surface.

wisp (WISP)—a small, lightweight, thin strand of hair; light, fluffy curls.

witch hazel (WICH HAY-zul)—an extract of alcohol and water from the bark of the Hamamelis shrub; soothing and mildly astringent; used as an anesthetic and skin freshener.

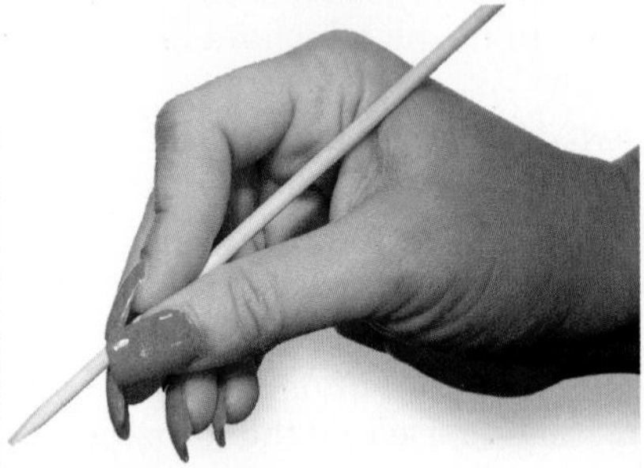

© Milady, a part of Cengage Learning. Photography by Dino Petrocelli.

wooden pusher

wooden pusher (WOHD-en PUSH-uhr)—a wooden stick used to remove cuticle tissue from the nail plate (by gently pushing), to clean under the free edge of the nail, or to apply products.

Wood's lamp (WOODZ LAMP)—filtered black light that is used to illuminate skin disorders, fungi, bacterial disorders, and pigmentation.

work ethic (WOHRK ETH-IK)—taking pride in your work and committing yourself to consistently doing a good job for your clients, employer, and salon or spa team.

work practice controls (WOHRK prak-tis con-trollz)—techniques, methods, and practices to minimize the risk of exposure to bloodborne pathogens or other potentially infectious material.

wrap (RAP)—to wind the hair on permanent wave rods.

wrap resin accelerator (RAP REZ-in AK-sell-er-aye-tor)—also known as *activator*; acts as the dryer that speeds up the hardening process of the wrap resin or adhesive overlay.

wrapping (RAP-ing)—winding hair on rollers or rods in order to form curls.

wringing (RING-ING)—vigorous movement in which the hands, placed a little distance apart on both sides of the client's arm or leg, working downward apply a twisting motion against the bones in the opposite direction.

wrinkle (RINK-ul)—a small ridge or furrow on the skin usually caused by the loss of elasticity in the tissue.

wrist (RIST)—also known as *carpus*; flexible joint composed of eight small, irregular bones held together by ligaments; the joint between the hand and arm.

written exam (RITT-en EX-am)—paper-and-pencil or computer-based testing covering theoretical concepts related to licensure area according to the laws specific to the state.

written agreements (RIT-en UH-gree-mentz)—documents that govern the opening of a salon or spa, including leases, vendor contracts, employee contracts, and more; all of which detail, usually for legal purposes, who does what and what is given in return.

X

xanthochromia (zan-thoh-KROH-mee-uh)—a yellowish discoloration of the skin.

xanthoma (zan-THOH-muh)—a yellowish-orange, lipid-filled nodule or papule in the skin, often on an eyelid or over a joint.

xanthomelanous (zan-tho-mel-A-nus)—those races having an olive or yellow complexion and black hair.

xanthosis (zan-THOH-sis)—a type of skin-related disease where one has an abnormal yellow discoloration of the skin, resulting from the accumulation of cholesterol within the skin cells.

X

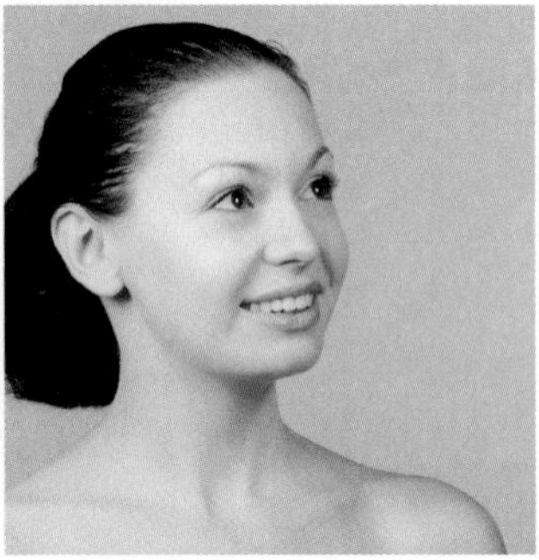

© Galushko Sergey/www.Shutterstock.com

xanthous

xanthous (ZAN-thus)—having yellowish skin tone.

xerasia (zuh-RAY-zee-uh; zuh-RAH-zhuh)—a disease of the hair marked by cessation of growth, dryness, brittleness and general lifeless appearance.

xeroderma (zee-roh-DUR-muh)—a disease in which the skin becomes dry, hard, and scaly.

xerosis cutis (zee-ROH-sis CUE-tiz)—the medical term for dry skin.

xyrospasm (ZY-roh-spaz-um)—also known as *shaving cramp*; a spasm of the wrist and forearm muscles; an occupational condition that may affect cosmetologists, estheticians, and barbers.

yak hair (YAK HAYR)—hair from the yak (a long-haired ox); this long, coarse, curly hair is used in the manufacture of inexpensive wigs, hairpieces, and hair extensions; it is often mixed with the soft hair from the angora sheep to add body and strength to angora hair.

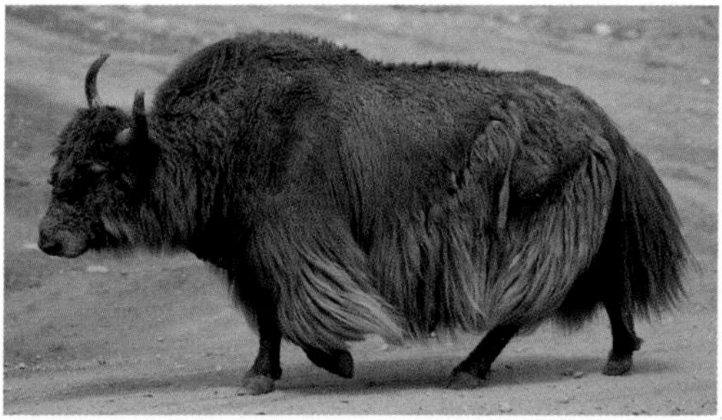

© Tan, Kim Pin/www.Shutterstock.com

yak hair

yard (YARD)—a standard English-American measure of length equal to 3 feet or 36 inches or 0.9144 meters.

yeast (YEEST)—a substance consisting of minute cells of fungi; used to promote fermentation; a high source of vitamin B.

yellow light (YEL-oh LYT)—a light-emitting diode that aids in reducing inflammation and swelling.

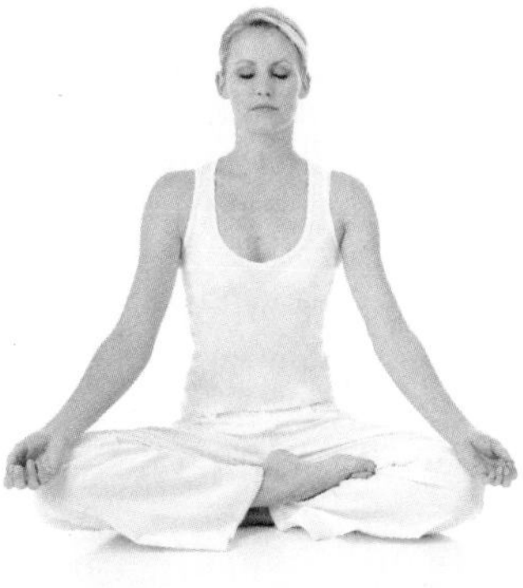

© VaclavHroch/www.Shutterstock.com

yoga

yin and yang (YIN AND YANG)—a Chinese philosophy often applied to personality theories; yin is the passive, negative, feminine force and source of heat and light; yang is the active, positive, masculine force and a source of heat and light.

yoga (YOH-guh)—a form of exercise that combines mental concentration, muscular control, breathing, and relaxation.

Zeis glands (ZYS-uz GLANDZ)—the sebaceous glands opening into the follicles of the eyelashes.

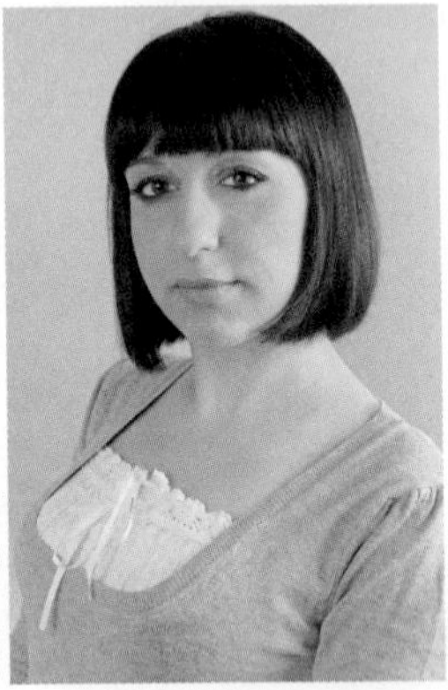

©Malivan_Iuliia/www.Shutterstock.com

zero-degree elevation

zero degree (ZEE-roh de-GREE)—also known as *zero elevation*; in haircutting, low elevation; hair is cut as it lays against the skin.

zigzag (ZIG-zag)—pertaining to short, sharp, angled partings used in haircutting, haircoloring, and roller setting.

zinc (ZINGK)—a white crystalline metallic element; used in some cosmetics such as powders and ointments; salts of zinc are used in some antiseptics and astringents.

zinc ointment (ZINGK OYNT-ment)—a medicated ointment containing zinc oxide and petrolatum; used for skin disorders.

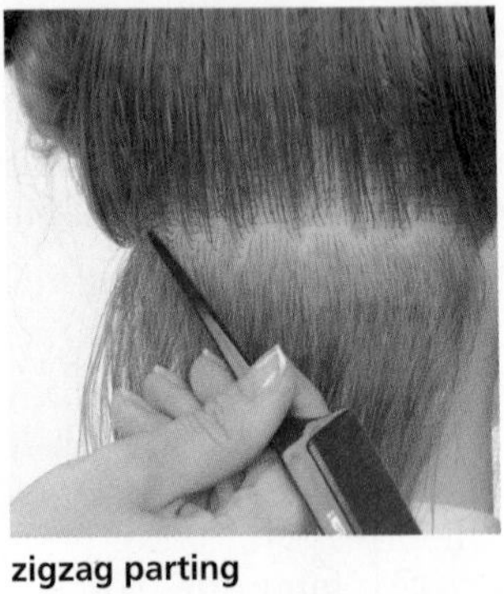

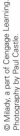

© Milady, a part of Cengage Learning. Photography by Paul Castle.

zigzag parting

zinc oxide (ZINGK AHK-syd)—a topical astringent and protectant; also a sunscreen.

zinc sulfate (ZINGK SUL-fayt)—a salt often employed as an astringent, both in lotions and in creams.

zinc sulphocarbonate (ZINGK sul-fuh-KAR-bun-ayt)—a fine, white powder; used as an antiseptic and astringent in deodorant preparations.

zoster, herpes (ZAHS-tur, HUR-peez)—an acute viral infectious disease affecting the skin and mucous membranes.

zygoma (zy-GOH-muh)—a bone of the skull that extends along the front or side of the face, below the eye; the molar or cheekbone.

zygomatic (zy-guh-MAT-ik)—pertaining to the zygoma (the molar or cheekbone).

zygomatic artery (zy-guh-MAT-ik AR-tuh-ree)—superficial temporal artery supplying blood to the orbit and orbicularis.

zygomatic bone (zy-goh-MAT-ik BOHN)—also known as *malar bones* or *cheekbones*; bones that form the prominence of the cheeks.

zygomatic nerve (zy-goh-MAT-ik NURV)—affects the skin of the temple, side of the forehead, and the upper part of the cheek.

zygomatic process (zy-goh-MAT-ik PRAH-ses)—the process of the temporal bone that helps to form the zygoma.

zygomaticus major muscles (zy-goh-MAT-ih-kus MAY-jor MUS-uhlz)—muscles on both sides of the face that extend from the zygomatic bone to the angle of the mouth. These muscles pull the mouth upward and backward, as when you are laughing or smiling.

zygomaticus minor muscles (zy-goh-MAT-ih-kus MY-nor MUS-uhlz)—muscles on both sides of the face that extend from the zygomatic bone to the upper lips. These muscles pull the upper lip backward, upward, and outward, as when you are smiling.

zygote (ZY-goat)—a diploid cell produced by the fusion of an egg and sperm; a fertilized egg cell.

APPENDIX

Contents

1. The pH scale.
2. The structure of the skin.
3. The layers of the skin.
4. The skeletal system (anterior and posterior views).
5. Bones of the cranium and face.
6. Bones of the neck, shoulder, and back.
7. Bones of the arm.
8. Bones of the hand.
9. Bones of the leg.
10. Bones of the ankle and foot.
11. Muscles of the head, face, and neck.
12. Muscles of the face.
13. Muscles of the anterior and posterior shoulder and arm.
14. Muscles of the lower leg.
15. Nerves and nerve branches of the head, face, and neck.
16. Nerves of the arm and hand.
17. Nerves of the lower leg and foot.
18. Arteries of the head, face, and neck.
19. Arteries of the arm and hand.
20. Arteries of the lower leg and foot.
21. The heart.
22. Blood flow through the heart.
23. Metric conversion tables.
24. A nutrition chart: Vitamins, minerals, and food sources.

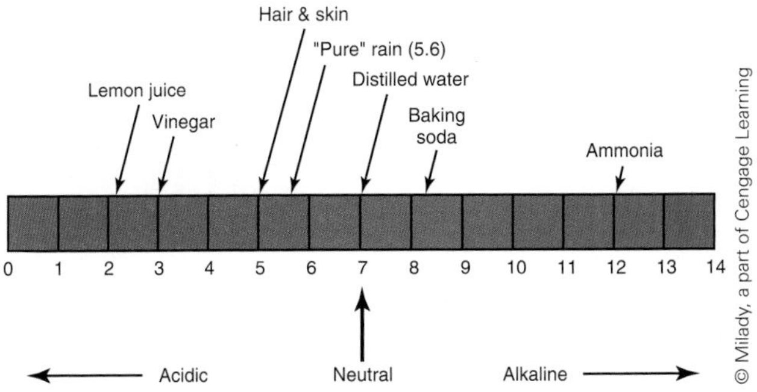

Figure Appendix-01 A pH scale is a measure of the acidity and alkalinity of a substance. It has a range from 0 to 14. A pH of 7 is a neutral solution, a pH below 7 indicates an acidic solution and a pH of above 7 indicates an alkaline solution. The pH scale is a logarithmic scale, meaning that a change of one whole number represents a ten-fold change in pH

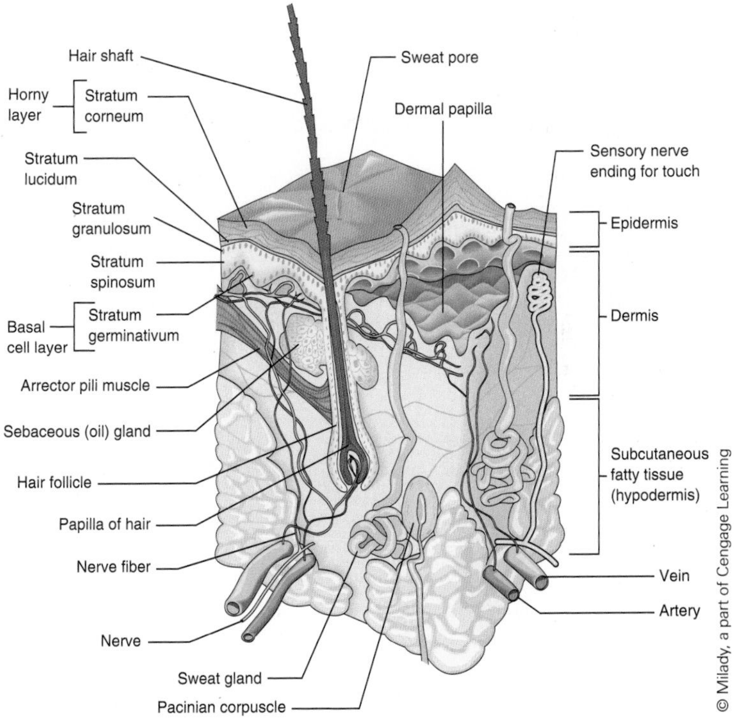

Figure Appendix-02 The structure of the skin

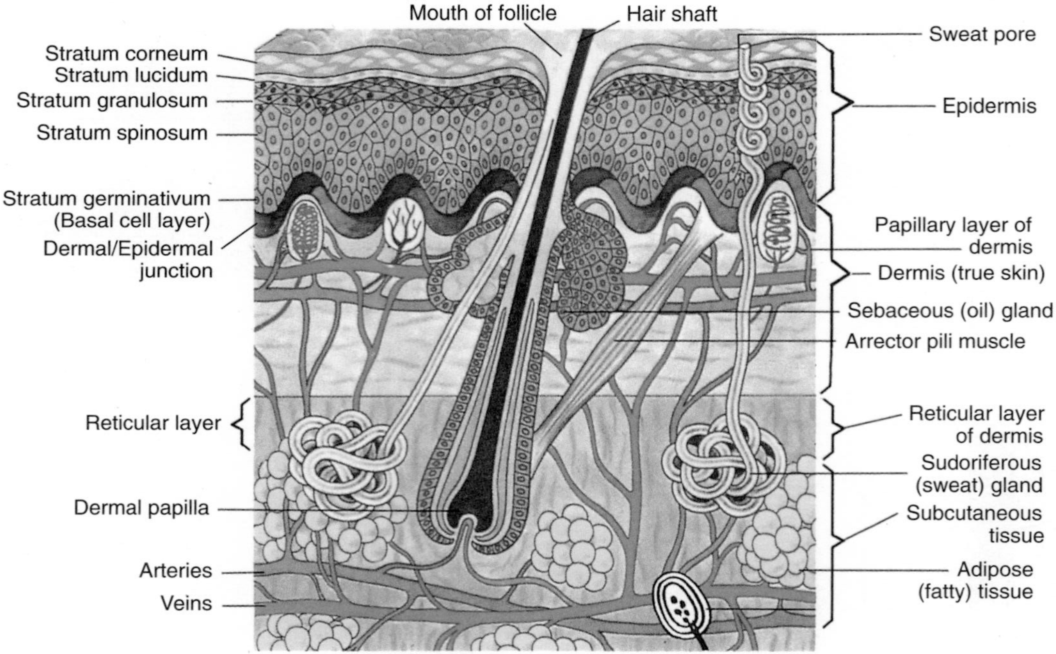

Figure Appendix-03 The layers of the skin

© Milady, a part of Cengage Learning

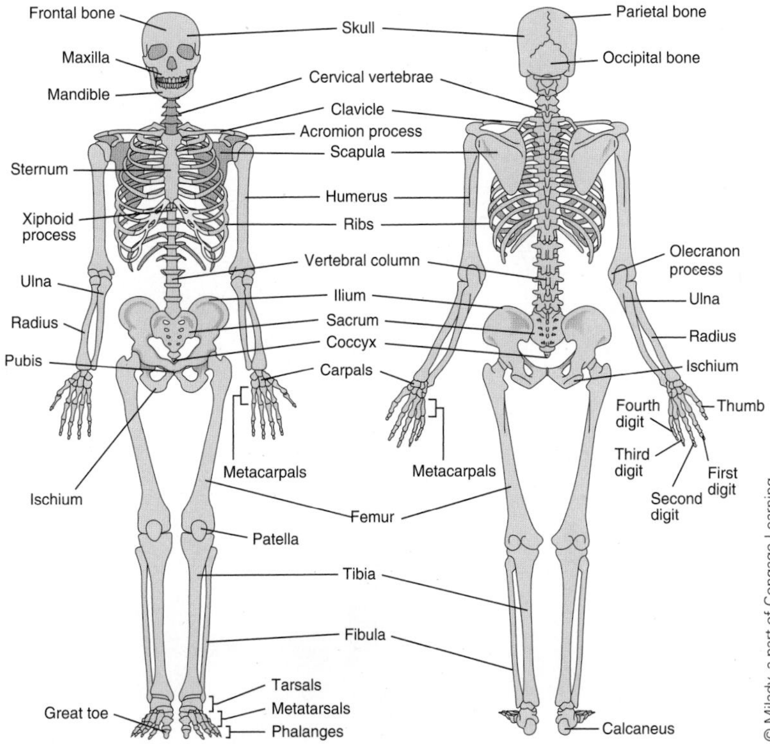

© Milady, a part of Cengage Learning

Figure Appendix-04 The skeletal system (anterior and posterior views)

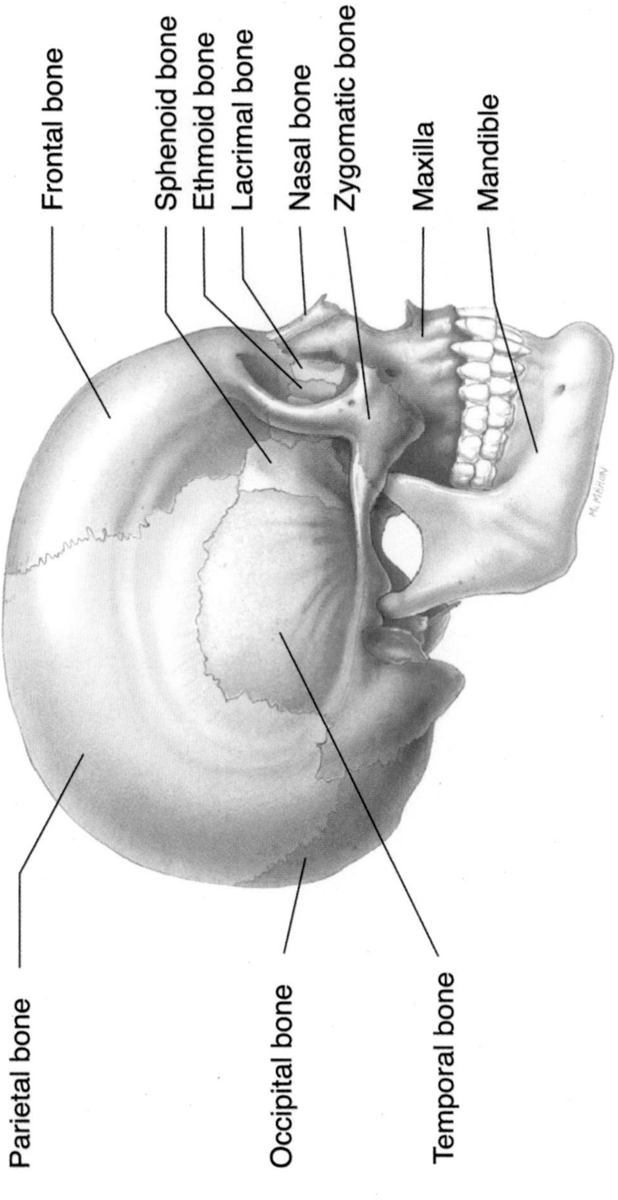

Figure Appendix-05 Bones of the cranium and face

© Milady, a part of Cengage Learning

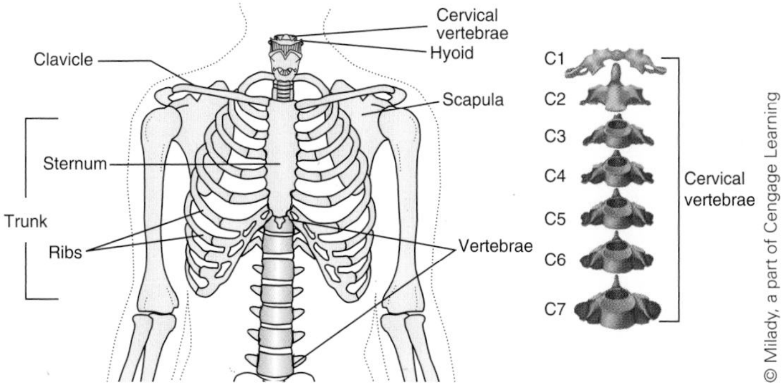

Figure Appendix-06 Bones of the neck, shoulder and back

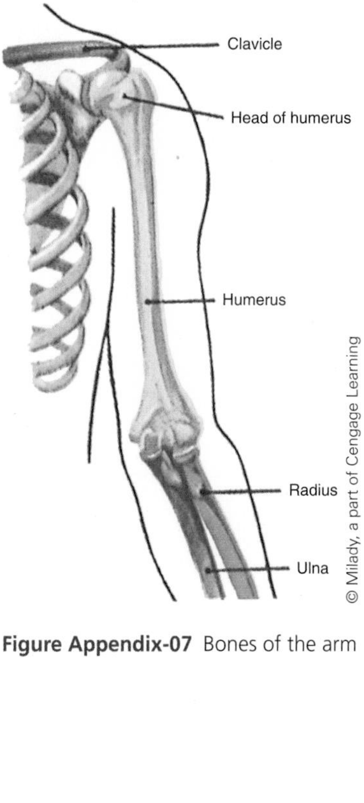

Figure Appendix-07 Bones of the arm

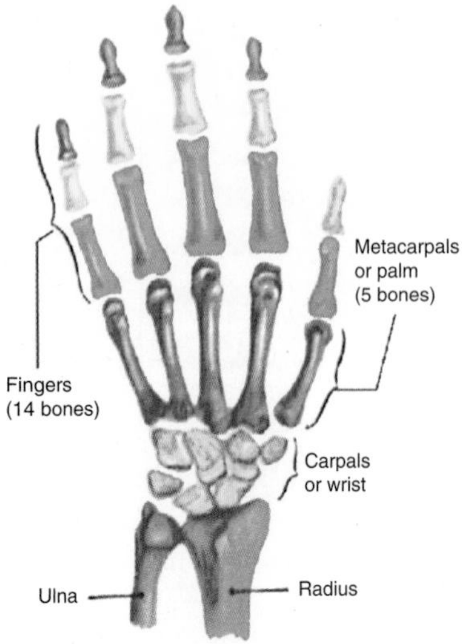

© Milady, a part of Cengage Learning

Figure Appendix-08 Bones of the hand

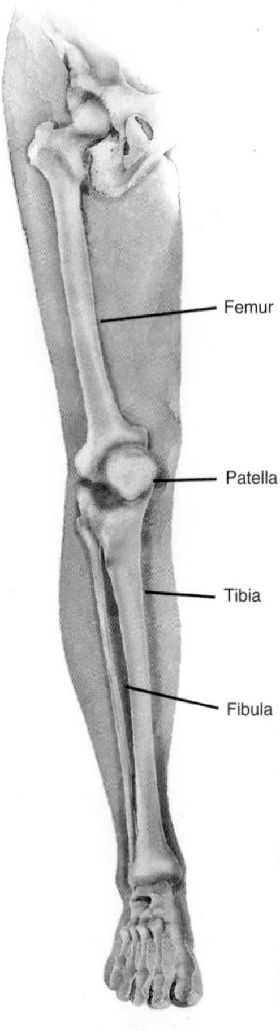

© Milady, a part of Cengage Learning

Figure Appendix-09 Bones of the leg

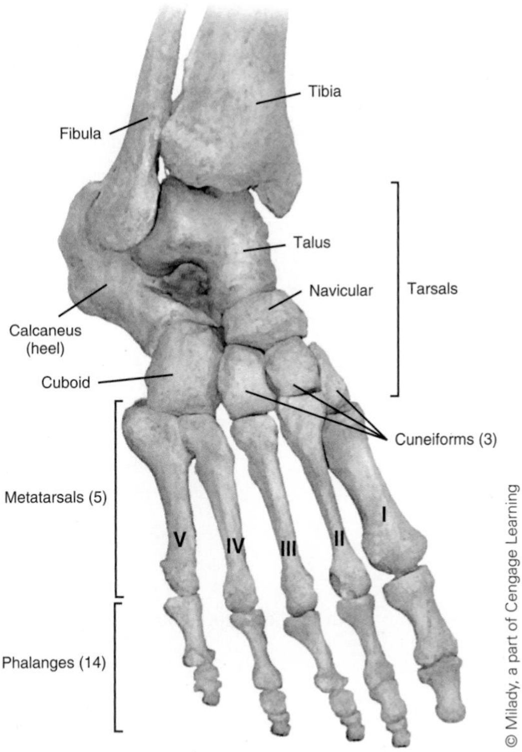

Figure Appendix-10 Bones of the ankle and foot

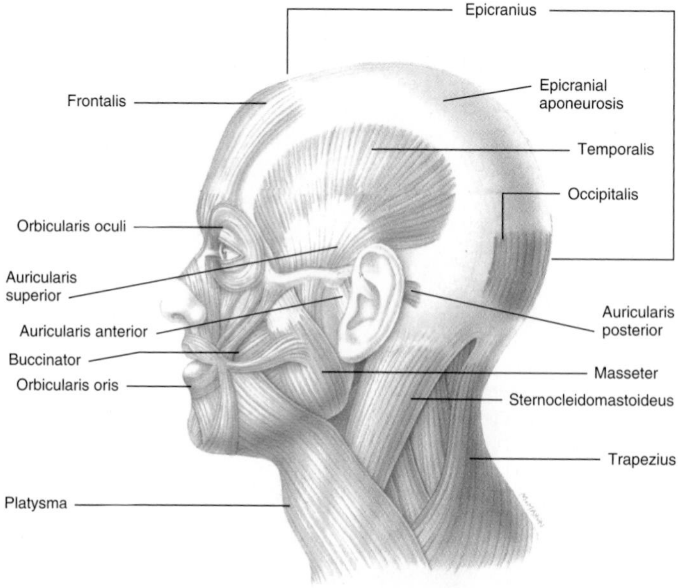

© Milady, a part of Cengage Learning

Figure Appendix-11 Muscles of the head, face and neck

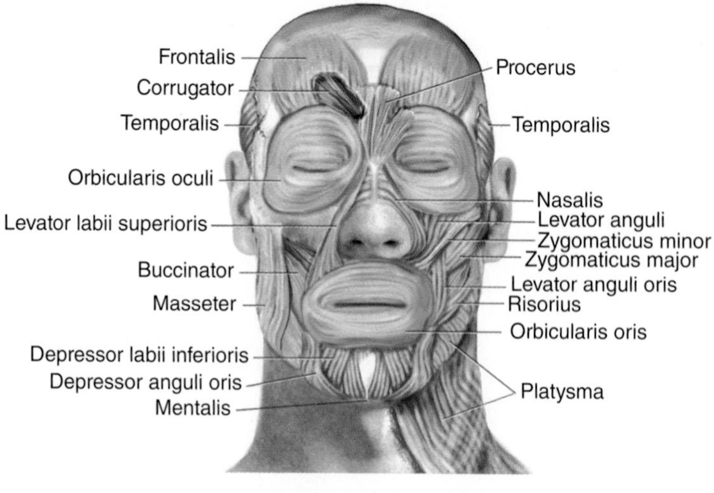

© Milady, a part of Cengage Learning

Figure Appendix-12 Muscles of the face

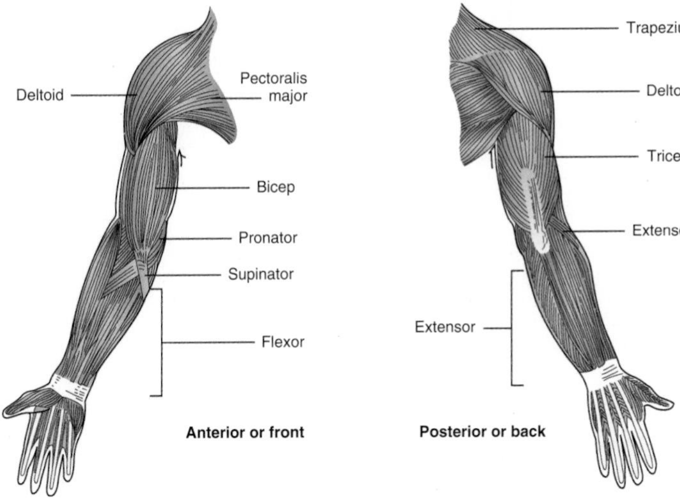

© Milady, a part of Cengage Learning

Figure Appendix-13 Muscles of the anterior and posterior shoulder and arm

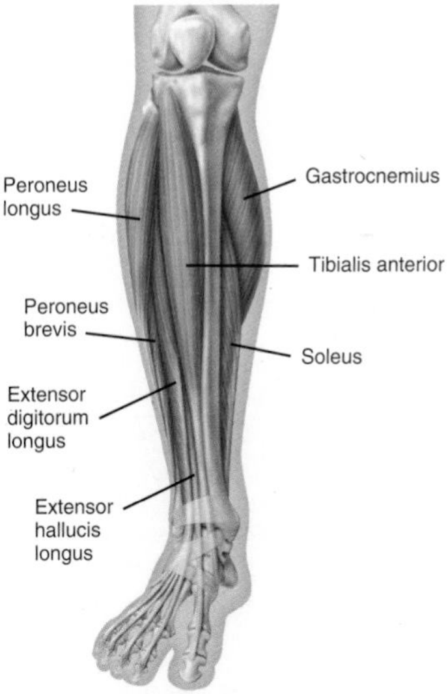

© Milady, a part of Cengage Learning

Figure Appendix-14 Muscles of the lower leg

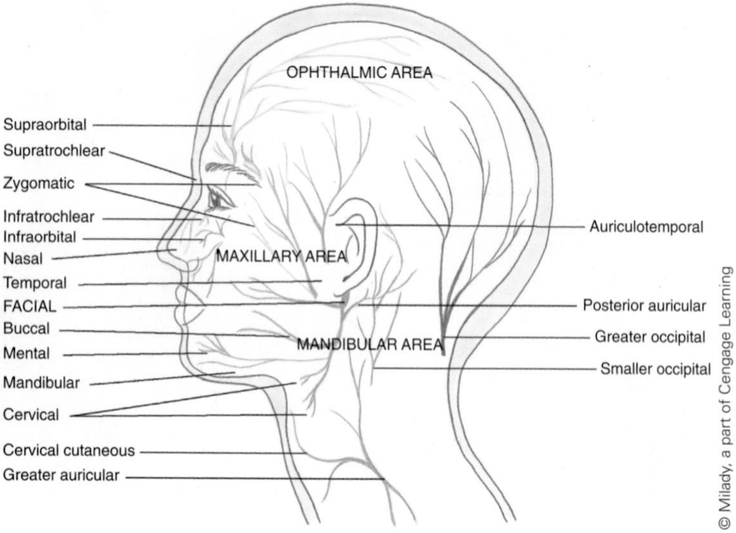

Figure Appendix-15 Nerves and nerve branches of the head, face and neck

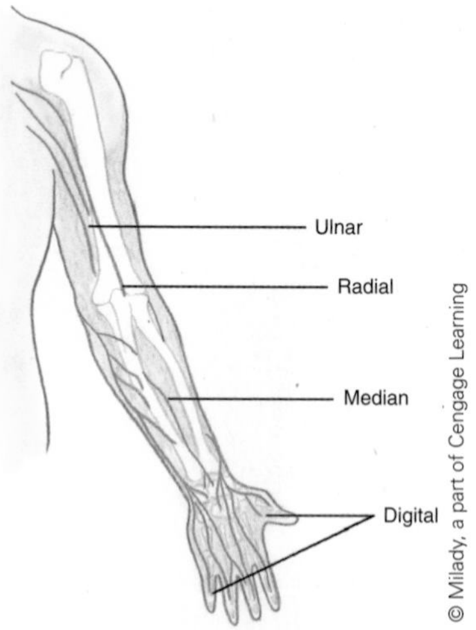

Figure Appendix-16 Nerves of the arm and hand

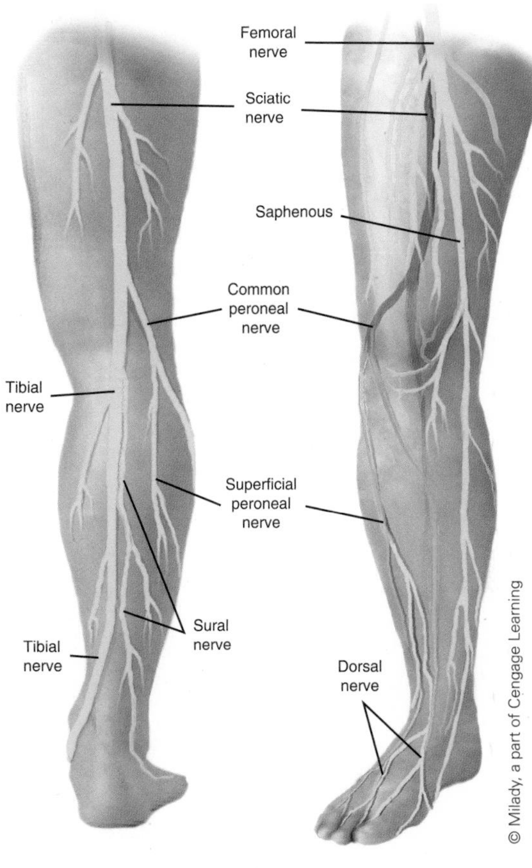

Figure Appendix-17 Nerves of the lower leg and foot

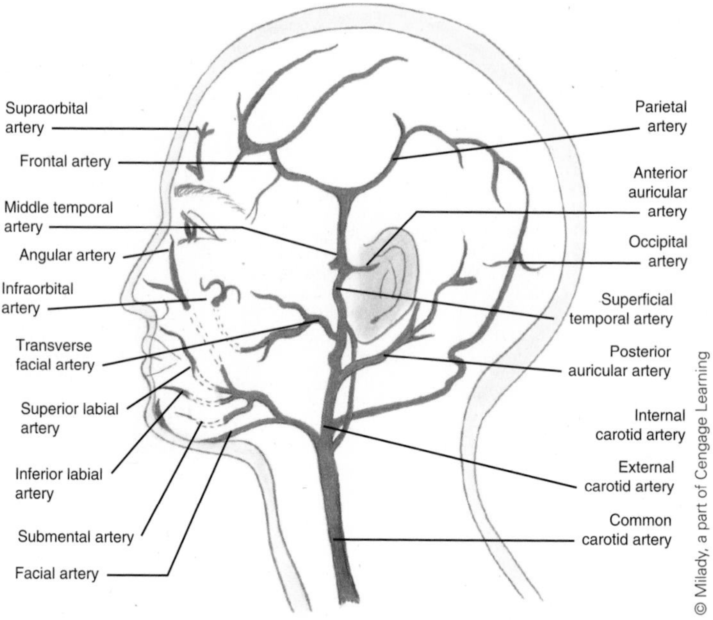

Figure Appendix-18 Arteries of the head, face and neck

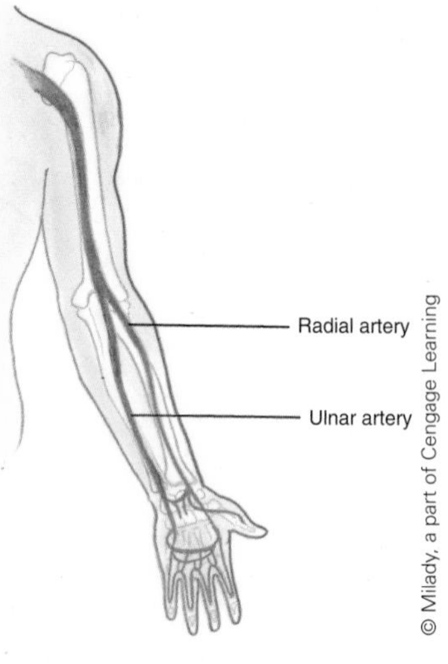

Figure Appendix-19 Arteries of the arm and hand

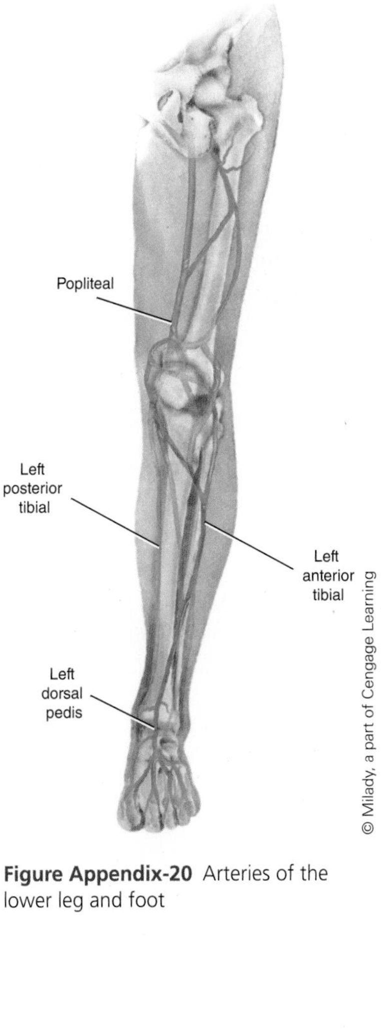

Figure Appendix-20 Arteries of the lower leg and foot

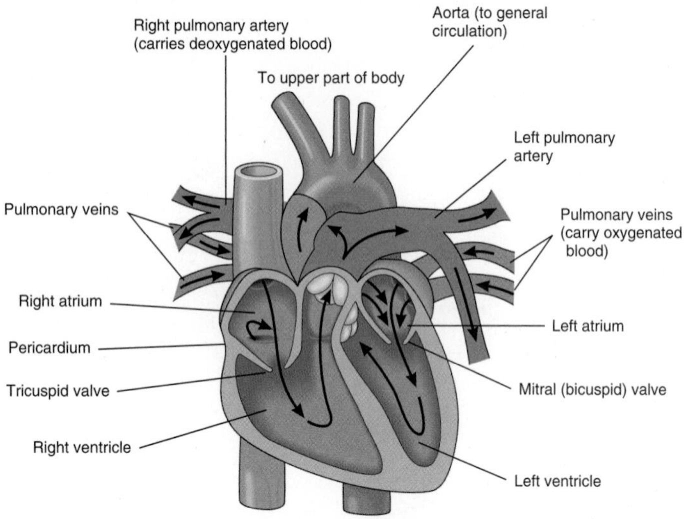

© Milady, a part of Cengage Learning

Figure Appendix-21 The heart

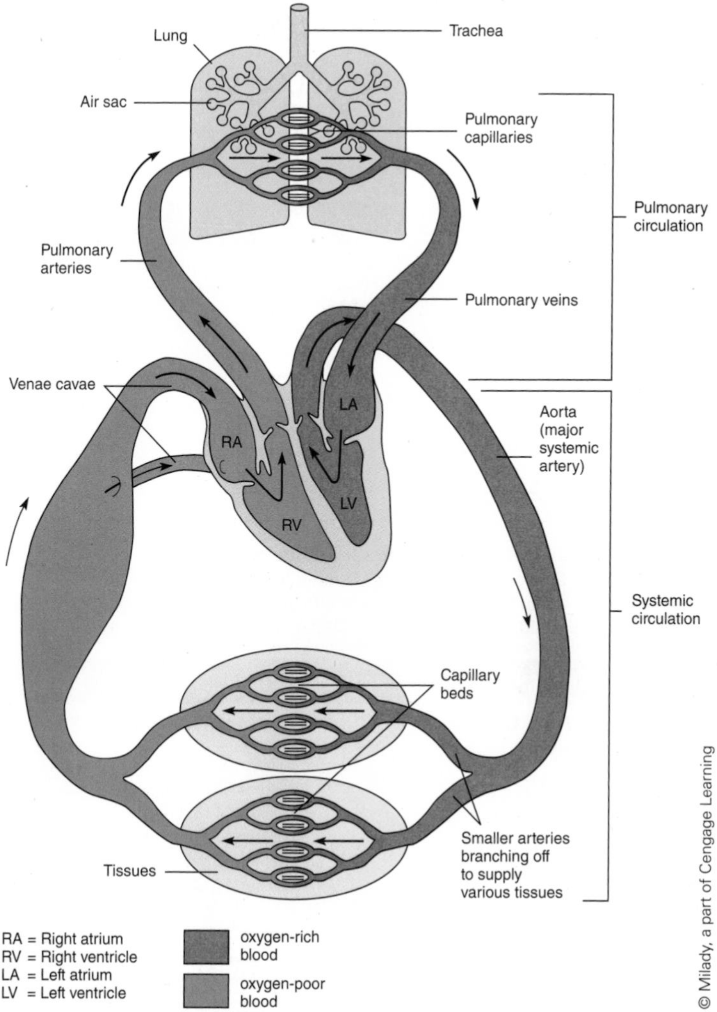

© Milady, a part of Cengage Learning

Figure Appendix-22 Blood flow through the heart

Metric Conversion Tables

U.S. MEASUREMENT–METRIC CONVERSION TABLES

The following tables show standard conversions for commonly used measurements.

Conversion Formula for Inches to Centimeters: (number of) inches × 2.54 = centimeters

Length	
Inches	**Centimeters**
⅛ inch (.125 inches)	0.317 centimeters
¼ inch (.25 inches)	0.635 centimeters
½ inch (.50 inches)	1.27 centimeters
¾ inch (.75 inches)	1.9 centimeters
1 inch	2.54 centimeters
2 inches	5.1 centimeters
3 inches	7.6 centimeters
6 inches	15.2 centimeters
12 inches	30.5 centimeters

Conversion Formula for U.S. Fluid Ounces to Milliliters:
(amount of) U.S. fluid ounce (fl. oz.) × 29.573 milliliters (ml)
Conversion Formula for U.S. Fluid Ounces to Liters:
(amount of) U.S. fluid ounce (fl. oz.) × .029573 liters (l)

Volume (Liquid)	
U.S. Fluid Onces	**Milliliters/Liters**
1 fluid ounce (⅛ cup)	29.57 milliliters/.02957 liters
2 fluid ounces (¼ cup)	59.14 milliliters/.05914 liters
4 fluid ounces (½ cup)	118.29 milliliters/.11829 liters
6 fluid ounces (¾ cup)	177.43 milliliters/.17743 liters
8 fluid ounces (1 cup)	236.58 milliliters/.23658 liters
16 fluid ounces (1 pint)	473.16 milliliters/.47316 liters
32 fluid ounces (1 quart)	946.33 milliliters/.94633 liters
33.81 fluid ounces (1 liter)	1,000 milliliters/1 liter
64 fluid ounces (½ gallon)	1,892.67 milliliters/1.8926 liters
128 fluid ounces (1 gallon)	3,785.34 milliliters/3.78534 liters

© Milady, a part of Cengage Learning

Figure Appendix-23 Metric Conversion Tables

A Nutrition Chart: Vitamins, Minerals, and Food Sources			
Vitamin RDA	**Natural Sources**	**Functions**	**Deficiency Symptoms**
A 5,000 IU	Yellow and green fruits and vegetables, carrots, dairy products, fish liver oil, yellow fruits	Growth and repair of body tissues, bone formation, vision	Night blindness, dry scaly skin, loss of smell and appetite, fatigue, bone deterioration
B-1 (Thiamine) 1.5 mg	Grains, nuts, wheat germ, fish, poultry, legumes, meat	Metabolism, appetite maintenance, nerve function, healthy mental state, muscle tone	Nerve disorders, cramps, fatigue, loss of appetite, loss of memory, heart irregularity
B-2 (Riboflavin) 1.7 mg	Whole grains, green leafy vegetables, liver, fish, eggs	Metabolism, health in hair, skin, nails; cell respiration; formation of antibodies and red blood cells	Cracks and lesions in corners of mouth, digestive disturbances
B-6 (Pyridoxine) 2 mg	Whole grains, leafy green vegetables, yeast, bananas, organ meats	Metabolism, formation of antibodies, sodium/potassium balance	Dermatitis, blood disorders, nervousness, weakness, skin cracks, loss of memory
B-7 (Biotin) 300 mcg	Legumes, eggs, grains, yeast	Metabolism, formation of fatty acids	Dry, dull skin; depression, muscle pain, fatigue; loss of appetite
B-12 (Cobalamine) 6 mcg	Eggs, milk/milk products, fish, organ meats	Metabolism, healthy nervous system, blood cell formation	Nervousness, neuritis, fatigue
Choline (no RDA)	Lecithin, fish, wheat germ, egg yolk, soybeans	Nerve metabolism and transmission; regulates liver, kidneys, and gallbladder	Hypertension, tomach ulcers, liver and kidney conditions
Folic acid (Folacin) 400 mcg	Green leafy vegetables, organ meats, yeast, milk products	Red blood cell formation, growth and cell division (RNA and DNA)	Gastrointestinal disorders, poor growth, loss of memory, anemia
Inositol (no RDA)	Whole grains, citrus fruits, yeast, molasses, milk	Hair growth, metabolism, lecithin formation	Elevated cholesterol, hair loss, skin disorders, constipation, eye abnormalities

Figure Appendix-24 A Nutrition Chart: Vitamins, Minerals and Food Sources

(Continued)

A Nutrition Chart: Vitamins, Minerals, and Food Sources			
Vitamin RDA	**Natural Sources**	**Functions**	**Deficiency Symptoms**
B complex (Niacin) 20 mg	Meat, poultry, fish, milk products, peanuts	Metabolism, healthy skin, tongue and digestive system, blood circulation, essential for synthesis of sex hormones	Fatigue, indigestion, irritability, loss of appetite, skin conditions
B complex (PABA) (no RDA)	Yeast, wheat germ, molasses	Metabolism, red blood cell formation, intestines, hair coloring, sunscreen	Digestive disorders, fatigue, depression, constipation
B-15 (Pantothenic acid) 10 mg	Whole grains, pumpkin and sesame seeds	Metabolism, stimulates nerve and glandular systems, cell respiration	Heart disease, glandular and nerve disorders, poor circulation
C Ascorbic acid 60 mg	Citrus fruits, vegetables, tomatoes, potatoes	Aids in healing, collagen maintenance, resistance to disease	Gum bleeding, bruising, slow healing of wounds, nosebleeds, poor digestion
D 400 IU	Egg yolks, organ meats, fish, fortified milk	Healthy bone formation, healthy circulatory functions, nervous system	Rickets, osteoporosis, poor bone growth, nervous system irritability
E 30 IU	Green vegetables, wheat germ, organ meats, eggs, vegetable oils	Red blood cells, inhibits coagulation of blood, cellular respiration	Muscular atrophy, abnormal fat deposits in muscles, gastrointestinal conditions, heart disease, impotency
F (no RDA)	Wheat germ, seeds, vegetable oils	Respiration of body organs, lubrication of cells, blood coagulation, glandular activity	Brittle nails and hair, dandruff, diarrhea, varicose veins, underweight, acne, gallstones
K (no RDA)	Green leafy vegetables, milk, kelp, safflower oil	Blood clotting agent, important to proper liver function and longevity	Hemorrhage
P (Bioflavonoids) (no RDA)	Fruits	For healthy connective tissue, aids in utilization of vitamin C	Tendency to bleed easily, gum bleeding, bruising, similar to vitamin C's symptoms

Figure Appendix-24 *(Continued)*

A Nutrition Chart: Vitamins, Minerals, and Food Sources			
Vitamin RDA	**Natural Sources**	**Functions**	**Deficiency Symptoms**
Calcium 1000-1400 mg	Dairy products, bone meal	Resilient bones, teeth, muscle tissue, regulating heart-beat, blood clotting	Soft, brittle bones; osteoporosis, heart palpitations
Chromium (no RDA)	Corn oil, yeast, clams, whole grains	Body's use of glucose, energy, effective use of insulin	Atherosclerosis, diabetic sugar intolerance
Copper 2 mg	Whole grains, leafy green vegetables, seafood, almonds	Healthy red blood cells, bone growth and formation, joins with vitamin C to form elastin	Skin lesions, general weakness, labored respiration
Iodine .15 mg	Iodized table salt, shellfish	Part of the hormone thyroxine which controls metabolism	Dry skin and hair, obesity, nervousness, goiters
Iron 18 mg	Meats, fish, leafy green vegetables	Hemoglobin formation, blood quality, resistance to stress and disease	Anemia, constipation, breathing difficulties
Magnesium 400 mg	Nuts, green vegetables, whole grains	Metabolism	Nervousness, agitation, disorientation, blood clots
Manganese 2 mg	Egg yolks, legumes, whole grains	Carbohydrate and fat production, sex hormone production, bone development	Dizziness, lacking muscle coordination
Phosphorus 800 mg	Proteins, grains	Bone development, important in protein, fat, and carbohydrate utilization	Soft bones, rickets, loss of appetite, irregular breathing
Potassium 2000 mg	Grains, vegetables, bananas, fruits, legumes	Fluid balance; controls activity of heart muscle, nervous system, and kidneys	Irregular heartbeat, muscle cramps (legs), dry skin, general weakness
Sodium 500 mg	Table salt, shellfish, meat and poultry	Maintains muscular, blood, lymph, and nervous systems; regulates body fluid	Muscle weakness and atrophy, nausea, dehydration

Figure Appendix-24 *(Continued)*

A Nutrition Chart: Vitamins, Minerals, and Food Sources			
Vitamin RDA	**Natural Sources**	**Functions**	**Deficiency Symptoms**
Sulphur (no RDA)	Fish, eggs, nuts, cabbage, meat	Collagen and body tissue formation, gives strength to keratin	N/A
Zinc 15 mg	Whole grains, wheat bran	Healthy digestion and metabolism, reproductive system, aids in healing	Stunted growth, delayed sexual maturity, prolonged wound healing
Selenium 055 mcg	Whole grains, liver, meat, fish	Part of important antioxidant: glutathione peroxidase	Heart damage, reduces body's resistance to chronic illnesses
Fluoride (no RDA)	Fluoridated water and toothpaste	Bone and tooth formation	Increased tooth decay

© Milady, a part of Cengage Learning

Figure Appendix-24 (*Continued*)